I0492330

Extraordinary Popular Delusions
& the Madness of Crowds Today:
Swastikas, Nazis,
Pledge of Allegiance Lies
Exposed by Rex Curry
+ Francis & Edward Bellamy

by Ian Tinny

Copyright © 2017

Dead Writers Club and Ian Tinny

(& Dr. Rex Curry upon whose research Tinny relied
along with research from the DWC)

All rights reserved

ISBN-13: 978-1981879328
ISBN-10: 1981879323

MADNESS

TABLE OF CONTENTS

MADNESS

1. POP DELUSIONS

Popular delusions are exposed to reveal the following: The Nazi salute was performed by public officials in the USA from 1892 through 1942. What happened to old photographs and films of the American Nazi salute performed by federal, state, county, and local officials? Those photos and films are rare because people don't want to know the truth about the government's past.

Public officials in the USA who preceded the German socialist (Hitler) and the Italian socialist (Mussolini) were sources for the stiff-armed salute (and robotic chanting) in those countries and other foreign countries.

Explore how the "ancient Roman salute" myth originated from the city of Rome in the state of New York (not Italy), Francis Bellamy's hometown. Learn about Mussolini's strange gift to the city of Rome, NY: a statue of two human male infants suckling on a female wolf. That statue remains on display in Rome, NY.

See how Boy Scouts and Girl Scouts helped spread the Nazi salute and the swastika to Germany and elsewhere.

Learn how the word "fascist" is related to the word

"faggot."

Discover how the military salute was the origin of the Nazi salute.

Read why the Pledge of Allegiance would not be performed by anyone (other than kooks) if the truth were taught in school.

Find out who you are, what you are, and how you got to be that way. Also learn who you should blame: your teacher (and the government's schools).

Debunk myths about Adolf Hitler, Joseph Stalin, Mao Zedong, Francis Bellamy (and his cousin Edward Bellamy), Fascism, Unionism, Socialism, genocide, swastikas, the Pledge of Allegiance to the flag, the cliche' "under God," Christianity, ancient Rome, military socialism, crony socialism, and the military-socialism complex.

This book presents a new kind of history that is not taught in schools. It recounts the mass murders committed by German socialism, Soviet socialism, and Chinese socialism as three aspects of a single history, in the time and place where they occurred: Eurasia (where they all held power) and beyond. It examines the influence of the USA (and its "Christian Socialism") on those horrors.

The Second World War is "The Socialist War" (WWS or World War S) because its two main culprits (Stalin and Hitler) were both self-declared socialists.[1] German socialists and Soviet socialists joined in a pact to divide up Europe, invading Poland together, and spreading World War II.

But before the socialist pact and its war even began,

---

[1] World War I was also a "socialist war" in that it was started by a socialist too: Gavrilo Princip.

Josef Stalin had killed millions of his own citizens—and kept killing them during and after the war. After his alliance with Hitler, Stalin switched his alliance to America's president, the socialist Franklin Delano Roosevelt.

Before Hitler was finally defeated, Hitler had murdered six million Jews and nearly as many other Europeans. At war's end, both the German and the Soviet killing sites fell behind the iron curtain, leaving the history of mass killing hidden away.

After the war, America's wartime ally (Stalin) continued killing, and he assisted Mao Zedong, who expanded socialism's mass slaughter by millions more. It all amounted to the socialist genocide (of which the Holocaust was a part): ~50 million people slaughtered under Soviet socialism; ~40 million under Chinese socialism; ~12 to 20 million under German socialism?

Hitler's regime is often labeled a "police state." The term applies equally well, and for longer terms, to the regimes of Stalin and Mao.

This book unmasks the influence of American socialism upon the totalitarian reichs of Stalin, Mao, and Hitler. These symbols are deciphered: S 卐 SS Z 卐 VW ⚡ T ✿ D t X + † ✙

The Nazi salute and Nazi behavior originated in the USA's Pledge of Allegiance in government schools (socialist schools). The daily ritual (and its notorious gesture) began in 1892, decades before its influence reached Germany and Adolf Hitler. The pledge was written by an ex-minister as part of a conspiracy to impose government (socialist) schools and to spread "military socialism" and "Christian socialism" in the USA and worldwide.

G-schools (government/socialist schools) will not

teach students about the American Nazi salute, nor about the socialist dogma that motivated Francis Bellamy, author of the pledge.

G-schools cover up German socialism and its relationship to American socialism. The USA's G-schools teach students to refer to Germany under Hitler with the terms "Nazi" and "Fascist" and "Third Reich." Hitler did not refer to his movement as "Nazism," nor as "Fascism," nor as the "Third Reich."[2] Orwellian over-use of the terms "Nazi" and "Fascist" and "Third Reich" is a deceitful lesson to trick students into supporting the word that Hitler DID use in a glowing manner to describe his own ideology: SOCIALISM.

Stalin Mao and Hitler all used and glorified the same word: Socialism.

Why is there so much ignorance about Stalin, Mao, and Hitler and the words they used? One reason is that no one reads PRIMARY sources when studying the topics.

Primary sources are hidden by g-schools in the USA because they do not want Americans to learn the pledge's embarrassing past and the political ideology behind the pledge and the government's schools.

Why does the USA continue to have a flag worshipping ceremony that occurs every morning in the government's schools? Why does the USA (the "land of the free") have schools operated by the government? How did the USA impose socialist schools and synchronized chanting along with so many other

---

[2] And audio and film recordings of Hitler's many speeches contain no examples. If any written or recorded example ever was found, then the solitary example would merely prove that Hitler made a deliberate decision to never use the term ever again and to instead continue with "socialism."

emblems of all police states? This book explains the origin of the USA's authoritarianism; why the problem exists globally; and how to protect yourself from it.

2. FRANCIS BELLAMY

Francis Julius Bellamy (May 18, 1855 to August 28, 1931) claimed to be the author of the Pledge of Allegiance. He was born in Mount Morris, New York; however, his parents moved to Rome when Bellamy was five years old. That was the city of Rome in the state of New York (not in Italy).

In the house of his parents, and while residing in Rome (NY), Bellamy was educated at a school known as the "Rome Free Academy" (RFA). The Rome Free Academy continues to operate in Rome, NY.[3]

Bellamy's connection to Rome, NY, is important because it was the origin of the "ancient Roman salute" myth (that the stiff-armed gesture used in the early Pledge of Allegiance is a gesture from the ancient Roman Empire) that was debunked by Dr. Curry.

Because Bellamy was from Rome, NY, the term "Roman salute" was used to refer to the gesture for Bellamy's Pledge of Allegiance (both the original gestures and the stiff-armed gesture - the classic Nazi salute - that developed from Bellamy's initial gestures).

People from the city of Rome in the state of New

---

[3] The school's logo includes two fasces symbols.

York were referred to as "Romans" during Bellamy's life (and they continue to refer to themselves as "Romans" today). Francis Bellamy himself was referred to as a "Roman" because of his connection to Rome, NY. One example of that is the headline: "Roman Lived to See U.S. Adopt Famed Flag Salute" from the Utica Observer newspaper (August 28, 1936).[4] That example (one of many) demonstrates how the flag salute became misnamed the "Roman salute" and confused with Italy's ancient Rome. As time went by, some confused people believed that the "Roman salute" referencing the city in New York, was instead a reference to ancient Rome in Italy.

Bellamy continues to reside in Rome, NY (he is buried in the Rome cemetery).

The early stiff-armed gesture in the USA's Pledge of Allegiance was not from ancient Rome. There was no such thing as an "ancient Roman salute."[5] The modern Roman salute myth evolved from the USA's Pledge of Allegiance.

Many cities in the state of New York have names reminiscent of classical history (Albany, Ithaca, Syracuse, Troy, and Utica), and that is why New York is the "Empire State" with the "Empire State Building" because it is a reference to the time period of the ancient Roman Empire.

---

[4] Another example: "Roman shares Pledge of Allegiance lessons, message nationwide" (Rome Sentinel April 11, 2017). Also: "Here are the backgrounds of some notable New York Romans, past and present -FRANCIS BELLAMY..." (Observer Dispatch newspaper in Utica, NY on Aug. 4, 2015).
[5] unless one counts the middle finger salute, mentioned by Suetonius and Martial, as the true Roman salute. That would be a better salute for the pledge and flag.

MADNESS

In 1901, Bellamy traveled to Rome, Italy, and met privately with King Victor Emmanuel III, the man who would later (1922) appoint the long-time socialist leader Mussolini as Prime Minister of Italy.

As Bellamy's Nazi salute spread, so spread his government (socialist) schools, and so spread the use of the fasces symbol to represent socialism.

The "Rome Free Academy" school that Bellamy attended continues to operate in Rome, New York, and the school's logo includes two fasces. The official seal of the United States Senate (adopted 1886) includes a pair of crossed fasces. Two fasces bestride the U.S. flag behind the podium in the U.S. House of Representatives.[6] The fasces style is used in the Lincoln Memorial (with his hands, Lincoln is caressing two leather-bound faggots poised at knee height at the right and left front of his chair). A fasces is on the bronze George Washington statue (1882) in front of Federal Hall National Memorial in Manhattan, New York City. The fasces appears on the

---

[6] The Congressional fasces might have inspired the socialist Mussolini in his use of the symbol, just as the gesture to the U.S. flag was the origin of Mussolini's salute. For example, U.S. presidents (and members of Congress) might have used the stiff-armed gesture to the flag within the chambers (all such photos have probably been destroyed). Newsreel footage and photographs show President Woodrow Wilson standing with the fasces symbols on the walls behind him before and during WWI ("the war to make the world unsafe for everything"). Is there a photograph of Wilson performing the American Nazi salute before the fasces and the flag?

Swastikas also decorate the walls of Congress, as shown in a New York Times photograph of former Representative Mick Mulvaney, confirmed as White House Budget Director (photo by Stephen Crowley, "Popular Domestic Programs Face Ax Under First Trump Budget" web article by Sharon LaFraniere and Alan Rappeport on 2/17/2017).

U.S. dime from 1916. The fasces is central to the emblem (1883?) of the Knights of Columbus, a group that altered the Pledge of Allegiance in 1954 with the insertion of "under God." The fasces style (as a bundle of arrows) adorns the U.S. quarter (1932) and resembles the emblem on the hat worn by Mussolini in a notorious photograph.

Mussolini was so impressed with the Roman and socialist themes in the U.S. that he honored Rome, NY with a statue of the "Capitoline Wolf" (upon which the fabled Romulus and Remus are shown suckling. It represents the socialist goal of every human suckling at the public/government teat -the wolf). The peculiar monument stands in front of The Beeches Inn in Rome, NY, where it is adorned with a plaque displaying a fasces and the phrase "New Rome." Mussolini made similar gifts to Cincinnati, Ohio, and to Rome in the state of Georgia (in 1931). An engraving on one of the statues reads "Anno X" ("Year 10" in Latin), referencing Mussolini's tenth year in power. In Georgia, a bronze plate on the monument prominently displays the fasces symbol. Romans believed that the father of Romulus (the mythical founder of Rome) was Mars (the god of war) and their belief abetted the dogma of "military socialism" (including Bellamy's version).

Mussolini learned the Bellamy salute when he was a powerful socialist leader. No "ancient Roman" influence (real or imagined) was mentioned by Bellamy, nor by James Upham (the person who assisted Bellamy in creating the Pledge's gesture), in their descriptions of how the Pledge and its salute was written.

Francis Bellamy never used the term "ancient Roman salute" when describing his pledge's salute.

The phrase "Roman salute" did not exist at the time

that Bellamy and Upham worked on the pledge (Dr. Curry's pedagogy is supported by the Oxford English Dictionary in this etymological regard). The concept/term "ancient Roman salute" was dreamed up decades after Bellamy wrote the pledge of Allegiance.

Francis Bellamy clearly explained that his pledge began with a military salute that was then extended out toward the flag. In practice, the second gesture was performed palm-down with a stiff-arm when the military salute was merely pointed out at the flag by bored children forced to do Bellamy's programmed chanting daily in government schools. That is how the straight-arm salute developed from Francis Bellamy's salutation and its use of the military salute (and how the USA's pledge salute led to the Nazi salute).

An instructor at George Mason University (GMU) wrote a short item for the American Philological Association (APA) questioning whether the so-called "ancient Roman salute" ever occurred in any Roman art or text. The item noted that the salute occurred in early silent films: the American "Ben-Hur" (1907), the Italian "Nerone" (1908), "Spartaco" (1914), "Cabiria" (1914).

All film examples of the early American Nazi salute are mild compared with the daily grind of government schools brainwashing children from 1892 to perform the gesture (with clockwork orange droning) under threat of violence for 12 years of their lives. Adult babies were also forced to perform the embarrassing gesture at events.

In response to the APA blurb about the GMU teacher, Dr. Curry publicly announced his discovery that the original U.S. flag salute (1892) predated and inspired the use of the gesture in the later films. The pledge's early Nazi salute had been unknown to the GMU instructor when he wrote about the films.

The GMU teacher did not know that in 1901 Bellamy traveled to Rome, Italy, and met with King Victor Emmanuel III, the man who would appoint the long-time socialist leader Mussolini as Prime Minister of Italy.

Dr. Curry pointed out that the earliest film -Ben Hur-had at least three directors, of which two had been born and raised in the U.S. That means they attended schools where they were likely forced upon threat of violence to perform the American Nazi salute and intone the pledge on cue daily. One director was from Canada, but had moved to the U.S. at a young age and lived in the U.S. long enough to observe the bizarre U.S. practice toward the flag before he and the other directors incorporated it into the film "Ben Hur."

The GMU teacher went on to author a confusing book that was debunked before it was published by the vexillologist Dr. Rex Curry. He does not dispute Dr. Curry's hypothesis that the Pledge of Allegiance was the origin of the Nazi salute and Nazi behavior. GMU's instructor mentions neo-classical artwork by Jacques Louis David, but he does not state that David's Horatii was the origin of the Roman salute myth.

In the Horatii painting, three brothers are reaching for weapons (swords) with their fingers and thumbs separated in a grasping gesture (and the two figures in back are reaching with their left hands).

GMU's instructor states that Horatii is the "starting point for an arresting gesture that progressed from oath-taking to what will become known as the Roman salute," which actually states nothing, and is an apparent reference to his own "starting point" for writing his book. He does not contend that the painting was the origin of the Nazi salute, nor that it was the origin of the "ancient Roman salute" myth.

The GMU book leaves readers with suspicion that GMU's teacher is unaware that Hitler and his supporters did not call themselves "Nazis"; that they did not call themselves "Fascists"; that "Third Reich" was not one of Hitler's slogans; that they called themselves "socialists"; that Hitler's emblem signified "S" letter shapes for "socialism." Is the GMU instructor ignorant or is he intellectually dishonest in hiding what Hitler's supporters called themselves: SOCIALIST?

The GMU teacher's book seems written to evade any comparison of Bellamy's socialism to the socialism touted by Mussolini and Hitler.

Hitler enjoyed American movies and had his own private cinema. Hitler could have viewed early movies showing the American socialist salute in fake "Roman" scenes. The documentary "Hitler's Private World: Revealed," shows him talking animatedly about his love for cinema (his tastes included Mickey Mouse). He also teased Eva Braun about a screening in his cinema at the Berghof, and he stated, "I understand you didn't like the movie last night. I know what you want. You want Gone with the Wind."

The GMU teacher quoted the untrustworthy book "Hitler's Table Talk" and Hitler's alleged statement: "I'd read the description of the sitting of the Diet of Worms, in the course of which Luther was greeted with the German salute." The GMU teacher had no idea what "description" the quote referenced. Another amazing discovery by Dr. Curry is that the quote's "description" refers to "Luther at the Diet of Worms" by the Belgian painter Émile Delperée (1882). The painting does not show the "German salute" just as David's Oath of the

Horatii does not show it. The person who wrote the quote was lying or misremembered the painting.[7]

The GMU teacher also quoted Hitler's alleged statement: "It was in the *Ratskeller* at Bremen, about the year 1921, that I first saw this style of salute." The GMU teacher was unaware that, about 1921, Ernst Hanfstaengl moved from the USA to Germany and instructed Hitler on propaganda rituals that were used in America. Hanfstaengl heard for the first time a speech by Hitler in a beer hall. According to author John Toland (p. 128 of his biography of Hitler), the first encounter between Hitler and Hanfstaengl was on 22 November, 1922 at the Kindlkeller, a large L-shaped beer hall. Hanfstaengl as the importer (and/or promoter) of the American Nazi salute is likely.

The GMU author was debunked also by Michelle Borg at the University of Sydney: "The author first turns to the early form of the Pledge of Allegiance, which originally included an entirely similar gesture to the one that came to be used by Fascists and Nazis. This uncomfortable association is not explored in depth; [He] simply asserts that the gesture had no political or historical connotations in the United States."

Borg's critique applies to Wikipedia too, depending on the date and time that Wakipedia is examined. It also applies to almost all media in the USA. They ignore the gesture entirely, or they pretend that the gesture had no political or historical connotations in the USA and no influence outside the USA.

How can anyone ignore more than a century of hypnotic brainwashing in government schools in the

---

[7] The Diet occurred in response to Martin Luther and his 95 theses, supposedly nailed to the door of All Saints' Church.

USA, Boy Scouts and Girl Scouts, modern Olympics, other sporting events, political rallies, parades and more? How does anyone ignore the persecution, bullying, and violence used to dictate the gesture and the mechanical chanting? How is it ignored today?

Fictitious Roman scenes in early silent movies only added to the "Roman" salute myth that developed from Bellamy's flag salutation (and his pledge preceded those films by more than a decade).

That the myth of the "ancient Roman salute" did not exist when Bellamy wrote his pledge (and for decades thereafter) also means that the concept of the "Roman salute" did not even exist when Jacques-Louis David painted his "Oath of the Horatii." Thus David was NOT thinking of a real or imagined "Roman salute" when he painted the Horatii, nor did David ever use the term "Roman salute" (again also see the Oxford English Dictionary).

The Horatii lie (that the Horatii painting was the origin of the "Roman salute" myth) is a very recent lie. It first appeared on Wikipedia (~2006) after Dr. Curry's discovery that the Pledge of Allegiance was the origin of the Nazi salute. The Horatii disinformation was deliberately fabricated by a liar to bury Dr. Curry's revelation that the pledge was the origin of the Nazi salute, to hide the pledge's shameful past, and to side-step the influence of American socialists (e.g. Edward Bellamy, Francis Bellamy) and of the USA's pledge upon German socialism and global socialism.

Research produces no examples in history of anyone asserting that the Horatii painting was an example of an archaic Roman salute, nor that it inspired the "Roman salute" myth. For example, Armand-Charles Caraffe, the artist who painted "The Oath of the Horatii" (in 1791), did not mis-interpret David's 1784 painting as an "ancient Roman salute."

David's painting did not inspire France in 1784 nor any time thereafter to legislate the gesture in a pledge or in any real life situations. Nor did any French adopt the gesture in that century, nor the next. Bellamy and the USA were the origin of the gesture's actual use in France, which occurred much later. The gesture did not become common in France until people in France were inspired by the long-time socialist leader Mussolini, whose gesture originated from the long-time socialist leader Francis Bellamy from the USA. For more information on the first wave of the gesture in France (from 1924-1933) and the second wave of the gesture (1933-1939) see books written by Robert Soucy.

David's painting did not inspire the gesture in the U.S., as evidenced by the lack of the gesture before 1892 and Bellamy's Nazi salute. The gesture is not shown in these examples of "saluting" that predate 1892: Frank Leslie's Illustrated Newspaper, v. 52, 1881, p. 68 wood engraving "Washington, D.C. - an incident of the inauguration - ex-confederate soldiers saluting President Garfield"; Harper's weekly, 1862 March 29, illustration "A Thrilling scene in east Tennessee--Colonel Fry and the Union men swearing by the flag"; Harper's Weekly, 1863 June 6, illustration "Registered enemies taking the oath of allegiance at the office of Gen. Bowen, at New Orleans" from a sketch by Mr. J.R. Hamilton.

From 1892, French children in the USA had been brainwashed to accept government (socialist) schools along with Nazi salutes and Nazi behavior therein. The conditioning continued for decades, as shown in a photograph of preschool age children performing the initial gesture of the old pledge salute at L'Ecole maternelle francaise in New York, New York (dated June 6, 1944, D-day, and photographed by Howard Hollem, Edward Meyer or MacLaugharie). The children were taught to render the Bellamy salute toward the French flag -not the U.S. flag- in the New York school. Bellamy was no bel ami to the French. He spread his socialism and his pledge worldwide. He desired to "Americanize" foreigners in the U.S. (and by "Americanize" Bellamy meant "teach them about Bellamy's socialism and worship of government").

An Americanization rally was held on April 27, 1917 at City Hall in New York City. A photograph shows children dressed in costumes of different countries (including France) with flags of the different countries as a woman stands with an American Flag on the steps of City Hall (Bain News Service). The children are rendering the first part of the gesture in the early Pledge of Allegiance.

Another breath-taking photograph of the same NYC rally shows that "Americanization" meant teaching a sea of thousands of students from government schools to render the Nazi salute to the U.S. flag and to chant mechanically in unison on command (the photo is entitled "1917 American School children saluting the Flag Stars and stripes Washington High School New York").

From 1892, the city of New York, and the state of New York, were the main distribution centers for Nazi salutes and Nazi behavior ("Americanization"), long before Camp Siegfried in Yaphank in the 1930s.

On April 23, 1911, the front page of the French publication Le Petit Journal was a colorful romantic drawing of a crowd of men, some with their hands outstretched in different forms (one holding a hat in the air). The title is described as "Conscripts taking an oath to follow the example of those who perished during the war of 1870." Is it as fictional of a scene as David's Horatii? The drawing appears to be influenced by him. It also appears to have been influenced by Bellamy. Perhaps some of them are Americans who joined the Escadrille Américaine (and flew swastika planes) for the French Air Department or some other part of the French military. Unlike David's painting, all the men who gesture appear to use their right hands. 1911 is nineteen years after 1892 for anyone who is keeping score.

The same liar who created the Horatii/Roman salute deceit had, until he was debunked, previously claimed that the stiff-armed salute was an actual ancient Roman salute, and he posted the lie that Roman statues displaying "adlocutio" (a gesture made by a person speaking) showed "the ancient Roman stiff-armed salute."

Wikipedia continues to mislead readers about the "ancient Roman salute" lie in articles that vary in quality from "confusing" to "deceptive." Liars on wikipedia parrot journalists in the old media: They will not write about the pledge's influence on socialism in Germany and elsewhere, and they will delete any information in that regard. They also do not dispute the information in this book (they merely suppress it).

The newly substituted Horatii falsity has been mindlessly repeated by many people (as the adlocutio lie was repeated and still is) because wikipedia glorifies itself as an encyclopedia, even though it is merely an anonymous bulletin board where anyone can post anything (exemplifying popular delusions and the madness of crowds).

It should be needless to say (but for wakipedia) that

Bellamy was not influenced by Jacques-Louis David's painting "Oath of the Horatii." According to Bellamy, his pledge's gesture resulted when he was with James Upham and Upham specifically suggested gestures for the pledge that Bellamy had penned. Upham suggested the military salute followed by the arm outstretched with the palm upward (which was similar to saying "Here is the flag").

It was the use of the military salute (at the beginning of the original Pledge of Allegiance and then extended outward toward the flag) that resulted in the classic Nazi-style gesture.

From the pledge's breech birth in 1892, the stiff-armed gesture grew in popularity and was used during meetings of fraternal organizations, including the Masons. Bellamy and Upham were Masons and they both specifically promoted the use of the pledge (and its straight-arm salute) by fraternal organizations and by the Masons.

The American Nazi salute spread beyond the USA's pledge when it was adopted for sycophantic chanting to state flags. Texas imposed its state "Pledge of Allegiance" in 1933. The 1933 description of the flag was extremely detailed and included precise instructions for the colors of the stripes, blood red, azure blue, and white, were said to impart the "lessons of the Flag: bravery, loyalty, and purity." In the same year that German socialism achieved dictatorship, Texas imposed the American socialist Nazi salute to its flag of "white purity" (reminiscent of Hitler's description of his flag's emblem in Mein Kampf). In 1933, the Hitlergruß (Hitler greeting) was mandated for civilians in Germany under a decree from Wilhelm Frick, the Reich Minister of the Interior.

Soon thereafter, in 1935, Georgia imposed the American Nazi salute and bizarre incantation to its state flag. Rhode Island out-Nazied them all when it imposed the American salute for its pledge to the state's flag in 1910 (its source was the State Department of Education).

America's Nazi-style behavior continued and now 17 states have a formal pledge or salute to state flags (Kentucky, Ohio, North Carolina, Louisiana, South Dakota, Oklahoma, Mississippi, Michigan, South Carolina, New Mexico, Virginia, Arkansas, Georgia, Tennessee, Texas, Alabama and Rhode Island). It is extremely difficult to find any photographs or film footage of the early state flag salutes of Texas, Georgia, or Rhode Island.

Germans learned American behavior via old films, WWI, newsreels, and the widespread use of the straight-arm salute by Germans who had studied or lived in the USA; via Americans who also studied or lived in Germany; via German-American groups in the USA (including the German-American Bund); via the Boy Scouts (who spread both the American Nazi salute and also the swastika symbol); via the official Olympic salute (another exposé, infra, by Dr. Curry is that the "official Olympic salute" was from the USA's Nazi salute from the Pledge of Allegiance).

In February 1939, supporters of German socialism attended a German American Bund rally at New York's Madison Square Garden. The gathering included innumerable U.S. flags. Today's writers demonstrate their ignorance of the American socialist's gesture when they describe the "shocking Nazi salutes" that occurred among the German socialism fans at the event. Some of those "shocking Nazi salutes" were used for the pledge to the U.S. flag. Which Nazi salutes are the usual gesture for the Pledge of Allegiance and which aren't? It is impossible to know from still photographs of the rally. Modern descriptions of the event are funny in that regard.

On May 23, 1941, Madison Square Gardens hosted the America First Committee (AFC). The event included the American flag's Nazi salute. In a photograph, the American socialist leader Norman Thomas performs the gesture that originated from the American socialist leader Francis Bellamy. Similar to Bellamy, Thomas was a Christian Socialist. Thomas was a Presbyterian minister and that provides an intriguing comparison to both Bellamy and to Martin Niemoller. Thomas was a six-time presidential candidate for the Socialist Party of America and performed America's Nazi salute a great deal (1928, 1932, 1936, 1940, 1944, 1948 -perhaps he dropped the Nazi salute in 1944 and 1948). Thomas co-founded the AFC and helped bring many socialists into the AFC's movement. In 1941 at Madison Square Gardens, Thomas was joined in his Nazi gesture by Democratic and Socialist Senator Burton Wheeler, Charles A. Lindbergh, and novelist and socialist Kathleen Norris.

General Hugh Johnson enjoyed the American Nazi salute while head of the socialist "National Recovery Administration" created under the socialist President Franklin D. Roosevelt (see the photograph of him speaking at the 44th Congress of American Industry at the Waldorf-Astoria in New York City on Dec. 6, 1939).

Socialists continue to proudly remind Americans that the daily pledge was written by a socialist. Of course, socialists remain blissfully ignorant of its relationship to German socialism and the notorious stiff-armed gesture.

They never repeat that part of the story after they are informed of it.

From 1892 through 1942, public officials (including U.S. presidents, congressmen, governors, state legislators and everyone down to the local dog catcher) performed the American Nazi salute.

In 2015, news outlets reported secret home movie footage from 1933 showing the "Nazi salute" performed by Edward the VIII and the future Queen Elisabeth (at seven years old). No American news reporter was aware that public officials in the USA performed the gesture from 1892 through 1942 and beyond.

Before WWII, it was not illegal for citizens of the USA to support the National Socialist German Workers' Party or Hitler's political campaigns.

The National Socialist German Workers' Party (NSGWP) began in 1920, achieved electoral breakthroughs in 1930, imposed dictatorship in 1933, and invaded Poland in 1939 as allies in socialist imperialism and colonialism with the Union of Soviet Socialist Republics in a pact to divide up Europe, spreading World War II, and leading to the socialist Wholecaust (of which the Holocaust was a part).

The pledge's stiff-armed salute existed from 1892 (three decades before the NSGWP) and continued in the USA throughout the existence of the NSGWP. It was the origin of the Nazi salute.

So the question remains unaddressed by Wakipedia, the traditional media, et cetera: which of the following had more influence? (1) The Horatii painting, or (2) decades of brainwashing with the gesture for the Pledge of Allegiance in and out of government schools (socialist schools) with threats, expulsions, persecutions, beatings, arrests, and even lynchings for those who refused (because clownish chanting is considered so important)?

If teachers had begun each day (from 1892) by holding up the Horatii painting and commanding students to mimic it or be punished, then that would be persuasive evidence. But that is not what happened.

David never asked people to pantomime his painting; Bellamy specifically DID ask people worldwide to perform his ritual. He also wanted everyone to impose socialism. He DESIGNED his salutation to be performed by everyone everywhere. Bellamy wanted his ritual to be learned by everyone who would later be involved with the movies Ben-Hur, Nerone, Spartaco, and Cabiria. He WANTED German socialists and Italian socialists and everyone to do it. Bellamy wanted children of foreign parents to render his vow in socialist (government) schools. Laws were imposed to make it so in the USA and elsewhere.[8] There is no evidence that Bellamy ever objected to any of it.

How many millions of people were forcefully indoctrinated with the American Nazi salute and robotic chanting in socialist schools for years of their lives (and then less often as adults)? The answer could be calculated approximately by researching the number of children who were educated in the US schools annually after 1892.

Did socialists in Italy and Germany fail to witness for

---

[8] Homeschooling is illegal in Germany today under a law that existed under Hitler's German socialism. Some families have sought asylum abroad in order to home-school their children. Immigration laws in some countries delay or prevent people from fleeing Germany's socialist schools (just as immigration prevented people from fleeing German socialism under Hitler).

decades the required daily outlandish intonation in the US schools that was seen by German and Italian families that came and went from US schools, parades, sports, public meetings, events? The American Nazi salute was specifically taught to immigrants to "Americanize" them and those immigrants included people of all ages who would attend night schools and day schools everywhere, including New York City, the "melting pot" of the world. The photograph "Students Saluting Under American Flag" from Getty Images (with credit Bettmann) shows such a scene and includes middle-aged adults (# 514702244). Future Nazis and others learned the gesture from the same source as did millions of U.S. students in schools over the span of decades: rote learning.

Or did foreigners also overlook everything about the pompous pledge ritual in newspapers, newsreels, movies, WWI, and WWII? Did they miss all the bombastic public officials from city, county, state, and federal levels, who grew up ~1892 and thereafter (including presidents, congressmen, etc.) who boastfully performed the gaudy gesture and hypnotic chanting publicly? Where are those photos and films today of the embarrassing old pledge gesture and public officials performing it?[9] Did any Germans or Italians ever see

---

[9] For example, a researcher reported that the Library of Congress claims that it possesses no photographs or film of President Franklin Roosevelt performing the Pledge of Allegiance (FDR was a three-term president). EVER. A search of the FDR library also provides no photo or film of FDR during the pledge ritual. This is all the more peculiar because a popular myth about FDR is that he "started" and promoted the hand-over-the-heart gesture in order to replace the American Nazi salute. There appear to be no photos of FDR doing either one.

those, or did the USA's Pledge of Allegiance never have any impact on anyone, anywhere, at anytime? Not even one Italian was ever aware of it? Not even one German was ever aware of it? Is that the position of wakipedia, the trad media, and the GMU writer? If they concede that the pledge must have had some influence on someone, somewhere, at sometime, then who, where, and when? How much?

Why is it so important for them to camouflage the shameful pledge and its putrid past?

They could point to earlier depictions of people holding their arms in the air, and they could declare all of them to be the "ancient Roman salute" (even depictions that predate Rome) and it would be equally as wrong. Ancient Egypt has depictions of people with arms raised. Prehistoric cave drawings do too.

The following is a quiz regarding these two salutes (students are invited to pick "A" or "B" as the best answer to the questions that follow below):

A. The German usage of the stiff-armed gesture under the socialist Hitler.

B. The Italian usage of the stiff-armed gesture under the socialist Mussolini.

Question 1: which usage was more well-known at the start of the modern Olympics in 1896?

Question 2: which usage was more well-known when the first film studios were built in 1897?

Question 3: which usage was more well-known at the turn of the century on January 1, 1900?

Question 4: which usage was more well-known during

World War I (1914-1918)?

Question 5: which usage was more well-known before Mussolini used the gesture in Italy?

Of course those are all trick questions because the question's topics predate (sometimes by decades) the two answers. But the situation changes by adding another choice for the answer: the American use of the gesture. That additional answer is in the following list of quiz answers (students are invited to pick "A" or "B" or "C" as the best answer to the previous questions):

A. The American utilization of the stiff-armed gesture under the socialist Bellamy's Pledge of Allegiance.

B. The German utilization of the stiff-armed gesture under the socialist Hitler.

C. The Italian utilization of the stiff-armed gesture under the socialist Mussolini.

The socialist Bellamy created the Pledge of Allegiance in 1892. The answer to questions 1 through 5 (above) is "A" from the three choices: The American usage of the stiff-armed gesture under the socialist Bellamy's Pledge of Allegiance.

Here is another question: which of the three utilizations above (A. B. or C.) lasted the longest? Most people answer incorrectly that the Hitler salute lasted longer because Hitler died later than Mussolini, and the U.S. Congress amended the flag code in 1942 so that it no longer mentioned the extended-arm gesture. But the question is tricky because all Americans did not immediately follow the flag code. Some Americans did not want to follow the flag code. The long-standing use of the stiff-armed salute in the USA persisted for more than a decade after 1942.[10]

The lifeless droning to the flag on cue in government schools (socialist schools) continues to this day, along with persecution of students who refuse (although the gesture was changed to hide the pledge's uncomfortable past).

Here is the "life-span" of the gestures:
1. Socialist Bellamy ritual 1892-1942 (and beyond, even beyond WWII. And the pledge lives on today).
2. Socialist Hitler ritual 1922?-1945.
3. Socialist Mussolini ritual 1919?-1943.

As the figures show, the Socialist Bellamy salute had about three decades of more impact preceding the Socialist Hitler salute and the Socialist Mussolini salute. It also outlived them. How many millions of people were forced daily to do the American Nazi salute and robotic chanting in socialist schools for years of their lives?

Wakipedia, the old media, and the GMU writer all expose their own dark side: they love the pledge and want to divert attention to the old "irrelevant" arm gesture. They don't want anyone to know that the topic concerns more than the mere gesture; the topic is about government repeatedly mandating a programmed ritual

---

[10] It might continue to occur, considering some reports that Latin classes (in high schools etc) sometimes have "Roman Olympic" events where students are taught (mis-taught) the "ancient Roman salute" and then perform it. They are never taught that it was the early American flag pledge's gesture.

of mechanized vocalizing on cue in government schools (socialist schools) and at the command of government officials.

Wakipedia, the old media, and the GMU writer adore the pretentious ritual and its abuse of children in the US today. They focus on the mere arm gesture in order to mask the real problem: the modern police state ritual and their love of it. The bigger problem is the authoritarian American ritual that was borrowed by German socialists, and that continues daily in the US, and that they continue to support in the US. They will not talk about their role in that.

We don't need any government education. We don't need any thought control. Under socialism, everyone is just another brick in the wall.

3. EDWARD BELLAMY

Francis Bellamy was cousin and comrade of Edward Bellamy (March 26, 1850 to May 22, 1898). At the age of 25, Edward contracted tuberculosis (TB), and it would eventually end his life. He suffered TB's effects throughout his entire adult life. Around 1879, he abandoned the daily grind of his journalism work, and pursued literary work with fewer demands upon his health.

In 1888, after years of study and suffering, Edward's literary work led to the publication of "Looking Backward," an international bestseller.

Ten years later (1898), in his hometown of Chicopee Falls, Massachusetts, Edward Bellamy died at 48 years of age from TB. His lifelong home was designated a National Historic Landmark in 1971.

There are many parallels between Bellamy's socialism and his lesser disease, TB. TB was called "consumption" because it seemed to consume people with long relentless wasting. Bellamy caught TB in his twenties. Bellamy might have caught TB when he lived in Germany (1868-1869) where he also caught his socialism illness.

Tuberculosis was used as a metaphor for political

decay by the socialist Adolf Hitler in his book "Mein Kampf" over two decades after Bellamy's death.

Tuberculosis (TB) remains a major deadly infectious illness today in developing countries that suffer under socialism. It infects two billion people or one-third of the world's population. Nine million new cases of the disease, resulting in two million deaths, occur annually, mostly in backward socialist countries with bad sanitation, where the "industrial revolution" was obstructed by the socialist pandemic. TB deaths compare with the number of deaths under the socialist Wholecaust (of which the Holocaust was a part).

Edward's book "Looking Backward," spawned "Nationalism" clubs worldwide (including Germany). Both Bellamy boys were self-professed socialists who supported the movement, its "Nationalist" magazine, and the Nationalist Educational Association (the NEA - named to deliberately mimic the National Education Association in the USA).

Francis Bellamy used his position with the National Education Association (NEA) to promote "military socialism" -the dogma that he touted with his cousin. In 1892, Bellamy became chairman of the National Education Association's executive committee for a National Public School Celebration plan that would lead to Bellamy writing the larger program that contained the smaller part known as the "Pledge of Allegiance."

The Bellamy "Nationalism" movement was so large that in 1935, Columbia University surveyed the scholars Edward Weeks, Charles Beard, and John Dewey regarding the most influential books and they all ranked Edward Bellamy's book "Looking Backward" (1888) nearly as influential as Karl Marx's "Das Kapital" (1867). Back then, they intended that as a compliment, not as a condemnation.

Although the German philosopher Marx published his book "Capital" in 1867 (the year before Edward Bellamy's trip to Germany), it was not translated into English until after 1886 (ideas in "Capital" had been promoted in newspapers and pamphlets in English. Marx's bizarre conspiracy theory, "Communist Manifesto," was published in 1848).

Marx's Communist Manifesto[11] was printed initially only in German, even though the prelude announced it was to be published in English, French, German, Italian, Flemish, and Danish. After Marx's death in 1883,[12] the German socialist philosopher Friedrich Engels authored prefaces for five editions between 1888 and 1893. Among those is the 1888 English edition, translated by Samuel Moore. It has been the standard English-language version.

The distribution and influence of the English translation of "Capital," and of the main English translation of "The Communist Manifesto" both

---

[11] It is a rape manual that is also known as "A Series of Unfortunate Events" and "It's OK to Be a Lazy Fuck."

[12] Marx's tomb in Highgate Cemetery, London, UK is a Stalinist monstrosity. Marx is depicted as a reverse Santa Claus; he gave EVERYBODY coal (tiny pieces) and expropriated everything from them. During life, Marx wanted to be a wealthy (capitalist) writer, but failed. In death, Marx has had more success as a capitalist: his burial plot is located on private property and his followers are charged an entry fee. Marx chose to purchase the grave even though there were state-provided alternatives for him at that time. Although some followers have complained about his capitalist repose, none, of course, has taken the effort required to "socialize" it (to have government steal money via taxes to pretend that it is "free"). Two attempts have been made to blow it up. Engraved on the tombstone is "#NotRealSocialism™"

coincided with Bellamy's book of 1888.

There are similarities among the "Communist Manifesto" (by the socialist apologist Marx from Germany) and "Mein Kampf" (by the socialist apologist Hitler from Germany) and "Looking Backward" (by the socialist apologist Bellamy from the USA). They share pompous attitudes about the lives of others, and child-like concepts of economics.

Bellamy's book touted "Military Socialism" and the "Industrial Army" at the same time that Marx's Communist Manifesto touted the "Industrial Army" (and it is mentioned in Capital). Both books urged that government schools (socialist schools) be imposed in order to enforce the "Industrial Army" and socialism.

From 1868-1869 Edward Bellamy spent a year in Dresden, learned to speak and write German, attended lectures and studied German socialism. While Bellamy was in Germany, many unions were formed, and so was the German People's Party (Deutsche Volkspartei). Edward's brother Frederick wrote that Edward's letters to him were full of German socialism which "he had read and studied much at home." (see Sylvia E. Bowman "The Year 2000").

In November of 1888, Edward Bellamy hired an interpreter to translate "Looking Backward" into German (see the biography by Arthur Morgan, p. 65). The German translation not only promoted National Socialism in Germany, it also promoted National Socialism in America and cultivated those Americans who later supported the USA's German-American Bund movement that supported German National Socialism.

In 1891, German-language editions of Bellamy's book were advertised in the USA, proclaiming that the novel "Lays the foundation of the Nationalist

Movement." The advertisements coincided with the "Nationalist" magazine of Edward Bellamy, published by the "Nationalist Educational Association."

A weekly publication that promoted Bellamy ideas was combined in advertisements with the book "Capital" by Marx as a package deal (see The New Nation, 1891-94. Marx's book was the translation by Dr. Edward Aveling).

Advertisements listed together the books of Karl Marx, Edward Bellamy, and Charles Bellamy (another one of Edward Bellamy's brothers).

The writer Gail Collins stated: "...far more American workers read Looking Backward than ever made it through Marx..." (Tomorrow Never Knows, The Nation, Vol. 252, Issue # 2, January 21, 1991).

Merritt Abrash described the Bellamy philosophy as Marxism Americanized (see Looking Backward: Marxism Americanized, In M.S. Cummings & N.D. Smith (Eds.)., Utopian Studies IV (pp. 6-9). Lanham, MD: University Press of America (1991).

The book "Edward Bellamy Abroad" by the author Sylvia E. Bowman states that Edward Bellamy's book was translated into every major language including German, Russian, and Chinese. Bowman's book is 543 pages long, and details the Bellamy inspiration to bloodthirsty socialists worldwide.

Bowman's book devotes an entire chapter (55 pages) to describe Edward Bellamy's influence in Germany, including the years leading up to the formation of the National Socialist German Workers' Party (Nazis). Despite her examination of Bellamy's life, Bowman is another example of an author who failed to make the discoveries made by Dr. Curry and described in this book.

Hitler was a big supporter of the Nationalist movement. In "Mein Kampf," he uses the words "Nationalist" and "Nationalism" many times (over 45 times?) and states in words reminiscent of Francis Bellamy's pledge program: "The spirit of nationalism and a feeling for social justice must be fused into one sentiment in the hearts of the youth. Then a day will come when a nation of citizens will arise which will be welded together through a common love and a common pride that shall be invincible and indestructible forever."

Edward Bellamy's Nationalist Clubs published newspapers, including one entitled "The Arena." In 1891, Francis Bellamy promoted socialism in an article entitled "Socialism versus Anarchy" published in the Arena newspaper.[13]

The book "The Pledge of Allegiance" by Dr. John W. Baer states that in the Pledge of Allegiance, Francis Bellamy is expressing the ideas of his first cousin (Edward). Francis was a vice president of the Christian Society of Socialists, affiliated with Edward's Nationalist movement (Francis worked as a lieutenant in the campaign to impose their "military socialism" upon the entire U.S. economy).

The book "Looking Backward" (by Edward Bellamy) was written in 1888 and described a fantasy about life in the year 2000. It is a totalitarian society where all private transactions are outlawed; where the government places all men in an "industrial army" (a Bellamy phrase) explicitly modeled on the military; where the government has taken over all schools as a government monopoly for the "industrial army" system to achieve

---

[13] According to the author Timothy Kubal, in "Cultural Movements and Collective Memory: Christopher Columbus and the Rewriting of the National Origin Myth."

"military socialism" (a Bellamy phrase); where everything is nationalized. All in this paragraph was portrayed as a utopia. The Bellamy cousins admired the military, and said it was very efficient, and they wanted the military system to be imposed upon all of society.

The Bellamy dogma continues to be promoted by the "Edward Bellamy Memorial Association." The association owns and occupies his home at 93 Church St, Chicopee, MA 01020. The association operates part of the house as a museum, renting out the other to obtain financial support.

Edward Bellamy's house is used by another group that continues to support the Bellamy dogma: the Theosophical Society (TS), a group created by Helena Petrovna Blavatsky from Russia, the leading theoretician of Theosophy who claimed to be an occultist and a spirit medium.

Believe it or don't, the Theosophical Society continues to exist (as of this writing) all over the world. There is a group holding meetings twice per month in Saint Petersburg, Florida.

4. GEORGE T. BALCH

Francis Bellamy and Edward Bellamy had help in their campaigns to impose government schools (socialist schools), Christian Socialism, Military Socialism, flag fetishism, and servile chanting in unison and on command (with embarrassing gestures). The Bellamys were helped by Colonel George Thacher Balch and by Captain Wallace Foster.

Balch (October 2, 1828 - April 15, 1894) was usually known as Colonel George T. Balch but he has also been referred to as Captain Balch and Brevet Lieutenant Colonel Balch. Balch worked with Captain Wallace Foster. After Balch died, Foster continued to promote flag fetishism until Foster's death in 1919.

In 1890, two years after Edward Bellamy wrote about Military Socialism in "Looking Backward," and two years before Bellamy started his pledge with a military salute, Balch used the military salute as a flag gesture on page 34 of Balch's book about patriotism. The title page states "Methods of Teaching Patriotism in the Public Schools" (hereinafter "Meth Teaching") and adds "Being an extract from an address delivered before the teachers of the Children's Aid Society of the City of New York by Colonel Geo. T. Balch, Auditor of the

Board of Education of the City of New York, June 28, 1889." It has 109 Arabic numeral pages (over 150 total pages, including 41 Roman numeral pages with a lengthy preface in which Balch explained that he intended to triple the length of the book with two more sections). This first third of his book Balch entitled "Emotional Patriotism" (a more accurate title would have been "Emotional Masturbation," especially in regard to the onanistic pledge that continues in schools today). [fap. fap. fap.]

Page 34 of Balch's book contains these instructions for the military salute to the flag:

Thereupon, at a second signal, the whole school will rise, and after a brief pause, until the utmost stillness reigns, at the command, "Salute the flag!" given by the Principal in a clear voice and a deliberate manner, each scholar—raising the extended right hand to the forehead (palm down), in unison with a like movement by the Principal—will salute the flag in military fashion.

Balch supported his scheme by citing then-new flag fetishism in the Navy from order # 374 signed by the Secretary of the Navy and directing all persons to salute the morning and evening colors (that "salute" is presumed herein to be the military salute).

Balch's military salute for students might have been used in only two schools (at the time his book was published) as evidenced by the following quote concerning a related scheme to use flags as awards: "The plan just sketched for using the flag as a reward for individual good conduct has recently been tried in two schools of the Children's Aid Society with the most marked success." (p 26).

Balch's was involved with 21 schools in New York City (schools operated by the Children's Aid Society). Not content with voluntary aid societies, Balch had the same yearning that all socialists (including the Bellamys) have: use the government to force his schemes on everyone everywhere. Balch wanted the government to take over education. It was the same yearning that motivated the militant socialists Stalin, Mao, Hitler, et cetera in their use of flags, nationalism, patriotism, and government/socialist schools.

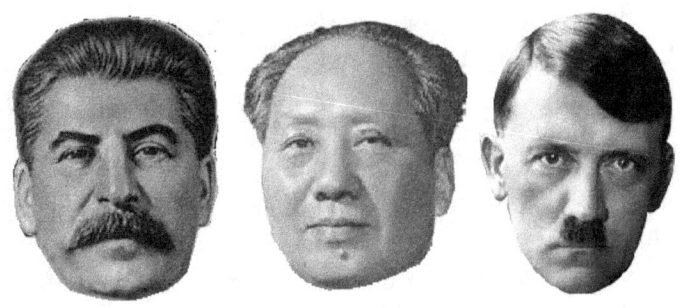

Balch's gesture in the quote above was the military salute alone and nothing more. Francis Bellamy's gesture was an initial military salute that was then extended outward to gesture at the flag. In its actual use, the second part of the Bellamy gesture was (because of the military gesture at the beginning) sometimes performed with a stiff-arm, in a manner that would become known as the "Nazi salute."

When Francis Bellamy and James B. Upham collaborated on the flag salutation in 1892, Bellamy was aware of Balch's pledge and Bellamy said so in writing ("The Story of the Pledge of Allegiance to The Flag" by

Francis Bellamy, reprinted by the University of Rochester Library Bulletin: The Story of the Pledge of Allegiance to the Flag, Volume VIII, Winter 1953, Number 2). Bellamy only mentions the words of Balch's pledge. It is not clear whether Bellamy or Upham were aware of the military salute mentioned in Balch's 1890 book.

Balch said that he was inspired in 1888 when he observed a teacher and students conducting a small patriotic ceremony in a classroom while Balch was working as the auditor of New York City's public schools.

After Balch died in 1894, there were multiple editions published (until 1909?) of another book in which he is mentioned and might have been involved: "A Patriotic Primer for the Little Citizen." The edition of the primer that was examined for research here was dated 1898 and only contained Foster's name for the front and copyright. There was a quotation attributed to Balch near the front of the book, and another Balch quotation within the body of the book. It is unclear from the publication the extent of Balch's participation. The introduction in the book states:

In consideration and in memory of the late Col. George T. Balch, the author dedicates the "American Patriotic Primer for the Little Citizen" to our boys and girls attending the public schools, with a fervent wish that their love for their country and flag may increase day by day and graduate them noble, generous, law-abiding, loyal American citizens. - W.F. [Wallace Foster]

Inside the front cover is a photograph of Balch with

this description: "Author of Teaching Patriotism in the Public Schools" [note again that it does not state that he is the author of "A Patriotic Primer for the Little Citizen"].

The printed text in the book appears to contain no hand gesture for children to use toward the flag. The military salute from the 1890 Meth Teaching book is not mentioned. The back cover contains an illustration that shows a woman holding the flag and the Balch/Foster pledge in front of two children; the boy appears to be waving his hat in his left hand; the girl appears to be waving or acclaiming with her right hand with the palm up.

Another version of the primer (also dated 1898 and marked "Third Edition") contains text of the Balch/Foster pledge ("We Give Our Heads and Our Hearts to God and Our Country! One Country! One Language! ONE FLAG!) surrounding the outside of a photograph that shows a woman holding the flag in front of six children; all six children are literally pointing at the flag with their index fingers extended on their right hands. That photograph clearly indicates that the Balch/Foster pledge was at one time performed by pointing at the flag as the ultimate gesture. It is a gesture that kindergartners can probably pull off without screwing it up.

There are few photographs, and perhaps no film footage of the Balch/Foster hand gesture(s) to the flag. There are many photographs (most remain hidden) of the Bellamy salute, as well as old film footage showing clearly how the initial military salute was extended outward to point at the flag in the classic hard stiff-armed palm-down Nazi gesture.

Page 70 shows that Foster (and Balch?) was aware of

Francis Bellamy's Pledge of Allegiance. Bellamy's salutation is printed in the Balch/Foster book. It is without any description of the hand gesture that was provided in the Youth's Companion in 1892. This is the reference in the 1898 Balch/Foster primer:

I pledge allegiance to my flag, and
The Republic for which it stands—
One Nation indivisible,
With Liberty and Justice for all.
> —Frank Bellamy.

Here is another excerpt from the 1898 primer (p 16):

64. What do we mean by the salutation of the Flag? The mark of respect among all nations is uncovering the head, the expression of love is to touch the heart. Hence we have been taught to say—as we touch, first our foreheads, and next our hearts— "We Give Our Heads! —and Our Hearts! —TO God! and Our Country!"

In a country where people from many nations are gathered together to enjoy the inestimable blessings which America offers, we little citizens think it right and just that the American principles, the American language and the American Flag Should be Supreme Over all Others, and so we complete our salute with the words, "One Country! —One Language! —One Flag!

[No military salute or hand gesture is described]

On page 20 of the book, the military salute is mentioned in a question for students:

"42. How do the officers and men of the United States army and navy salute the flag? By raising the extended right hand to the forehead, palm downward."

On page 21 the practice of uncovering and bowing the head is mentioned:

"44. What should we all do on passing the schoolhouse flag or in a military camp, or on boarding a United States war vessel? Uncover and bow the head. It will be appreciated, and you will be honoring the flag of your country."

The book went through several printings by 1909.

It is not clear when Balch or Foster switched from the military salute alone, to the gesture toward the flag (without the military salute).

The page opposite Balch's photograph (in an 1898 third edition) states this: "Boys and girls, off with your hats as the teacher goes by, and reverentially bow or salute them whenever you have the opportunity, for true teachers are the guardian angels of the Republic. - W.F." This quote helped take the American Nazi salute outside of the pledge and into gesturing toward other people decades before Hitler's German socialism. What happened in government schools did not stay in government schools.

In March, 1912, the Teachers Magazine, page 274 (Teachers Magazine for Primary Grades. Ives-Butler Company) describes an extended arm gesture and attributes it to Balch. It is not clear from the article when the hand gesture was added. The author of the article is not listed. The article claims to repeat material from Balch (who had died 18 years before in 1894). It is probable that in 1893, before Balch died, the only students performing Balch's pledge (with a military gesture, or without a gesture, or with some other gesture) were the students who attended New York City's twenty-one Children's Aid Society schools (the schools with which Balch was most involved). The following is from the 1912 Teacher's Magazine:

THE PLAN EXPLAINED TO THE CHILDREN.

"In May and June, 1891, these schools were all visited and addressed on the subject of "Why children in the public schools should salute the Nation's flag and how they should salute it." In connection with the address, the pupils were exercised in the necessary movements and in the words. The address and the drill were adapted in language and form of expression (as near as it is possible for age to adapt itself to youth) to the measure of the comprehension of the children. That they enjoyed it was evident from their great interest and their enthusiasm. At that time the only words used were, 'We give our heads and our hearts to our country!" Observing, however, that the Italian and German flags were used in a few of the Schools, and appreciating how important were the first impressions, that it was American citizens we were endeavoring to mold and shape, and citizens of no other nation, in October of 1891, the words, "one country, one language, one flag." were added. —

"The words finally agreed upon were these: "We give our heads and our hearts to God and our country! One country, one language, one flag!"

THE DRILL.

"The manner of executing it is as follows:

"The pupils have been assembled and are seated. The flag borne by the standard-bearer is before the school. At the signal (either by a chord struck on the piano, or in the absence of a piano from a bell), each child seizes the Seat preparatory to rising.

"Second Signal. —The whole school rises quickly, as one person, each one standing erect and alert.

"Third Signal. —The right arm is extended, pointing directly at the flag. As the flag bearer should be on the platform where all can see the colors, the extended arm will be slightly raised above the horizontal line.

"Fourth Signal. —The forearm is bent so as to touch the forehead lightly with the tip of the fingers of the right hand. The motion should be quick but graceful, the elbow being kept down and not allowed to stick out to the right. As the fingers touch the forehead, each pupil will exclaim in a clear voice, 'We give our heads'—emphasizing the word 'heads.'

"Fifth Signal. —The right hand is carried quickly to the left side and placed flat over the heart, with the words: 'and our hearts!" uttered after the movement has been made.

"Sixth Signal. —The right hand is allowed to fall quickly but easily to the right side; as soon as the motion is accomplished, all will say, "to God and our country!"

"Seventh Signal. —Each child, still standing erect but without moving, will exclaim: "One country!" (emphasis on country).

"Eighth Signal. —The children, still standing motionless, will exclaim: 'One language!" (emphasis on language).

"Ninth Signal. —The right arm is suddenly extended to its full length, the hand pointing to the flag, the body inclining slightly forward, supported by the right foot slightly advanced; the attitude should be that of intense earnestness, the pupil reaching, as it were, toward the flag, at the same time exclaiming with great force: 'One flag.'

"Tenth Signal. —The right arm is dropped to the side and the position of attention recovered.

"Eleventh Signal. —Each child seizes the seat preparatory to turning it down.

"Twelfth Signal. —The school is seated.

"Flag Bearer. —The color bearer grasps the staff at the lower end with his right hand and a foot or more (according to the length of the staff) above the end of the staff with his left hand. The staff is held directly in front of the middle of the body, slightly inclined forward from the perpendicular. At the fourth signal the flag will be dipped, returning the salute; this is done by lowering the left hand until the staff is nearly horizontal, keeping it in that position until the tenth signal, when it will be restored to its first or nearly vertical position.

Balch's "one country, one language, one flag" cliché was similar to Bellamy's "one nation, indivisible" phrase in that they both reference the War of Northern Aggression and the fact that no state would be allowed to leave, and that mass murder would be used to force all states to stay in the United Socialist States of America.

They are reminders of Germany's "Deutschland über alles!" (Germany above all), a phrase from the song "Deutschlandlied" by August Heinrich Hoffmann in

1841, nearly a half-century before Hitler was even born (but 13 years after Balch was born), and expressing hopes for the eventual reunification of the ~30 German states.

They are reminders of the German National Socialist poster: Ein Volk, ein Reich, ein Führer ('One People, One Nation, One Leader'). The slogan's impact was huge in 1938, with the Anschluss ('union'), when Germany joined in union with Austria, and kept going into other nations thereafter.

Evidence in the earlier publications (1890, 1898) about Balch indicate that Bellamy's gesture (1892) was performed in the Nazi-style in advance of any Nazi-style gesture promoted by Balch (as described in the questionable 1912 article).

There is additional evidence of Balch's standard military salute in the Youth's Companion (hereinafter YC), a weekly magazine published in Boston. On August 29, 1889, the YC printed the article "Teaching Patriotism" which knocked the flag rituals advocated by the "gentleman of New York" (Balch had delivered an address on June 28, 1889 to the teachers of the Children's Aid Society in New York City. Balch's book would be published in 1890). YC said that the rituals were better suited for the military. The YC article is evidence that Balch was merely touting the military salute.

The YC article's "military" remark also refers to Balch's desire that government/socialist schools ape the military system with three types of metallic badges (for scholars, teachers, and principals), drills, rituals, color guards, standard bearers, signal flags, the use of small flags as rewards daily for good conduct by students, scholar's flags, class flags, school flags, the use of the flag as a semaphore, weekly reports and much more, including these chapters: "Permissive and mandatory legislation" and "Voluntary vs. compulsive patriotism" and "How shall the loyalty of a school to American institutions be ascertained and tested?"

"Test Day" is every day for golems in government schools (socialist schools) as each morning begins with the inverted IQ test: the Pledge of Allegiance piped in by Big Brother over the class intercom [mic feedback]. The pledge ensures that student IQ's are low enough to maintain submission to socialism.

It is a reminder of the science fiction short story "Examination Day" by Henry Slesar: A student is worried about an upcoming IQ test at the government (socialist) school, and his parents assure him that he will do fine, even though they too are worried. SPOILER ALERT: the IQ test identifies all who are "too intelligent" and results in their executions.[14]

The Pledge of Allegiance was Slesar's "Exam Day"

---

[14] Lenin, Stalin, Mao, Hitler, Pol Pot, and others understood that they had to identify everyone who was too intelligent to be duped by socialism. Everyone with an IQ that high had to be killed. That is why mental health experts recommend psychiatric evaluations of all socialists, both real and imaginary.

For example, the socialist professor Malcolm Caldwell become a cheer-leader for Pol Pot and traveled to Cambodia to experience the socialist utopia and was murdered on the day he met his idol. This comic tragedy writes itself. Believe it or not, one of Caldwell's ridiculous books was published *posthumously*: "Kampuchea: A Rationale for a Rural Policy." In it he wrote that KR socialism "opens vistas of hope not only for the people of Cambodia but also for the peoples of all other poor third world countries." Before he got himself killed in Cambodia, clown Caldwell had visited North Korea and repeated lies to glorify Kim Il-Sung.

every day because student dissenters were expelled from socialist schools, persecuted, and beaten; and adult rebels were arrested, imprisoned, and lynched.

Everyone should be thankful that "Meth Teaching" did not order children to wear armbands and waive Balch's book about like Mao's little red book. Instead of teaching, Balch promoted flag waiving and state worship similar to the socialists Stalin, Mao, Hitler.

Later, in 1892, the YC would promote an expanded military salute for Bellamy's Pledge of Allegiance.

Shortly after the YC article about him, Balch mentioned the Youth's Companion and Balch repeated at length (over three pages) the YC's flag promotion in his "Meth Teaching" book (1890). Starting on page 78 of Balch's book:

On the 9th of January, 1890, The Youth's Companion, published in Boston, Mass., which has a circulation of 33,645 copies in the State of New York, and of nearly half a million in the United States, made public the following offer:

THE FLAG AND THE PUBLIC SCHOOLS.

The Youth's Companion, in one of its issues of more than a year ago, set forth the idea of the flag and the public schools. The idea is becoming popular, and the American flag can now be seen floating over many a patriotic school.

The Youth' s Companion now asks the privilege of floating an American flag (at its own expense) over one public school-house in each of the forty-two States.

Which one of the schools in each State shall have the flag?

The scholars in any of our public schools, wishing

to secure the flag for their school, can compete for it in the following manner:

They are invited to write an essay, of not more than 600 words in length, on " The Patriotic Influence of the American Flag when Raised over the Public Schools."

These essays are to be handed to their teacher for examination. The essay selected by the teacher as the best may be forwarded to The Youth's Companion on or before April 1, 1890.

Each essay sent to us must be accompanied by the name of the school, the author, and the town and State.

The school in each State sending us the best essay on the subject will receive from us, free of all expense, a regulation bunting flag, nine by fifteen feet in size—forty-two stars.

The awards will be made as soon after April 1st as possible, in season for the schools to dedicate the flags on the Fourth of July, 1890.

As soon as the award of the flags has been made, The Youth's Companion will publish the names of the schools receiving them, also the names of the writers of the essays.

Perry Mason & Co., Publishers The Youth's Companion, Boston, Mass.

In April last the award of the flag for the State of New York was made by the publishers of The Youth's Companion in accordance with the agreement set forth in the foregoing notice; the flag going to Grammar School No. 63, situated at North Third avenue and 173d street, in the Twenty-fourth Ward of the City of New York, of which Mr. John H. Myers is the Principal. The following is the essay thus declared to be the best of all from the Empire State:

"THE PATRIOTIC INFLUENCE OF THE AMERICAN FLAG WHEN RAISED ABOVE A PUBLIC SCHOOL."

It shall be my object in writing on this subject, not to prove that this influence should be exerted over the older people so much, but over the boys—for two reasons: first, because being a boy, I am able to judge more accurately of the feelings of a boy; and secondly, because those who are boys now, will, in future time, be the great men of our nation —the presidents, the statesmen, the soldiers, editors, the clergymen, etc.

On coming to school and seeing the "Stars and Stripes" floating in the breeze over the school-house, what boy would not pause in admiration and think of the glorious battles in which this same beautiful banner had so triumphantly waved—at Stony Point, Saratoga, at the mast heads of Paul Jones' gallant ships, at Fort McHenry, from which the idea of our beautiful song, "The Star Spangled Banner," was taken—all through the Mexican War, and later still in the bloody battles of the "Rebellion," at Murfreesboro, Gettysburg, and on the victorious "Monitor."

And it must be a mean-spirited and unpatriotic boy indeed, who would not be willing to fight under a flag for which so many brave men have fought and died.

And then he would think what that flag represented—a country, not like Russia or Turkey, where the people are compelled to bow to the will of one man, who has but to say the word and one's head is severed from his body, or the individual is compelled to conform to some particular creed in which the despot believes—but a country where everybody is free! free to worship God as he please, free to elect the men who govern him; a country which protects him where he is now—which protects the schools and floats its flag over them as a sign of such protection, the school where some of the happiest, and, maybe, some of the bitterest hours of his life have been spent.

A country where men have equal chances to win in the struggle of life; and, as he thinks of all these glorious privileges, do you suppose for a minute that he would stand by and calmly see that emblem of freedom torn down?

No!!! the very thought rouses his ire! And as he enters school he remembers the words of the poet—
"Forever float that standard sheet!
Where breathes the foe but falls before us?
With Freedom's soil beneath our feet,
And Freedom's banner streaming o'er us."

And as he thinks of these words, he vows, with one all-concentrating and all-hallowing vow, that, Almighty God helping him, he will never, never, NEVER see the flag dishonored.

And every one of us from the utmost depths of his soul, echoes—
"AMEN!"
Louis V. Fox,
Grammar School No. 63.
April 1st, 1890.

Louis V. Fox cited Russia under the Czar as an

example of despotism in 1890, two decades before the socialist Czars Lenin and Stalin would make their predecessors seem angelic in comparison.[15]

In 1890 the U.S. government filled a boy's head with the same evils it spreads today: never-ending violence and warfare so rabid that it inspires kids and kidults to violence against anyone who "dishonors" a piece of cloth. Fittingly mixed up, of course, with prayerful invocations of God.

Fox and Balch probably did not consider Jehovah's Witnesses to be true Christians. And they probably did not care about Muslims nor anyone else who did not want to salute and bombinate on command. Anyone who refused was not a "True Christian" as far as they were concerned.

"Christian Socialists" share blame for the concept "desecration of the flag" (treating the flag as a sacred religious object) and for laws that criminalize "desecration of the flag." Government schools created snowflake generations that threaten violence against anyone who "disrespects" any Chinese-made American flag. "Scared" and "sacred" both have the same letters and one is used to inculcate the other. Balch is one of many examples of why that iNsaNitY existed then, and why it continues today.

The Balch books glorify violence and war for small children. The following is another example from the Balch/Foster book "A Patriotic Primer for the Little Citizen" –

Gen. Benjamin F. Butler's famous Flag Order No.

---

[15] The pock-marked little squirt Stalin has been compared to Empress Catherine II of Russia. The gray blur (Stalin) turned the USSR into a gray blur too.

10, 5th, 1862.

Wm. B. Mumford, a citizen of New Orleans, before a military commission, having been convicted of treason, in tearing down the United States flag from a public building of the United States for the purpose of inciting other evil-minded persons to further resistance to the laws and arms of the United States, after said flag was placed there by Commodore (flag officer) Farragut, of the United States navy.

"It is ordered that he be executed according to the sentence of the said military commission, on Saturday, June 7th, inst., between the hours of eight a.m., and twelve m., under the direction of the provost-marshal of the district of New Orleans; and for so doing this shall be his sufficient warrant."

The primer does not provide the following information: When Mumford was taken to be hanged and was permitted to deliver a final speech. He spoke of his patriotism for the Confederacy and his love for what he considered the true meaning of the U.S. flag, which he had fought under in the Seminole and Mexican-American wars. After Mumford was hanged, Confederate Governor of Louisiana Thomas Overton Moore issued a statement declaring Mumford a hero and a model. Louisiana schools taught the opposite of what the Balch/Foster primer taught in NYC.

Children had a role-model of violence and war in the life of Balch. Born in 1828, Balch promoted Military Socialism and Christian Socialism before the Bellamys did. Because they promoted the deadly dogma of socialism, the Bellamys share some blame for the dearth and death of millions globally, although neither one of the Bellamys personally killed people. Balch did both.

Balch attended West Point Military Academy and after graduation in 1852, he was commissioned a lieutenant of artillery for the Union. In 1861 he was with the artillery at Fort Pickens, in Pensacola, FL. Soon after, the War Department directed him to the Ordnance Bureau in Washington, D.C.

Balch was a proud killer for the USA's worst mass-murderer: President Abraham Lincoln. Balch (and the Killer-In-Chief Lincoln) did it for "One Nation! One flag!" The war was called the "War of Rebellion" (in the primer). On the topic of slavery, Balch's chant was silent. Balch did not want the South to have a different piece of cloth. That would be disrespectful.

Balch was considered a success in the most socialistic institution of all: the military. It provides food, clothing, shelter, jobs, training (schooling), et cetera and causes people like Balch to imagine that the same system can be imposed on EVERYONE in regular society to provide food, clothing, shelter, jobs, training (schooling), et cetera. The militant socialists Stalin, Mao, and Hitler had similar imaginations. In 1863, conscription (slavery) was imposed for the North's most socialistic institution: the military.

Balch's boss was killed on April 15, 1865. After the nation's worst murderer was murdered by John Wilkes Booth, the latter exclaimed "Sic semper tyrannis!" (Thus always to tyrants!).[16]

Later, Balch promoted the display of a portrait of the country's most prolific killer in every classroom. It is a

---

[16] The phrase remains on the seal of the state of Virginia.

It was on the T-shirt worn by Timothy McVeigh after he attacked the federal government in response to Waco and Ruby Ridge.

practice that continues to occur in some schools today. China has a similar practice: the Chinese government embarrasses everyone with ubiquitous portraits of that country's most prolific killer (Monster Mao, another economic illiterate) in schools, on buildings, on paper money, and everywhere, as a national role model. What a government of socialist sickos! Similar behavior occurred under the socialists Stalin and Hitler.

Balch used a military title (colonel) when he worked at schools, in his publications, and through much of his life.

Did he continue to dress in uniform so as to help youngsters fantasize about shooting, stabbing, and killing as they were led in military salutes and flag drills?

Balch was concerned that immigrant children were potential criminals. But it was acceptable if they were taught to travel to other states or foreign lands to commit mass murder for their government. Or to violently attack (or execute) anyone who disrespected its flag.

Nothing in his books mentions self-defense against violence for students on the streets of New York City, nor defense of the family or home from criminals.

When Balch said he wanted to promote patriotism and government schools (socialist schools), he meant it and, like so many socialists, he would kill you to do it. When he said he wanted you to remain in the Union and worship the federal government, he meant it, or else! It is the ultra-violence of socialism.

Balch was also worried about native Americans ("Indians" in the primer), even though, technically speaking, they were not foreigners (in fact the opposite). They had a language and behavior that was foreign to Balch. He wanted to teach them to venerate the US flag and to laud it in "one language!" (American?).

A chapter entitled "We, of necessity, killed a great many women and children," mentions Balch fulfilling his career goals in regard to the Sioux near Fort Pierre, South Dakota in the book "The First Sioux War: The Grattan Fight and Blue Water Creek, 1854-1856" by Paul Norman Beck.

Balch died on April 15, 1894. His obituary states that his body was taken to Troy, NY for burial (the home town of his wife). Troy, NY, was named in 1789 after the famous city popularized in Homer's Iliad. As the state of New York was settled, cities were often given names from classical history. Troy follows the NY pattern of Syracuse, Rome, Utica, Ithaca, or the towns of Sempronius and Manlius.

Troy (Hisarlik, Turkey, in Asia Minor, aka Ilium) was the site of excavations of Greek/Trojan remains in the 1870s. The archaeologist Heinrich Schliemann discovered scrawls that he labeled "swastikas" in that area. Thereafter, a swastika fad developed in the USA, Germany, and other parts of the world, with the symbol used on jewelry, clothing, architecture, printing, pottery, and more.

Rome, NY (not in Italy) was where Francis Bellamy was raised. After his pledge spread, its stiff-armed gesture became known as the "Roman salute." After Bellamy died in Tampa, FL on August 28, 1931 at the age of 76, his cremated remains were buried in Rome, NY.

Here are some words and concepts to look for in Balch books: corporate; Christian; Christianity; Christianizing; religion; religious; religious songs; degeneracy; free; free education; free schools; public schools; day schools; industrial schools; patriotism;

military; socialism; race; flags.

Some Americans believe that everyone has always enjoyed hoisting flags and droning obediently in unison on command. Not so. Here is a comment from Foster in 1910: "Oklahoma seems to have been overrun with this class of undesirable citizens, who have entered the schools and refuse to allow patriotic organizations to display the Stars and Stripes in or over the school, or to introduce patriotic instructions in the schools where they are teaching." (p 310 of the Journal of the 28th National Convention of the Woman's Relief Corps, Auxiliary to the Grand Army of the Republic, Volume 28, Part 1910 by Woman's Relief Corps (U.S.). National Convention).

Many historians (ALL historians besides Dr. Rex Curry?) portray Bellamy and Balch as benignly trying to put a flag in (or over) school houses. The other historians ignore the bigger point: They were trying to impose SOCIALISM in education and beyond. They wanted government to take over all schools. What is it about writers that causes them to portray the Bellamys and Balch/Foster as cute flag-pushers but not socialism-pushers? Are they avoiding how government/socialist schools imposed segregation by law and taught racism as official policy? They do not want to discuss how American socialists wanted (and continue to want) more "Military Socialism" imposed on all of society in order to provide single-payer food, single-payer clothing, single-payer shelter, single-payer schools, assigned jobs, and everything?

Balch spent much of his career in a system that imposed segregation by law and taught racism as official policy: the military. The Bellamys and Balch/Foster both glorified the violent military system and government/socialist schools, two socialist institutions that continued to impose caste systems via segregation by law, while teaching racism as official policy, in a manner that would be culturally appropriated by German socialists decades later. The legacy of the Bellamys and Balch/Foster in the USA outlasted German socialism.

5. PLEDGE OF ALLEGIANCE DRILLS

Francis Bellamy's Pledge of Allegiance was published first in the Youth's Companion Magazine in 1892. That article shows the following: The original pledge began with a military salute for the phrase "I pledge allegiance...." and then the right-arm military salute was extended outward toward the flag for the rest of the pledge so that the right arm was held aloft at an angle directed at the flag, as if to signify, "There is the flag."

The following paragraph is an excerpt showing the pledge as printed for the first time in the 1892 edition of the Youth's Companion Magazine:

At a signal from the Principal the pupils, in ordered ranks, hands to the side, face the Flag. Another signal is given; every pupil gives the Flag the military salute - right hand lifted, palm downward, to a line with the forehead and close to it. Standing thus, all repeat together, slowly: "I pledge allegiance to my Flag and the Republic for which it stands; one Nation, indivisible, with Liberty and Justice for all." At the words, "to my Flag," the right hand is extended gracefully, palm upward, towards the Flag,

and remains in this gesture till the end of the affirmation.; whereupon all hands immediately drop to the side. [end of excerpt]

The impact of the military salute as the origin of the Nazi salute is visible in old film footage of children performing the Pledge of Allegiance. Film footage shows conclusively that the military salute was, in practice, extended straight outward to point at the flag (with the palm down).

The original Youth's Companion article along with other research led to more discoveries by Professor Curry:

(1). Due to the way that the pledge used the gestures sequentially, the military salute led to the Nazi salute. The Nazi salute is an extended (outstretched) military salute. Although the original Youth's Companion description directed that the palm be turned upward, that was not the case in practice. Historic photographs and film show that in practice the palm was down because the awkward pledge was performed casually with the initial military salute perfunctorily stretched straight out toward the flag (palm down, because the military salute is palm down in the USA, although it is not palm down in the British army and in some other countries).

(2). The straight-armed salute of the early Pledge of Allegiance was the source of the salute of the National Socialist German Workers' Party (Nazis).

(3). The gesture was neither an ancient Roman salute nor an ancient Olympic salute, and was not ancient in any way.

(4). Photographs and films show that eventually the military salute was dropped entirely from the chanting ritual. Perhaps teachers and parents were disturbed by the military part, if not by the whole pledge. Perhaps it was considered disrespectful to the military – a euphemistic way of saying it was creepy to have children pretending to be in the army. When the military salute was abandoned, nothing remained but the classic Nazi salute.

The above explains why the media, schools, history museums, and other so-called "educational" outlets, will never show film footage (nor photographs) of the early Pledge of Allegiance. Due to general political considerations, they do not want to show the pledge's shameful past (and its shameful present, and its shameful future).

The following is a list of persons who are immortalized in photographs or film performing the early American pledge salute:

General Hugh Johnson (Director of National Recovery Administration under President Franklin Roosevelt)
Senator Burton Wheeler (Socialist and Democrat w the America First Committee, or AFC)
Charles A. Lindbergh (aviator; w AFC)
Norman Thomas (Presidential Candidate six times for Socialist Party & w AFC. A Christian Socialist).
Kathleen Norris (novelist and socialist)
Lois Wilson (film actress)
Margaret Hamilton (film actress)
Katherine Alexander (film actress)
Virginia Weidler (film actress)

MADNESS

Peter Holden (film actor)
Peter Miles (film actor)
Darryl Hickman (film actor)

6. WAR OF REBELLION AGAINST SOCIALISM

Which is more similar to the swastika flag: the Confederate flag or the U.S. flag? Which is more of a sign of racism?

The Confederate flag is a popular answer in government schools (socialist schools), with students who are ignorant of the history of the U.S. flag, its Pledge of Allegiance, and the Bellamys.

That answer changes when students learn that the U.S. flag and its Pledge of Allegiance were the origins of the Nazi salute and Nazi behavior (e.g. obsequious chanting). The pledge is disrespectful to citizens. It was also the origin of the Nazi salute and Nazi behavior under the swastika flag.

The government (socialist) schools that Bellamy promoted imposed segregation by law and taught racism as official policy. Racism in socialist schools permeated all areas, including hiring teachers, and the creation, location, and maintenance of schools.[17] Those racist

---

[17] Under German socialism, all academics (including university level) were civil servants and thus subjected to the official racism of the socialist educational system under Hitler. Many academics were dismissed from their jobs.

policies even outlasted German national socialism. Some observers argue that official segregation and racism continues today in the socialist schools, albeit in ulterior ways. Age segregation continues.

Within the racist schools, segregated classrooms of black children were forced to perform the Nazi salute and to drone slavishly together at the ring of a bell for 12 years of their lives. People who refused were expelled, beaten, imprisoned, and even lynched. It is impossible to quantify the damage that was done (and that continues to be done) by socialist racism.

Even after some school segregation ended, the government continued its racism and used forced busing to destroy black neighborhoods.

The U.S. continues to hold the worst world records for imprisoning blacks and otherwise ruining their lives with felony convictions for victimless crimes and fabricated arrests.

Nondiscrimination laws make it illegal for businesses to say they won't hire Mexicans, but immigration laws make it illegal to hire almost any of them - even if Americans want to hire them and they want to work - just because they happen to have been born in Mexico. Of course, the same official discrimination and segregation is mandated against the Chinese, and the Irish, and the other seven billion people on earth. Laws in the U.S. specify who Americans can marry, hire, live with, work with, rent to, et cetera. Socialism imposes discrimination and bigotry, while socialists pretend to embrace tolerance and diversity.

Francis Bellamy and Edward Bellamy admired how the military had killed so many Americans during the War for Southern Independence. It was the source of their Nationalism and their national socialism. The phrase "one nation indivisible" in Bellamy's salutation reveals his perception of the war: not against slavery, but to "preserve the union" by reversing the South's declaration of independence.

After the War of Northern Aggression, the pledge enabled Christian Socialists to lead a daily witch hunt for disloyalty within government schools (socialist schools) each morning at the ring of a bell.

Bellamy did that despite the history that is celebrated each 4th of July: when slaveholders seceded from their country (slave-holding Britain) and soon thereafter the "damn Yankees" waved the red, white, and blue flag over their seceded slave-holding rebel land.

Bellamy wanted everyone to bombinate his Pledge of Allegiance to the nation and its flag - a flag that had flown over a nation of slavery since the flag's creation so long ago.

Here are numbers of slaves under the US flag:

1790 - 697,897[18]
1800 - 893,041
1810 - 1,191,364
1820 - 1,538,038
1830 - 2,009,050
1840 - 2,487,455
1850 - 3,204,313
1860 - 3,953,760[19]

---

[18] Before 1790, some of the first slaves in America were Europeans. Shipwrecked Europeans were taken as slaves by natives (e.g. the Calusa and Timucua in Florida). Before that natives took each other as slaves.

[19] These numbers are small compared to the number of people enslaved under the confederation of Stalin, Mao, Hitler (SMH) and other socialists. The numbers are small

People complain that the formation of the USA was flawed because the original Constitution recognized slavery (despite the objections of some American revolutionaries). Yet, slavery continues to exist in the USA and remains in the Constitution. The Thirteenth Amendment states: "Neither slavery nor involuntary servitude, **except as a punishment for crime whereof the party shall have been duly convicted**, shall exist within the United States, or any place subject to their jurisdiction." [emphasis added].

The U.S. sets world records for modern slavery and especially against blacks (often imprisoned for non-violent capitalist activity under modern prohibition). Prisons and military bases are "socialist utopias" that provide food, clothing, shelter, medical care (and little freedom). The U.S. has so much utopian socialism.

Louisiana State Penitentiary (LSP) is a huge prison farm, the largest maximum security prison in the U.S., and is known as "Angola" after the African country the slaves of this former (?) plantation originally came from.[20]

---

compared to the number of people murdered by SMH and other socialists. Socialism is bizarre because it kills so many of its slaves. It is a confederacy of dunces.

People react differently to the public display at a rally of a Soviet socialist flag, as compared with a German socialist flag. My Chairman is better than your Fuhrer! My socialist is better than your socialist! How strange. Many who are offended by the confederate flag don't mind the flags of Soviet socialism nor Chinese socialism, both symbols of millions more killed.

[20] Africa has a long history of slavery, including Africans enslaving other Africans and selling them to non-Africans (e.g. Europeans going to America).

Further back in history, Hebrews were allegedly slaves to Africans in Africa. There are pyramids there, monuments of

LSP was and is a slave planation under the U.S. Constitution. All prisons are.

In November 2016, voters wrestled with whether to remove an amendment from Colorado's state constitution that was similar to the U.S.'s 13th Amendment. Some supporters of the old slavery clause argued that it only refers to forcing inmates to work with little or no pay (that caging a man for decades does not enslave him?). Courts have ruled that the presence or lack thereof of similar state constitutional amendments

---

slavery, that should be torn down.

Slavery is practiced in Mauritania, Mali, Niger, Chad and Sudan. Around 11-21-2017, Zimbabweans celebrated the ouster of longtime Marxist socialist President Robert Mugabe. Around that same time, blacks were being sold by auction in Libya. So, Lincoln did not "end slavery."

"Blacks were not enslaved because they were black but because they were available. Slavery has existed in the world for thousands of years. Whites enslaved other whites in Europe for centuries before the first black was brought to the Western hemisphere. Asians enslaved Europeans. Asians enslaved other Asians. Africans enslaved other Africans, and indeed even today in North Africa, blacks continue to enslave blacks." -attributed to Thomas Sowell

"I was a slave," said Lily Tang Williams of her life in China under Mao.

Romanian socialism under Ceausescu sold ethnic Germans and Jews. West Germany paid ~$20,000 for each German exported, and Israel paid a similar amount for each Jew who made the Exodus from socialist slavery.

Boxer Cassius Marcellus Clay, Jr., named after an abolitionist who freed his inherited slaves, changed his name to Muhammad, a slave owner/trader.

Was Obama a descendent of slave owners on his mother's side and of slave sellers on his father's side?

Africa has a long-history of racism and color discrimination among Africans.

Socialism is slavery. Capitalism is self-ownership.

does not prevent such slavery. Removing such clauses does not stop slavery in the US. The amendments are merely embarrassing clauses that point out modern domestic slavery. Removing such clauses will only dupe people into ignorance.

The USA's long-standing slavery was expanded to include everyone when another slave amendment -the 16th amendment (ratified February 3, 1913)- supplemented the 13th amendment and allowed Congress to impose a Federal income tax. The IRS was created in 1862, a year before 1863's emancipation proclamation purported to end slavery.

It's amazing that in the 21st century there are socialists who say "taxation ISN'T theft." They sound like people defending slavery in 1860. The 21st century is the softcore version of 20th century socialism. Being even more subtle, it may persist longer.

Today, the average American family head will be forced to do twenty years' labor to pay taxes in his or her lifetime. When you ask statists, "How much should we give?" they only answer "More! more! more!" If stealing 100% of the product of a person's labor is slavery, then at what percentage is it not slavery?

Socialists sometimes say that socialism exists when the means of production are owned by the government. They don't want you to know that when they say "the means of production" they mean YOU.[21]

---

[21] Socialists also seize the "means of reproduction" especially in regard to women. China did this with its "one-child" violence which not only controlled adult women but also resulted in massive infanticide, mostly of female newborns.

In news on 12/12/2017, Ji Hyeon-A said that in North Korea she was forced to undergo an abortion without medication at a local police station. She said that North Korea

Some Confederacy groups begin their meetings with the Pledge of Allegiance to the US flag. I am not making this up. Many spectators find that hilariously oddball. Perhaps it is not so odd.

The U.S. flag resembles the First Confederate national flag (not the Confederate battle flag with the "X" letter shape of the St. Andrew's cross). The first Confederate national flag contained three horizontal stripes of equal height, alternating red and white, with a blue square two-thirds the height of the flag as the canton. Inside the canton are white pointed stars of equal size, arranged in a circle, pointing outward, and representing the seceded states. As secession spread, the flag contained thirteen stars representing thirteen seceded states (similar to the thirteen seceded states and stars on the original flag of these united states of America).

Today, whenever the First Confederate national flag is flown (instead of the Confederate battle flag), students from the government's schools are ignorant of the flag. If the First Confederate national flag replaced the Confederate battle flag, years would pass before most

---

does not allow for mixed-race babies.

Romanian socialism banned contraceptives and abortions. The "plan" called for higher birth rates (the opposite of Chinese socialism's contemporaneous one-child tyranny). Ceausescu proclaimed in 1985: "The fetus is socialist property... Those who refuse to have children are deserters." The government forced all women between the age of 18 and 40 to have a monthly gynecological exam to assure that no one robbed socialism by having a secret abortion. The policies made Romania infamous for abandoned babies.

Stalin also imposed abortion bans, legal barriers to divorce, and, by and large, continued women in the role of homemakers and childcare.

students from government schools understood what the flag was and that a substitution of flags had occurred.

Southerners in the Confederate States of America (CSA) believed they embodied the ideals of the American Revolution, and the earlier secession in 1776.

Abraham Lincoln's Gettysburg Address said the soldiers sacrificed their lives "to the cause of self-determination - that government of the people, by the people, for the people should not perish from the earth." H.L. Mencken said: "It is difficult to imagine anything more untrue. The Union soldiers in the battle actually fought against self-determination; it was the Confederates who fought for the right of people to govern themselves." The Lincoln red pill is hard to swallow for most Americans.

The name of the racist German socialist Karl "Whitey" Marx appeared with 58 other names (as part of the International Workingmen's Association or IWA a.k.a. the First International, and probably all white) upon a letter congratulating the white racist Lincoln upon Lincoln's re-election (the letter was written between November 22 & 29 of 1864). The letter references "the Negro" and laments how "the white-skinned laborer" in the USA was distracted by Lincoln's war and was thus unable "to support their European brethren in their struggle for emancipation; but this barrier to progress has been swept off by the red sea of civil war." The white-skinned laborers were now "free" to "emancipate" their European comrades into socialism under its future leaders: Lenin, Stalin, Hitler, Mussolini et cetera. None of the 58 signatories traveled to the USA to fight for "the Negroes" as they were too busy emancipating their own enslaved European "white-skinned laborers."

Marx, the man behind the worst slavery (not emancipation) and the worst red seas of blood in history, promoted his deadly dogma to the Union's Killer-In-Chief, the man who presided over the worst mass killing of Americans in history. Lincoln set (and holds) the US record for deaths of people he considered to be his own citizens residing in the US (650,000 deaths) in the nation's deadliest mass shooting.

In what other ways did Marx (May 5, 1818 - March 14, 1883) influence Lincoln (February 12, 1809 - April 15, 1865) his contemporary? Marx's racist views had been touted in the USA from 1848 or before (16 years before the IWA letter to Lincoln) when Marx's "Communist Manifesto" had been published on February 21, 1848 (Lincoln was president from March 1861). Marx's Das Kapital was not published until 1867.

In November 1848, the abolitionist leader Frederick Douglass spoke against antebellum socialists who argued "that wages slavery is as bad as chattel slavery." Douglas considered Marx's view "arrant nonsense." Socialists were annoyed that abolitionists diverted attention from the greater struggle of northern laborers (and global laborers) against capitalism and "wage slavery" (Socialists have maintained this lame claim ever since. The same "wage slavery" argument is literally repreated today by socialists). Abolitionists interfered with Marx's fight for the coming future of comprehensive socialist slavery on everyone everywhere (and the true wage slavery that only exists under socialism).

Socialism, as touted by Marx and the International Workingmen's Association, attracted many thousands of supporters throughout the USA. The large immigration of German workers had a big impact on the politics of the North in the years before the War of Northern Aggression.

Lincoln's mass slaughter impressed another white racist German socialist criminal. Hitler praised Lincoln in Mein Kampf: "[T]he individual states of the American Union . . . could not have possessed any state sovereignty of their own. For it was not these states that formed the Union, on the contrary it was the Union which formed a great part of such so-called states" (page 566?). Hitler and Marx understood Lincoln's true motivation: forcing states and people into a union. Slavery.

Hitler joined with the Soviet socialist Stalin in a confederation to spread their socialism by violently taking over other states, and forcing others to remain within their control, expanding slavery by millions for decades. Modern socialist plantations were then expanded by Mao in China.

Those tactics were popularized in 1848 when the German socialists Karl Marx and Friedrich Engels wrote The Communist Manifesto (published in German on February 21, 1848). The "Demands of the Communist Party in Germany" (March 1848) demanded the unification of Germany (In 1848 there were many sovereign states - Empires, Kingdoms, Grand-Duchies, Duchies, Free Cities, et cetera, - in the German Confederation. They had descended from the settlement at the Congress of Vienna held in 1815 at the end of the French Revolutionary and Napoleonic wars).

The German socialists Marx and Engels exported German socialism to China, the Union of Soviet Socialist Republics, and worldwide.

Another reminder of the Germans Marx and Hitler, came from Eric Foner, the socialist/Marxist professor of history who has spent much of his career at Columbia University. Foner cited Lincoln on behalf of the preservation of the Union of Soviet Socialist Republics.[22] Foner denounced the secession movements in Latvia, Lithuania, Estonia, and Georgia, and called upon Mikhail Gorbachev to suppress them with the same ruthlessness Lincoln showed the South. According to Foner, no "leader of a powerful nation" should tolerate "the dismemberment" of Soviet socialism. "The Civil War," Foner explained gleefully, "was a central step in the consolidation of national authority in the United States." And then: "The Union, Lincoln passionately believed, was a permanent government. Gorbachev would surely agree." Modern American socialists boastfully repudiate the Lincoln cultists' myth about slavery and they declare that Lincoln's so-called "Civil War" was the violent suppression of independence, exactly what Foner wanted to see under Soviet socialism.

Foner and his colleagues promote "The Lost Cause of Socialism," a set of revisionist beliefs that describes the socialist cause as a heroic one against great odds despite its collapse. The beliefs endorse the virtues of the socialists Stalin, Mao, and/or Hitler, et cetera, viewing their dogma as an honorable struggle for the collectivist leviathan, while minimizing or denying the central trait of slavery under socialism. Aspects of it did win acceptance in some parts of academia. The Lost Cause myth helps white socialists such as Foner deal with the shattering reality of catastrophic defeat and impoverishment in a struggle they had been sure they

---

[22] In his book "Lincoln Unmasked," the author Thomas DiLorenzo exposes a February 1991 article by Foner in "The Nation" called "Lincoln's Lesson" regarding these issues.

would win. Socialists emerged from the USSR's collapse thoroughly beaten but largely unrepentant. The Lost Cause helps them rationalize how the "majority group" (socialists) persecuted marginalized groups and killed 100 million people (equal to having the "Civil War" relived over 160 times, which would span 640 years, so that it would still be going on and would never stop until the year 2501); and socialism enslaved even more than that.

During and after the disintegration of Soviet socialism, many monuments to slavery, slaveowners, and the socialist war (statues of Lenin, Stalin, Marx, etc) were torn down.

In "The Story of American Freedom," Foner[23] observes that the Pledge of Allegiance from Francis Bellamy (another socialist, Lincoln cultist, and apologist for the War of Northern Aggression) was quickly joined with the practice of standing for the playing of "The Star-Spangled Banner" as well as the observance of Flag Day. Patriotism is the last refuge of scoundrels. The less an academic amounts to, the more he loves the flag.

Lincoln and socialism inspired Francis Bellamy and Edward Bellamy. The Bellamy comrades wanted everything to be taken over by government. The pledge of servility put everyone on the road to serfdom. They are one of the origins of modern feudalism, crony socialism, and the military-socialism complex. Edward

---

[23] Foner is yet another historian whose dogma made it impossible for him to discover that the socialist Bellamy was the origin of Nazi salutes and Nazi behavior. Foner is also another historian whose dogma makes him reluctant to now ever mention Dr. Curry's discoveries, nor to address the pledge topics as a question. He would prefer that no one ever hear about it.

Bellamy's internationally best-selling socialist book "Looking Backward" portrayed their goal as a utopia.

The Bellamys wanted the government to take over all schools as a government monopoly in order to create the "industrial army" system to achieve "military socialism" (a Bellamy phrase). The Bellamys touted "military socialism" (the phrase they used to describe their dogma) because they so admired how the military harmed the South. They wanted the military system imposed on all of society as socialist cronyism.

The economist Walter E. Williams said "Prior to capitalism, the way people amassed great wealth was by looting, plundering and enslaving their fellow man. Capitalism made it possible to become wealthy by serving your fellow man."

The Pledge of Allegiance is a slave's pledge of allegiance to his master. Everyone should say "I am not your negro!"[24]

The salutation continues to be a daily witch hunt for disloyalty within g-schools at the ring of a bell.[25] Each morning, kids drink the Kool-Aid. Are you allegiant enough?

---

[24] The title of a 2016 film that is based on an unfinished book.
[25] The pledge is often left out of discussions of "Loyalty Oaths" (Wikipedia, depending on when one looks, is guilty of that). The US Supreme Court has upheld the constitutionality of mandatory loyalty oaths when those involved public officials and not private citizens.

7. HISTORY OF MASONS

Francis J. Bellamy and James Bailey Upham (the person who assisted Bellamy in creating the Pledge of Allegiance) were both Freemasons. Bellamy was a Mason in Little Falls Lodge No. 181, in Little Falls, NY (and a genuine Masonic Lodge website, the Grand Lodge of British Columbia and Yukon, openly and proudly boasts of his membership in Freemasonry). James Bailey Upham was a Mason in the Converse Lodge in Malden Massachusetts (Also see "Twenty-Three Words" by Margarette S. Miller).

Edward Bellamy's father-in-law was a Baptist minister who'd been forced out of his church for becoming a Freemason.

Freemasonry fit the Bellamy dogma of "military socialism." Regimentation and ritualism appealed to Masons like Francis Bellamy and James Upham. Freemasonry touts an intricate mythology, veiled in allegory, and manifested by pledges, uniforms, symbols, and flamboyant rituals.

Within the Masonic order, Upham was a Knights Templar, the most esteemed and discriminating order. The word "discriminating" is double entendre in that the Knights Templar is the only Masonic order that excluded (and still excludes) non-Christians (people they classify as Jews, Muslims and atheists), according to the book "To the Flag" by Richard J. Ellis (another book about the pledge with the glaring omission to ask or answer the question of the pledge as the origin of the Nazi salute).

The Order of the Knights Templar, also known as the American Rite, is the highest order in the York Rite, the largest Masonic organization in the United States. According to the book "The Pledge of Allegiance" by Dr. John W. Baer, it is equal to a thirty-third degree Scottish Rite Mason, the top of the Masonic hierarchy.

The Masons also exclude women and there is a separate "auxiliary" organization that accepts women and it is called the "Order of the Eastern Star" and its emblem is a star turned upside down.

Bellamy was a bigot. Bellamy's racism is shown in many examples, including these: "Where every man is a lawmaker, every dull-witted or fanatical immigrant admitted to our citizenship is a bane to the commonwealth," and "Where all classes of society merge insensibly into one another every alien immigrant of inferior race may bring corruption to the stock," and "...there are races which we cannot assimilate without lowering our racial standard, which should be as sacred to us as the sanctity of our homes."

Bellamy wanted the government to take over all schools and to stamp out individuality and force everyone to be the same (that is what Bellamy and other socialists meant by "equality"). When the government granted his wish, the socialist schools imposed segregation by law and taught racism as official policy.

The 1925 film "The Vanishing American" depicts segregated Native Americans being taught the Nazi salute and Bellamy's bootlicking vow in a government school.[26] An infamous photograph that is available on the internet shows African American children performing the Nazi salute and repeating Bellamy's Pledge of Allegiance in their segregated socialist school (1899 "Saluting the flag at the Whittier Primary School" Hampton, Virginia, photographer Frances Benjamin Johnston). Another photograph shows Jewish children giving the Nazi salute to the American flag with the caption "Irene Kaufmann Settlement Playground Opening Flag Raising, May 1934" (Rauh Jewish Archives at the Heinz History Center). Another infamous photograph shows segregated Japanese Americans performing the American Nazi salute shortly before they were placed in an internment camp (the photograph is by Dorothea Lange, a photographer who worked for the ominously titled Resettlement Administration (RA); for the FERA (forerunner of today's FEMA); for the Farm Security Administration (FSA); and under the auspices of the USDA).

During Bellamy's time (and today?), the Knights Templar and Masons, in general, lamented what they called capitalism's crass commercialism, selfish materialism, and excessive individualism. That view fit nicely with the socialist views of Upham and Bellamy.

That anti-capitalist view also fit Hitler and is expressed in Mein Kampf.

---

[26] "The Vanishing American" raises a question about the authenticity of the alleged native American Indian greeting of "How" with the raised flat palm of the right hand. Is the Indian greeting a myth that sprang from films that were influenced by the early Pledge of Allegiance? If native Americans did perform the "How" greeting, was it a corruption of the pledge gesture and "Hello" that they mis-borrowed from settlers?

"Mein Kampf" is usually translated into English as "My Struggle," however it could also be translated as "My Campaign," because Kampf is related to the word "camp" in the sense of a battlefield, a field, or an encampment, and is related to the following words: champagne (grapes from a field), campaign (war), champignon (mushrooms from a field), champion (battlefield victor), champ, camp (field setting), and campus. "Mein Kampf" is about Hitler's struggle for (his campaign for) socialism.

The title "Mein Kampf" is a reminder of German Chancellor Otto von Bismarck's "Kulturkampf" ("Battle for Culture") of 1871–78 and of Bismarckian socialism (aka State Socialism or "Staatssozialismus" in German), an established trend that Hitler expanded. Much of the Bismarckian socialism that Hitler supported had utilized cliché lies that are similar to the toxic culture of socialism imposed in the USA and everywhere: Health Insurance Bill of 1883; Accident Insurance Bill of 1884; Old Age and Disability Insurance Bill of 1889; Workers Protection Act of 1891; Children's Protection Act of 1903.

"Mein Kampf" refers to Freemasonry multiple times and always in a disapproving manner. Nevertheless, Freemasonry was involved in the formation of Germany's National Socialist Party. That involvement included Rudolf Glandeck von Sebottendorff (born Adam Alfred Rudolph Glauer in 1875) and Hermann Pohl (founder of the fraternity, the German Order Walvater of the Holy Grail).

Sebottendorff had been initiated into the Rite of Memphis, a Freemason group. Sebottendorf and Pohl established a fraternity in Munich known as the "Thule Gesellschaft," on August 17, 1918 (see "Anti-masonry

Frequently Asked Questions," Section 6, version 2.9, of the Grand Lodge of British Columbia and Yukon). It was originally called the "Studiengruppe für germanisches Altertum" (Study Group for German Antiquity).

On January 5, 1919, the Thule group merged with the Committee of Independent Workers, renaming themselves the Deutsche Arbeiter-Partei (the German Workers' Party). Adolf Hitler claimed he was the seventh member to join this group and he changed its name to the National Socialist German Workers' Party in 1920.

Sebottendorff authored the novel "Der Talisman des Rosenkreuzers" (The "Rosicrucian Talisman"; "Rosicrucian" combines the words "rose" and "cross").

Another of Sebottendorff's books "Bevor Hitler Kam" ("Before Hitler Came" 1933) was banned in Bavaria. That book stated that Hitler was influenced by the Thule Gesellschaft.

The Thule dogma was influenced by occultists such as Lanz von Liebenfels (1874-1954 and a promoter of Ariosophy), Madam Helena Blavatsky (who also used the swastika to promote Theosophy), and Guido von List (1848-1919).[27] List's pet words (Ariosophy, Aryan, Armanist) all evoked his occult socialist ideas of an aristocracy of enlightened leaders and List's central goal of a super socialist man, or the superior socialist society.

In 1899, Lanz founded his Order of the New Templars, and the name was inspired by the Knights

---

[27] Such ideas persisted for decades as shown by the book Hakenkreuz und Davidstern [Swastika and Star of David], Volkstiimliche Einfiihrung i. d. Geheimwissenschaften [A Popular Introduction to the Occult Sciences], by Anton Memminger (Wiirzburg, 1922).

Templar. In his related magazine "Ostara" he used the swastika as well as the kruckenkreuz (aka croix potent). Lanz' magazine was noticed by Hitler. In 1934, a year after Hitler came to power, Lanz claimed that the Order of the New Templars was the "first manifestation of the [German National Socialist] Movement…"

There are photographs of James Upham that show him wearing the uniform of the Knights Templar. Although Upham, Bellamy, and other Masons knocked crass commercialism and capitalism as part of their socialist ideology, they enjoyed sashes, gloves, belts, swords, plumes, and other rich regalia.

While Upham and the Bellamys promoted "military socialism," the Masonic uniform at that time (as worn by Upham) was modeled after the military and included various medals and badges that were similar to those adopted later by the National Socialist German Workers' Party.

One of the badges is called a Maltese Cross and others are what German socialists called the "Ritterkreuz" (Rider Cross, Knight's Cross, or Iron Cross).

It is doubtful that any Mason today would still wear Upham's uniform publicly because those symbols became almost as notorious as the swastika (Hakenkreuz or "hooked cross") under the National Socialist German Workers' Party.

The Freemasons suffer faults that are shared by other civic groups. A review of websites for most civic groups reveals ignorance of private property rights, supply and demand pricing, laissez-faire economics, free markets, individual rights, and capitalism.

A review of most civic groups reveals vague altruistic clichés that translate into active support for expanding government and various socialist schemes.

Freemasons begin meetings with the Pledge of Allegiance today. They do it because of Francis Bellamy and James Upham, both Freemasons and both socialists, who created the original 1892 chant.

Bellamy and Upham took advantage of the vague socialism of the Freemasons (and similar civic groups) to spread their dogma. It continues to happen even though the original straight-arm salute has been replaced.

In the past, the Masons excluded people that they defined as "negroes, mulattoes or women." The groups in many states would not admit people they classified as "cripples."

While freedom of association is an important right, those types of policies are pernicious when people support government institutions, because government institutions are utilized to impose such policies by force of law. That is what happened in the USA.

In the USA, the Bellamy and Upham dogma supported a government takeover of education in order to have children mimic the military and to produce an "industrial army" (a Bellamy term). The government's schools imposed segregation by law and taught racism as official policy. The USA's behavior was an example for three decades before the Nazis.

American socialism was similar to German socialism at that time because Jehovah's Witnesses, blacks, and the Jewish, and others attended government schools that dictated segregation, taught racism, and punished children who refused to perform the straight-arm salute and smarmy chanting of the pledge to the flag. There were acts of violence. The pledge made many Americans feel like Hitler at Passover. There were incidents in which government schools attempted to take children away from parents on the grounds of "unfit parenting" if the parents would not force the children to repeat the vow and perform the gesture.

The Mason's had (and have?) a practice of discriminating against many people to exclude them from their groups, but they did not exclude Germans. The Masons were (and are) an international organization.

It is important to remember that during all that time, German-American Freemasons attended racist and segregated government schools in the U.S. and saluted with a straight-arm salute toward the U.S. flag, as written by the self-proclaimed national socialists (and Masons) Francis Bellamy and James Bailey Upham. That was a long time before (and leading up to) the adoption of the salute by the National Socialist German Workers' Party.

The National Socialist German Workers' Party was influenced by German-Americans who were already national socialists in the United States. Some German-Americans joined the German American Bund movement (Deutsch-Amerikanischer Volksbund) to support national socialists in Germany before WWII. The bund began as the Friends of New Germany in Chicago in 1933. This group traced its roots to the Teutonia Society and National Socialist Party, both active in the USA during the 1920s.

There was much travel between the U.S. and Germany (the Hindenburg zeppelin disaster occurred in 1937 in New Jersey).

When Jesse Owens competed in the 1936 Olympics in Nazi Germany he performed the initial part of the American gesture to the flag (the military salute part), but did not perform the straight-arm gesture, as he did not want the gesture to be misunderstood as a salute to Adolf Hitler. Other photographs show U.S. athletes performing the American stiff-armed salute (the classic Nazi salute) at the Olympics in 1936 and at earlier Olympic games. The 1936 Olympics exemplifies how the American Nazi gesture had spread outside of the pledge itself and was being used as a general salute during the U.S. national anthem and the anthems of other countries.

In the past, the U.S.'s Nazi gesture had been adopted as the Official Olympic salute, and the Olympics had helped to spread the U.S.'s gesture globally.

The modern Olympics began in 1896, four years after Bellamy's pledge gesture in 1892. The following is a list of the locations where German socialists and Italian socialists and socialists worldwide witnessed the American Nazi salute both as a gesture during the National Anthem (for victorious US athletes) and as the official Olympic salute:

1896 Athens, Greece
1900 Paris, France
1904 St. Louis, USA
1906 Athens, Greece
1908 London, UK
1912 Stockholm, Sweden
1916 Berlin, Germany (Cancelled due to WWI)
1920 Antwerp, Belgium (No Germany)
1924 Chamonix & Paris, France (No Germany)
1928 St. Moritz, Switzerland & Amsterdam, NL
1932 Lake Placid & Los Angeles, USA
1936 Garmisch-Partenkirchen & Berlin, Germany

MADNESS

In 1896, the year of the first modern Olympic games, Hitler was 7 years old. Mussolini was 13. They (and their fellow socialists) had many opportunities to see photographs and films of Olympic rituals from the first Olympic game and all the games that followed. Their supporters had the chance to attend the games and view the rituals in person. Before the "notorious" Berlin Olympic games there were ten Olympic games during the time when the stiff-armed gesture was a commonplace American salute or was the official Olympic salute, or was both.

Hitler would have had the opportunity to see the gestures in Germany in 1916 but for the fact they were cancelled due to WWI. Despite the cancellation, extensive preparations were made in Germany for the 1916 Olympic games, making it likely that Olympic bureaucrats in Germany were aware of the official Olympic salute (if one existed at that time).

It is probable that Hitler and Mussolini (or some of their close supporters) learned during their years of saluting that the gesture was in widespread use in government schools in the US and had been in use for decades in the US before socialists in Germany and Italy picked it up.

It is unclear when the American Nazi salute became the official Olympic salute. That is a different issue from the presumption that Americans used the gesture (the US Pledge of Allegiance gesture) at the earliest games as a general salutation and/or as the American gesture for victorious US athletes on the awards podium during the National Anthem, or other instances when a country's national anthem was played (it is also unclear when the national anthem practice began at the Olympic games).

MADNESS

One claim holds that the Olympic salute (from the American Nazi salute) was used at the 1912 Stockholm games, but no further evidence has been found yet. If so, then it would be more clear that the official Olympic salute predated the salute of German socialists and Italian socialists and probably helped (with the pledge of allegiance) to influence that adoption of the salute by socialists in Germany, Italy, and elsewhere.

Perhaps the salute accompanied the appearance of the Olympic flag in 1914, in Paris. The flag might not have been hoisted in an Olympic stadium until the Antwerp Games in 1920.

Due to WWI, Germany was banned from the 1920 and 1924 Olympics.

In 1923, Hitler and his socialists protested violently against Jews, Frenchmen, and Americans participating in the German Gymnastics Festival in Munich.

In 1924, to commemorate their Olympic games, France issued four postage stamps with two of the stamps showing the classic American Nazi salute. There is also a medal that repeats the image on one of the stamps and it includes the inscription "Le Salut" (the reverse shows the Olympic rings, 18 x 27 mm with integral loop). A 1924 Olympic poster appears to show the gesture (or it shows half-naked males performing the Queen's parade wave and simultaneously caressing tenderly each other's left shoulders). It is interesting to note again that German athletes did not participate in the 1924 Olympics.

A 1936 poster features the Quadriga from the Brandenburg Gate, a landmark of the city of Berlin. In the background is the figure of a wreathed victor, his right arm appearing raised. In the 1936 poster, the salute is not clear because only part of the arm is shown.

There are disputes about whether the Olympic salute differed from the salute of the National Socialist German Workers' Party and the 1936 poster seems designed to obscure the issue.

In 1936, many of Jesse Owens' fans in the U.S. attended (and had attended) segregated government schools where the pledge was performed with the straight-armed gesture, and where they were required by law to vocalize it grovelingly on command in government schools (socialist schools). The U.S. practice of official racism and segregation in government schools even outlasted Germany's socialist party after its defeat in WWII, and into the 1960's and beyond.

In 1936, the military salute alone (as performed by Owens at the Olympics) was not the customary civilian salute to the U.S. flag. The 1936 Olympics and the war that followed all added to the 1942 interference by Congress regarding the flag ritual at that time. Congress eventually eliminated the military salute, and then eliminated the straight-arm salute shortly thereafter. Congress legislated in favor of the hand-over-the-heart. The gesture was not officially altered by Congress until 1942, after the beginning of WWII. That is when the modern hand-over-the-heart was enacted into law.

In some schools the boys and girls saluted differently. Boys began the pledge with the military salute while girls began the pledge with the hand over the heart. The difference might be explained by the fact that girls were not forced into slavery (conscription into the military) for the government's insane wars. When the hand-over-the-heart was enshrined in the flag code, Congress imposed the effeminate gesture for the pledge, and eliminated the masculine gesture. A 1920 photograph shows the differing boy/girl gestures at Central High School in Prince Georges County, Maryland (by photographer Theodor Horydczak).

Horydczak was from Poland, and could have been another of innumerable conduits for America's Nazi salute into Europe, assuming that Horydczak communicated about life in the U.S. with family or friends who remained in Europe.

In 1931, the Star-Spangled Banner was designated the national anthem (Mar. 3, 1931, ch. 436, 46 Stat. 1508). It is probable that Americans were already saluting the Star-Spangled Banner with the Nazi salute before Congress made it the national anthem in 1931. If they weren't, then they probably started saluting the Star-Spangled Banner with the Nazi salute after it became the official national anthem in 1931. That probability is high because on June 22, 1942, Congress directed that during the national anthem "when the flag is displayed the salute to the flag should be given" (Section 7, Pub.L. 77–623, 56 Stat. 380, Chap. 435, H.J.Res. 303, enacted June 22, 1942. WITH the extended arm).

In the law, Congress modified the "Bellamy salute" and directed that everyone present begin with the right hand over the heart and then extending the right hand, palm upward. The new statute eliminated Bellamy's initial military salute probably because someone in 1942 suspected that Bellamy's military salute was the reason for the classic stiff-armed Nazi salute with the palm down (a discovery made by Dr. Curry), instead of the "palm upward." In the early flag code, Congress confirms Dr. Curry's conclusion. The military salute was the origin of the Nazi salute.

It might answer the following question: why did the

military salute (from the forehead or from the heart) cease to be a common part of many daily school rituals? Answer: Because it was the origin of the Nazi salute. It was a remarkable way for the military salute to fade out of government schools (socialist schools).

The following is the specific quotation of how Congress commanded everyone to salute for the pledge in the first 1942 statute (the next paragraph, after the national anthem salute) to wit:

That the pledge of allegiance to the flag, "I pledge allegiance to the flag of the United States of America and to the Republic for which it stands, one Nation indivisible, with liberty and justice for all", be rendered by standing with the right hand over the heart; extending the right hand, palm upward, toward the flag at the words "to the flag" and holding this position until the end, when the hand drops to the side. However, civilians will always show full respect to the flag when the pledge is given by merely standing at attention, men removing the headdress. Persons in uniform shall render the military salute.

For persons in uniform the statute retains the military salute. The author of the statute knew that the military salute was "safe" as long as civilian sheeple were not directed to extend the military salute outward to point at the flag. Otherwise, the herd would transform the military salute into the hard stiff-armed American Nazi gesture (no matter what anyone else commanded). The morning pledge stupidity was more proof that government schools (socialist schools) produce dolts and must end.

That proof was augmented by the incompetency of the author of the statute; he failed to clarify what he meant by "right hand over the heart." For sheeple who understood Bellamy's original military salute, and who had been forced to perform in that manner all their lives, the "right hand over the heart" might mean that the long-standing military salute should be performed with "the right hand over the heart." This puzzle was not solved by the next alteration of the flag statute.

There are photographs showing the pledge beginning with the military salute over the heart. Some of those photographs predate 1942 by decades. The "Bellamy salute" had been modified in some locations to begin the initial military salute over the heart (perhaps because it was creepy to have children mimic soldiers, or because it was considered disrespectful of the military).

Only six months later, Congress altered the statute to entirely eliminate the extended arm gesture (the second part of the pledge's hand salute). Section 7, Pub.L. 77–829, 56 Stat. 1074, Chap. 806, H.J.Res. 359, enacted December 22, 1942. (WITHOUT the extended arm). To wit:

That the pledge of allegiance to the flag, "I pledge allegiance to the flag of the United States of America and to the Republic for which it stands, one Nation indivisible, with liberty and justice for all", be rendered by standing with the right hand over the heart. However, civilians will always show full respect to the flag when the pledge is given by merely standing at attention, men removing the headdress. Persons in uniform shall render the military salute.

Congress' earlier subtle attempt to stop the classic

stiff-armed American Nazi salute (by dropping the initial military salute, or by specifying "palm upward") had not worked as planned, it seems.

Part of the problem was that some sheeple do not immediately bend over every time Congress bleats. Some Americans did not want to change America's Nazi gesture and might have explained (with different words) "We've been requiring the American socialist's ritual daily in government schools (socialist schools) for decades before we exported it to German socialists and Italian socialists," adding "It's ours," and "They should stop, not us." The first two comments are largely correct.

Congress' six-month self-reversal regarding the Flag Code is an amusing reminder of the US Supreme Court's self-reversal in three years from Minersville School District v. Gobitis, 310 U.S. 586 (1940) to West Virginia State Board of Education v. Barnette, 319 U.S. 624 (1943) concerning the Pledge of Allegiance. Were the politicians influenced by the Gobitis case? Did Congress' tinkering with the pledge influence the U.S. Supreme Court's decision in Barnette that occurred six months after the alteration of the Flag Code in December 1942?

There is an alternative statutory interpretation of the Flag Code: Did members of Congress who passed the statute intend that the pledge begin with the military salute performed with "the right hand over the heart"? If so, then that would mean that the pledge continues to be performed incorrectly; that the statutory prescription for the pledge is the military salute performed with the right hand over the chest (see Professor Curry's analysis in this regard). There are old photographs that show this method. It is not excluded by statutory interpretation of the law's language.

The "military salute over the heart" interpretation is supported by photographic evidence in the Library of Congress (in the Prints and Photographs Division): an 1899 photograph from Washington, D.C. shows students performing the military salute over the heart; a 1942 photograph from Hollywood, CA shows students performing the military salute over the heart.

It is frightening to raise the question "Is the correct gesture for the pledge the military-salute-over-the-heart?" because that gesture might be adopted if knowledge of this issue spreads. Many military fanatics are aggressive in promoting the daily psychological operation (psyop) in government schools (socialist schools), they misperceive the pledge as quotidian homage to themselves, and many would prefer the modern ritual performed with the military-salute-over-the-heart (if not the classic military salute to the eyebrow).

8. AMERICA EXPORTS TO GERMANY

In "Mein Kampf" Hitler never mentioned the stiff-armed gesture.

The notorious gesture used by German socialists and American socialists was never referred to as the "Roman salute" by Hitler. The term "Roman" appears many times in Mein Kampf (along with various other references to ancient Rome and various uses of the word "Rome"), but the phrase "Roman salute" never appears as a description of the notorious stiff-armed salute, nor as any other description.

There are innumerable ways in which German socialists learned the American socialist salute.

From 1892 through 1942, public officials (including U.S. presidents, congressmen, governors, state legislators and everyone down to the local dog catcher) performed the American Nazi salute and were photographed and filmed doing so. Those photos and films are rare because people don't want to know the truth. Public officials in the USA who preceded the German socialist (Hitler) and the Italian socialist (Mussolini) were sources for the stiff-armed salute (and hypnotic babble) in those countries and other foreign countries.

A specific possible source of the gesture for Hitler was President Woodrow Wilson during World War I (WWI). Perhaps Wilson (and members of Congress) used the gesture during his appearances before Congress, where film footage and photographs show Wilson standing with the fasces symbol on the wall behind him[28] (providing inspiration to both the socialist Mussolini and Hitler). Newsreels and photojournalism of those events helped Wilson spread socialist ideas globally and led to Hitler, Lenin, Stalin, and World War II.[29]

Socialist leaders in the USA (e.g. Wilson) were using the gesture before socialist leaders in Italy and Germany aped them (along with bootlicking vows in unison on command in government schools (socialist schools)).

---

[28] e.g. see the fasces symbols on both sides of the U.S. flag in photos and film of Wilson's absurd "14 points" speech to Congress regarding WWI ("the war to make the world safe for Hitler, Lenin, Stalin and World War II"). Are there films or photos of Wilson (or other presidents or congressmen) performing the American Nazi salute before the fasces and the flag? The best evidence indicates that the fasces may have been there from 1857, so there could have been a lot of Presidents and members of Congress doing the Nazi salute in front of the fasces symbol. Any photos or film anywhere? Fasces symbolism appears also on the House of Representatives mace (from 1841) and inkwell (from ~1810-1820) and is boasted about on the House's website. It is interesting to note that the Chambers were remodeled in 1950 (at last check Wikipedia incorrectly implied that the Fasces first appeared in 1950, which would be startling if true as that was shortly after the defeat of the socialist Mussolini. A new version of the fasces replaced the old version in 1950. It is enough of a surprise that in 1950 the House *continued* the earlier Fasces theme on the wall behind the podium).

[29] See "Wilson's War: How Woodrow Wilson's Great Blunder Led to Hitler, Lenin, Stalin, and World War II" by Jim Powell.

President Wilson insisted that all school children recite the pledge, and he led them into doing so using the American Nazi salute. Flag fetishist Francis Bellamy lived through WWI and Wilson's flag fetishism. After World War II, the Bellamy salute that Wilson so loved became less popular. The mechanical incantation on command continued daily (with an altered hand gesture), and it haunts children to this day.

Another specific source for Hitler learning the stiff-armed salute and sadomasochistic chanting from the United States would be Ernst "Putzi" Hanfstaengl, one of Hitler's intimates, who attended schools in the USA.

During the time that Hanfstaengl was attending school in the USA, the straight-arm salute was used for various purposes, including: the National Anthem (the Star Spangled Banner); by American athletes during Olympic games and other sporting events; for school flags; and even as a general greeting, or for cheering during sports events (including Harvard football games).

About 1921, Hanfstaengl moved to Germany and heard for the first time a speech by Hitler in a beer hall. Hitler stated that the first time he saw the straight-arm salute he was in a beer hall and he described it as occurring at "about" the same time (as when Hanfstaengl claims that Hanfstaengl heard Hitler speak in a beer hall). According to the author John Toland (p. 128 of his biography of Hitler), the first encounter between Hitler and Hanfstaengl was on 22 November, 1922 at the Kindlkeller, a large L-shaped beer hall. Hanfstaengl as the importer is also consistent with the untrustworthy "Hitler's Table Talk" quote: "It was in the *Ratskeller* at Bremen, about the year 1921, that I first saw this style of salute." Hanfstaengl as one importer (or promoter) of the American pledge's Nazi salute is probable.

Of course, there were other Germans, et cetera, who had moved to and from the United States since 1892 (the start of the stiff-armed salute's use for the national flag). Walter K. Schroder's book "Stars & Swastikas: The Boy Who Wore Two Uniforms" explains that his family moved back to Germany (from New York) before WWII, when Schroder was 9 years of age. At 15 he was drafted into the German Army. Although Schroder was not the cause of Hitler adopting America's gesture, he is another published example of the influence of Americans in Germany during that time.

There were also movie depictions and other ways in which Germans would have been influenced by the early American raised-arm gesture.

Rudolph Hess published an article titled "The Fascist Greeting" in June 1928, claiming that German socialists used the gesture as early as 1921, before they had heard about the behaviors of the socialist Mussolini.

9. SWASTIKAS 卐 + 卍 ? SS + S + VW?

The swastika was a popular symbol in the United States during the time (1888, 1892, and beyond) that the Bellamy cousins were promoting their "industrial army" under their "military socialism" in their government schools (socialist schools) with their Pledge of Allegiance and its stiff-armed salute.

1869 is the year inscribed under Hakenkreuzes at the Abbey of Lambach-am-Traum in upper Austria where young Adolf Hitler (April 20, 1889 - April 30, 1945) would attend many years later as a student of the Benedictines while he resided in Lambach with his parents (1897/98). That may have been the first contact the Hitler youth had with Hakenkreuzes. He saw them on the four corners of the monastery, where they had been sculpted several years before, pursuant to orders of the abbot, Theodorich Hagen (Theoderich Hagn). Spaced around the carving were the letters "A" and "L" and "T" and "H." The "AL" stood for "Abbey Lambach" and the letters "TH" for Theodorich Hagen. The Hakenkreuzes were jokingly referred to as "Hagenkreuzes."

It is interesting to note that the four letters on the

Abbey emblem included the letters "A" and "H," the initials for Adolf Hitler ("AH"). When young "AH" became a student at Lambach, Father Hagen had already died, but the Hagenkreuzes lived on. On last checking, they remain there as of the date this was written.

In the 1870s, swastikology senselessness spread after the archaeologist Heinrich Schliemann discovered scrawls that he generously described as "swastikas" in his excavations of Greek/Trojan remains in Asia Minor at Troy (Hisarlik in Turkey). Most of the doodling was on spindle whorls. It is difficult to imagine how Schliemann's work led to lunacy about "swastikas" as profound signs of an "Aryan" race. Was the "Aryan" race also shown in the crude zigzags, circles, stars, dashes, dots, lozenges, and more that were present too? It would make more sense if Schliemann's "swastika" scrawls represented "spinning" on the spindle whorls, as Dr. Curry suggested.

The non-uniform scribbles that Schliemann found were not repetitions of the thick black hard-angled alphabetical trademark adopted by socialists in the late 1800s and thereafter. For example, a terracotta sphere showed thirteen forms with 'swastikal' symmetry in a band around the sphere's equator. Each form was so different that Dr. E. Brentano believed each form was a separate letter in a swastikal alphabet.

In 1875, the "modern-style" swastika was used by the Theosophical Society (TS), an international group that promoted odd racial theories (using the term "Aryan"). The leader of TS, Helena Blavatsky (1831-1891), used a "seal" (as early as 1875) that included a swastika at the top of seven symbols (for seven races). The swastika was in the classic "Nazi" form (on one point, as if drawn in a diamond, and in the "S" letter orientation. Note that many modern depictions of Blavatsky's seal show an altered swastika to conceal its earlier "Nazi" style). Two very DIFFERENT "swastikas" (one looks like a non-hooked fat cross) found by Schliemann at Troy prove that the Trojans and their ancestors were pure cracker Aryans, according to Blavatsky (Secret Doctrine volume 2, page 101).

In 1885, Helena Blavatsky of the Theosophical Society resided in Würzburg in the Kingdom of Bavaria. Austrian/German ultra-socialist Guido von List and his followers such as Lanz von Liebenfels, were influenced by Blavatsky's socialist ideas; their German version of thought became known as Ariosophy and influenced German socialists.

1888 brought the publishing of Edward Bellamy's socialist book "Looking Backward" and Blavatsky's book "The Secret Doctrine" (bearing the swastika seal on the cover). The Bellamy / Blavatsky love fest began. Blavatsky claimed to be telepathic, but in reality she was telepathetic. "The Key to Theosophy" authored by Blavatsky, was published in 1888 in New York and stated: "The organization of Society, depicted by Edward Bellamy, in his magnificent work 'Looking Backwards,' admirably represents the Theosophical idea of what should be the first great step towards the full realization of universal brotherhood."

In "The Secret Doctrine," Blavatsky wrote: "Mankind is obviously divided into god-informed men and lower human creatures. The intellectual difference between the Aryan and other civilized nations and such savages as the South Sea Islanders, is inexplicable on any other grounds." Blavatsky was anti-Semitic. She wrote, "But now Judaism, built solely on Phallic worship, has become one of the latest creeds in Asia, and theologically a religion of hate and malice toward everyone and everything outside themselves" (The Secret Doctrine page 471). She also stated that Jews were "degenerate in spirituality," although she still considered them Aryans (page 200). She used the term "Aryan" in a way that is a reminder of its etymological relationship (from Greek aristoi for "noble") to these words: aristocrat, aristocracy, Ariosophy, Aristotle, Ari, arch, Iran.

In 1889, swastikaphile Michael Zmigrodski, a Polish archaeologist, joined in the socialist silliness at the Paris Exposition with more than 300 drawings of various swastikas. He added to the claim that the mark represented an "Aryan race."

1889 Hitler was born (April 20, 1889).

1892 the Pledge of Allegiance was created by American socialist Francis Bellamy in the USA and it became the origin of the Nazi salute. The Theosophical Society helped popularize the swastika while promoting Edward Bellamy's socialist scheme. Americans would wear swastikas as jewelry and perform the Nazi salute (for the Pledge of Allegiance and more).

In 1894, the author Thomas Wilson's book "The Swastika, the earliest known symbol and its migrations" was published as a report of the U.S. National Museum.

From 1897-1898, Hitler might have been first exposed to the creative and commemorative use of Hakenkreuzes that decorated Lambach Abbey where he attended school.

In 1910, the Boy Scouts of America (BSA) was founded as part of the international Scout Movement. Boy Scouts in the USA wore medals bearing the swastika and performed the Nazi salute for the flag pledge and adopted (as did Girl Scouts, Brownies, Camp

Fire Girls) America's Nazi salute as their own salute. The handbook "Scouting for Boys" (p. 27, 4th edition, 1911 and also see "Scouting For Boys Ed. 3rd") displays the scout swastika badge and states, "'Swastika,' the Badge of Brotherhood. - Can be given by a scout of any rank (except a Tenderfoot) to anybody who has done him or the movement a good turn. It is a token of thanks. This badge entitles the holder to the assistance of any scout at any time. A scout on seeing a person wearing this badge will go up, salute, and ask if he can be of any service." Dr. Curry's research indicates that scouting might be the first direct association of the Nazi salute with the swastika.

Today, most people who read that swastika-salute quote (above) will not realize that the salute (in the USA) was the American Nazi salute triggered by the swastika and in the UK the salute was a modified Nazi salute.

The book repeats a dusty myth to explain: "In the old days the free men of England all were allowed to carry weapons, and when one met another each would hold up his right hand to show that he had no weapon in it, and that they met as friends" (p. 41).

Scouting For Boys Ed. 3rd was written for British scouts and the American Nazi salute was altered slightly so that three fingers are pointed outward instead of four: "Scout's Salute and Secret Sign - The three fingers held up (like the three points of the Scout's badge) remind him of his three promises in the Scout's promise."

It continues: "He always salutes an officer - that is, a Patrol Leader, or a Scoutmaster, or any commissioned officer of His Majesty's forces, army and navy — with the full salute. Also the hoisting of the Union Jack, the colours of a regimen, the playing of "God Save the

King," and any funeral." This quotation indicates that the scouts were saluting flags in the UK, another practice borrowed from the USA (where it began in 1892). The UK scout's "full salute" began as the "three-finger" salute in the military fashion (to the forehead), but it evolved into the Nazi fashion with the right arm outstretched toward flags and leaders (again following the USA practice). Old photographs of Sir Robert Baden-Powell show him saluted by scouts with their right arms stretched outward in the Nazi manner (with the three-finger hand gesture).

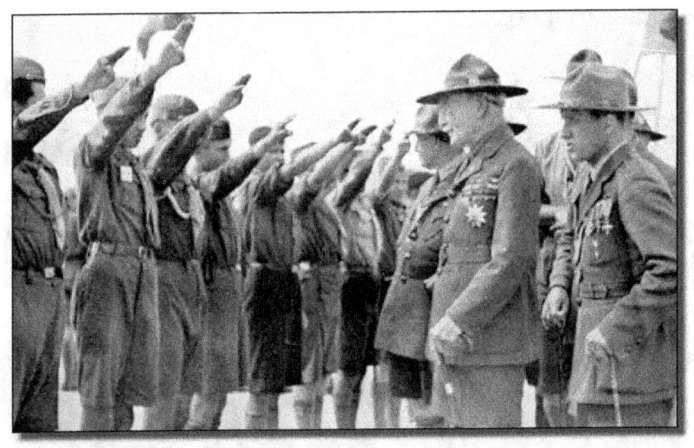

The evolution of the UK scout salute is a reminder of the evolution of Francis Bellamy's Pledge of Allegiance salute.

In a further eerie reminder of Hitler's occasional "half-salutes" to socialist "comrades" (years later), the scout book advises: "When a Scout meets another for the first time in the day, whether he is a comrade or a stranger, he salutes with the secret sign in the half salute." (The book explains: When the hand is raised shoulder high it is called "The Half Salute."

The preface to the third edition boasts: "It may be satisfactory to Scoutmasters and others to know that, thanks to their energy and to that of their boys, the Boy Scouts movement has made a large and rapid development during the time of its existence, not only throughout the United Kingdom, but also in almost every British Colony and in many countries beyond the seas, such as Germany, the United States of America, Russia, Argentina, Chili, etc."

After the 1924 Flag Day Conference, the "flag code" (with the raised-arm salute) was published in the Boy Scout Handbook.

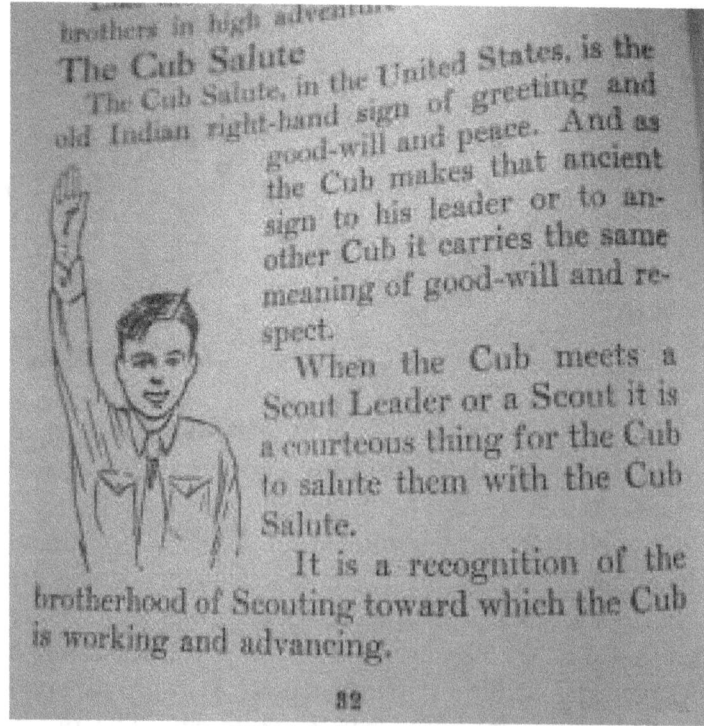

brothers in high adventure

The Cub Salute

The Cub Salute, in the United States, is the old Indian right-hand sign of greeting and good-will and peace. And as the Cub makes that ancient sign to his leader or to another Cub it carries the same meaning of good-will and respect.

When the Cub meets a Scout Leader or a Scout it is a courteous thing for the Cub to salute them with the Cub Salute.

It is a recognition of the brotherhood of Scouting toward which the Cub is working and advancing.

32

The original first printing of the Boy's Cubbook in 1930 continued to promote the classic American Nazi salute by Scouts, only worse: as a more general "greeting." It included an illustration of the gesture (p. 23). It is another scary parallel to the adoption of the gesture under German Socialists.

The 1930 printing was recalled by Boy Scouts of America (BSA) to change to the salute. The reason is found in the History of Cub Scouting, published by BSA in 1987 (p. 13): "The Boy's Cubbook for Wolf rank was published while the first packs were being chartered in April 1930. It was quickly revised to change the Cub salute. In the original edition, the salute was the Indian sign for peace, with right arm upraised, palm out. Apparently, leaders saw that the salute was disconcertingly similar to the Nazi salute of Adolf Hitler, who was beginning his rise to power in Germany en route to engulfing the world in war. The new salute was the familiar two-fingered touch of the right hand to the forehead." The 1987 explanation was almost as inaccurate as the original 1930 book. The 1987 version touts the American-Indian myth, and shows complete ignorance of the use of the gesture in the early Pledge of Allegiance.

BSA destroyed whatever original printings they had of the offending Cubbook.

It is disturbing to note that the Boy's Cubbook for "Wolf rank" (with the "Nazi" salute) was published while the first "Wolf packs" were being chartered in April 1930, just as Adolf Hitler was gaining power with the National Socialist German Workers Party, and spreading similar "wolf pack" and "stiff-armed salute" concepts in Germany.

Boy Scouts and Girl Scouts still use a remnant of the

early pledge. Scouts use a military-style salute that developed from the initial military salute of the Pledge. A stereotypical Scout website states that scouts should memorize the pledge, that the "denner" (den leader) should lead the group in the pledge at meetings, and the web site mimics government schools by providing the usual shallow propaganda about Francis Bellamy and the Pledge.

Another example of how Boy Scouts and Girl Scouts still use a remnant of the early Pledge of Allegiance is when the two-fingered or three-fingered gesture is sometimes extended upward and outward.

Scouts traveled internationally to spread their paramilitary practices and American military socialism. Was German socialism an evolution of "Lord of the Flies" with Boy Scouts gone bad?

Boy Scouts used the swastika and then American soldiers used the swastika as their insignia early in World War I, and up to 1941, against Germany. The symbol was used by Americans in the French Escadrille Lafayette; by the 45th Infantry Division; and on Boeing P-12 planes (e.g. the P-12B of the 55th Pursuit Squadron of the United States Army Air Corps. The squadron insignia at the time was a yellow swastika on a medium blue circle with a yellow surround. That was the squadron insignia until 4 May 1932).

A swastika emblem was used by the Krit Motor Car company (based in the USA from 1909-1916) on vehicles exported to Europe and used in World War I.[30]

---

[30] Some Krit emblems were astonishingly similar to some later German socialist swastikas. Some Krit emblems had a black swastika on a white circle with a red surround (and the surround contained gold lettering). Some German swastikas had a black swastika on a white circle with a red surround

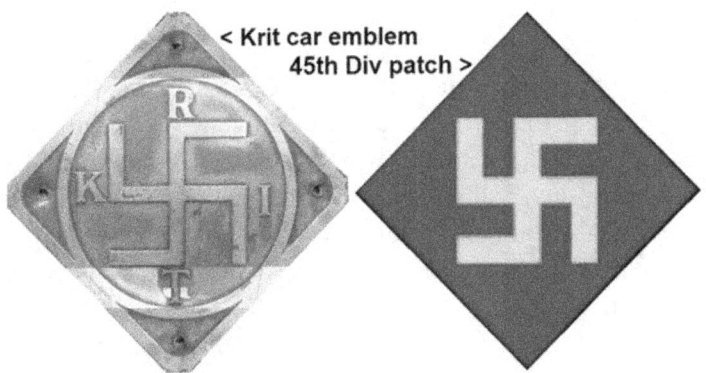

< Krit car emblem
45th Div patch >

An American postcard pre-dating World War II, and circa 1915 (World War I) shows the swastika joined with the U.S.'s flag. The postcard reads "May our glorious flag and this 'lucky star' guide you and keep you wherever you are." The swastika is the 'lucky star' under the U.S.'s flag. At that time, the flag was worshiped with the Nazi salute under threat of prosecution in schools that imposed segregation by law and taught racism as official policy.

Americans wore swastikas and performed the Nazi salute (for the Pledge of Allegiance and more), as part of the Boy Scouts, the Girl Scouts, the 45th infantry Division, and elsewhere.

(and the surround contained gold lettering of "NATIONAL-SOCIALISTICHE D.A.P.) designed as a lapel pin or tie pin. Americans wore swastikas on jewelry from Krit that boasted its eye-catching red-black-white emblem on lapel pins, tie clips and pins, cuff links, watch fobs and more.

The misleading documentary "The Dark Charisma of Adolf Hitler" (in which Ian Kershaw was the historical consultant / script consultant) shows a car in Germany with Hitler's Hakenkreuz on the front grill in a manner reminiscent of a Krit car (episode 1 at ~57:58; ep. 2 at ~1:24 and ~14:39).

On March 21, 1916, the French Air Department created the Escadrille Américaine (Escadrille N.124), later renamed the Escadrille Lafayette. It utilized American volunteers and was first deployed on April 20 in Luxeuil-les-Bains, France. In fighting Germans, the Americans would fly planes bearing large swastikas on the sides, in a pattern similar to that adopted decades later (in WWII) by Germany. The planes also bore smaller swastikas that appeared on the headdress of an American Indian Chief that was also used as insignia on planes. Photographs show the large swastika on SPAD planes (SPAD S.XIII?), French biplane fighter aircraft of World War I, developed by Société Pour L'Aviation et ses Dérivés (SPAD).

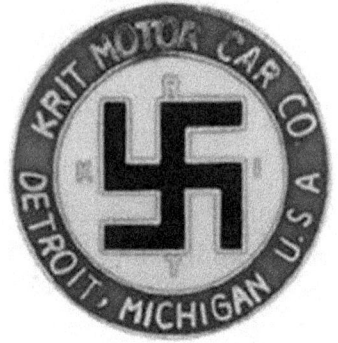 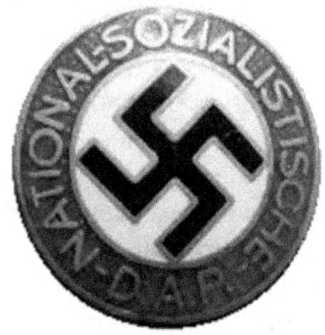

The French Escadrille's insignias are remarkably similar to insignias used later (after 1920?) in the USA by the 158th Field Artillery Regiment and by the 45th Infantry Division. The people who write about the 158th and the 45th seem ignorant of the Escadrille's insignias and any possible connection in the symbolism (they claim that the 45th Division's swastika "had been selected as a typical American Indian symbol." That supports the likelihood that the 45th Division's swastika was inspired by the French Escadrille, or that they have the same origin, perhaps from the earlier use by Boy Scouts). Were any of the Americans who served in the French Escadrille from the region (Oklahoma, Colorado, Arizona, and New Mexico) that would become the 45th Division? Had any of them been Boy Scouts?

It is incorrect to assert that the 45th Division's swastika is "a typical American Indian symbol" even though it might have been selected as such through ignorance. Perhaps it became "a typical American Indian Symbol" after Europeans brought it to America and began asking Native Americans to put it on pottery, baskets, and blankets[31] (compare that to saying that a horse image is "a typical American Indian Symbol"; a rifle is a "typical Native American" weapon; that horses are a "typical American Indian" mode of transportation; that horse hair pottery is "typical American Indian" pottery; that horse figurines and blankets are "typical American Indian" art. Native American Indians did not have horses and rifles until Europeans supplied them).

The "American Indian swastika" is overstated. That is why people who refer to the "Native American swastika" never name a tribe, and speak as if all tribes were one and the same. It is not clear what word would have been used by any American Indians for a "swastika."

---

[31] Something similar occurred with the "Ica stones" from the Ica Province, Peru. Some of the stones show carvings of dinosaurs alongside humans. From the 1960s Javier Cabrera Darquea popularized the stones, obtaining many from a farmer named Basilio Uschuya. Uschuya, after claiming them to be genuine ancient artifacts, admitted to creating the carvings because he knew that they were what customers wanted.

The hard right angles and the thickness of the 45th's swastika are not characteristic of any "typical" ancient (pre-European migration) American Indian symbol that might be described generously as a "swastika," nor in the 45th Division's area. For example, a 45th Division photograph of Captain Sidney P. Kretlow (see infra) bears a 158th Field Artillery Regiment emblem that includes an "Avanyu Azure" (also called Awanyu) to represent Arizona. Some people would call it a "swastika" even though it has only three arms and is oriented in the "Z" direction (the opposite of the 45th Division swastika) and is curved. There is little information available (such as its alleged age) concerning the Avanyu as represented by the 158th. Most other depictions of Avanyu show a long snake. The term "Avanyu" as applied to the 158th Regiment's insignia is confusing.

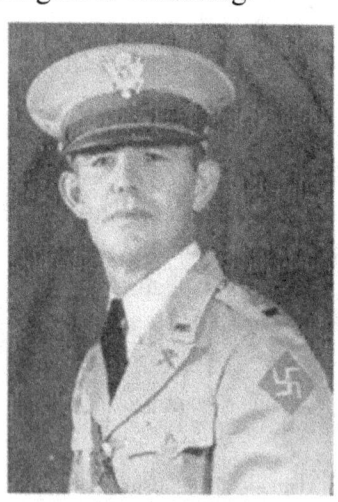

The USA's Military Swastika

A scene in the 1959 American film "Verboten" (by director Samuel Fuller) shows a wounded U.S. Army sergeant conversing with a German woman inside her residence. On the wall hangs a picture of Hitler wearing a swastika armband. The sergeant tells the woman that the swastika was an old American Indian sign that "Hitler took from us" and adds that the 45th infantry wore it "before Adolf got the idea."

The sergeant does not explain that the stiff-armed Nazi salute is Americana from the Pledge of Allegiance (from ~1892) that "Hitler took from us" and that Americans did it for decades "before Adolf got the idea" (and that some Americans continued to do it during WWII). That topic was... "verboten." The latter sentence about the pledge would have been more accurate than the former sentence about the swastika. The sergeant could have explained that Americans were wearing swastikas and doing the Nazi salute before Germans did it.

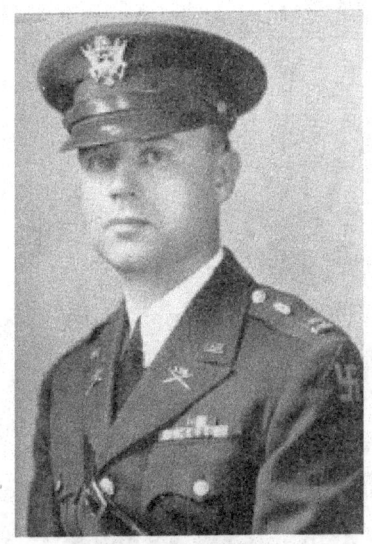

The USA's Military Swastika

A photograph - dated 1938- of Captain Sidney P. Kretlow shows the 45th Infantry Division's swastika on his left shoulder. The 45th Division's swastika is a reminder of the manner in which German socialists wore the tag on armbands on the left shoulder.

In the recent past, it was difficult to find any photograph of anyone in the 45th Division wearing the swastika. As of this writing, there is one website with photographs of 45th Division personnel in uniform, but many of the photographs are framed or cropped so that the swastika on the left shoulder is not visible.

It is important to view the manner in which the 45th Division swastika was worn on the left shoulder.[32] The swastika was oriented flat on one side (as if in a square, not a diamond). It is a reminder that German socialists altered their hooked cross so that it was oriented as if in a diamond, highlighting the "S" letter shapes for "socialist."

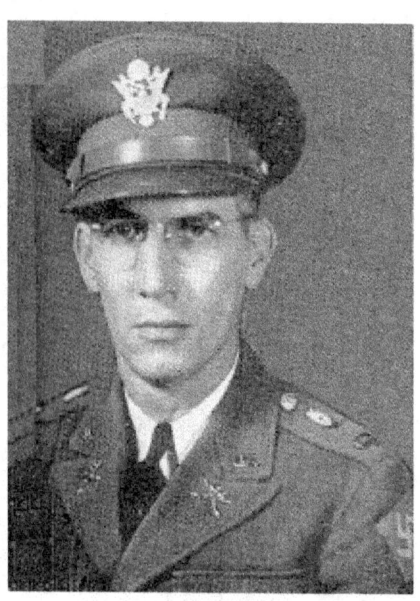

The USA's Military Swastika

During the time of the 45th infantry accoutrements, Americans wore swastikas on military uniforms and performed the Nazi salute (for the Pledge of Allegiance

---

[32] Three photographs should accompany this section. The photo on the left is often mis-identified as an officer under German socialism. That is how striking the similarity is.

and more).

A Freemasonry group -the Grand Lodge of British Columbia and Yukon- displays on its website a photograph of what it identifies as a Navajo Indian carpet (circa 1925) decorated with the Freemason hallmark (square and compass) between two swastikas. That Freemason site also boasts that Francis Bellamy, author of the USA's flag salutation, was a Mason. The site neglects to mention anything about the pledge's early Nazi salute and influence on Freemasons or on anyone.

In 1917, socialism was imposed in Russia (renamed the Union of Soviet Socialist Republics). After the revolution, socialism's first fake money (new paper rubles) displayed many swastikas[33] in the same "S" letter style for "socialism" emulated later by German socialists. In the case of the USSR the crossed "S" letters could have been interpreted as "Soviet Socialism."

To whatever degree the symbol meant "good luck," Soviet socialists shared with German socialists the belief (popular today) that socialism is "good luck" ("luck" is an appropriate term for people who lie about how everything is magically "free" - food, clothing, shelter,

---

[33] Swastika count: the 250 ruble banknote has 5 swastikas (dated 1917); 1000 ruble, 3 swastikas (1917); 5000 ruble, 3 swastikas (1918); 10,000 ruble, 3 swastikas (1918). The Tsar abdicated 2 March 1917. The provisional government lasted ~8 months (at that time Alexander Kerensky was a leader in the Socialist Revolutionary Party), until the Russian Social Democratic Workers' Party (RSDRP) took over in October 1917. The 250 note shows the double-headed eagle bereft of the crowns, scepter, and orb (with a cross atop). The notes printed in 1917 and 1918 were used in those years and thereafter.

healthcare, schools, goods, services, et cetera). It is good luck when people are able to locate necessities under socialism. Keep your fingers crossed! "Good Luck" is akin to putting "In God We Trust" on socialist money.

Soviet notes had many more swastikas than German notes. If swastika rubles remained in circulation until 1922 or 1923, then they would have overlapped the creation of the National Socialist German Workers Party (1920).

The hammer and sickle did not become the official symbol of the Russian Soviet Federated Socialist Republic until 1924. Socialism's obsolescence was symbolically frozen in time with old hand tools, as capitalism progressed into machinery for agriculture and industry.

In 1919 Soviet socialist ruble notes contained the German language: "PROLETARIER ALLER LANDER, VEREINIGT EUCH" ("Workers of all Lands, Unite!" Marx's commercial jingle in screaming capital letters)[34] to spread socialist hegemony to Germany.

A 1936 Deutsche Reichsmark (in the denomination 1000, and bearing the portrait of architect Karl Friedrich Schinkel) shows striking similarity to the 250 ruble note (1917). The similarities are: a centered swastika[35] of

---

[34] "Workers of the world Unite! You have nothing to lose but your ~~chains~~ food!" In ancient Rome the "proletarius" were citizens of the lowest class. They were propertyless people, exempted from taxes and military service, who "served the state" only by having children. The word "proles" is related to "offspring, progeny," and related to the modern word "prolific." Under modern socialism, they continue to be required to "serve the state" but they are no longer exempted from taxes and military service.

[35] The 250 ruble note has at least five swastikas (two on the

similar size and orientation, as a background decoration; coloring (green, blue, red, yellow on the ruble and on the Reichsmark); and intricate design flourish surrounding the swastika (to make counterfeiting difficult).

The first German banknote with the Hakenkreuz (pronounced more or less "HAHK-en-KROITS") in the background was the 100 Mark banknote issued on June 24, 1935 with a portrait of Justus von Liebig, a German Chemist.

Another hooked cross appeared in the background of the 10 Mark banknote issued on August 1, 1942, and bearing the portrait of a young female (a German Hitler Youth?).

It is another reason why the hammer and sickle should be as reviled as the hooked cross: both symbols were used under Soviet socialism.

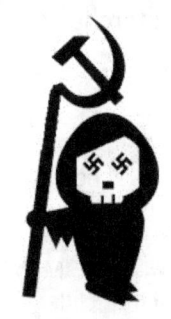

As noted earlier, Helena Blavatsky of the Theosophical Society (TS) claimed to be from an aristocratic Russian-German family and used the swastika in TS (1875) and later while working with the American socialist Edward Bellamy.

At the turn of 1918-19, and unmentioned in "Mein Kampf," Hitler wore a red brassard and supported the short-lived Bavarian Soviet Republic (or Munich Soviet Republic), according to Thomas Weber in the book "Hitler's First War."

Mein Kampf mentions Kurt Eisner, "Soldiers'

---

obverse; three on the reverse, and some of the swastikas are easily overlooked because they have numbers covering them. Some of the other ruble notes also have multiple swastikas.

Councils," and that time period.

There is something important that is not in Weber's book: Perhaps the Bavarian Soviet Republic experience played a role in the German National Socialist leader (Hitler) adopting a swastika style that had been used as a trademark of socialism by Soviet socialists on ruble currency (in 1917 and 1918).

The Bavarian Soviet Republic provides more evidence that Adolf Hitler used the swastika to signify crossed "S" letters for "socialism" under his National Socialist German Workers Party.

The swastika's Soviet replacement -the hammer and sickle- had similarities and it "freed" the earlier symbol for German socialists. Both symbols have two crossed pieces (the new Soviet symbol was a cross formed by a hammer and scythe). Both symbols include serpentine or sickle shapes. The hammer and sickle is referenced in Russian as: Серп и молот, serp i molot (Я).[36]

---

[36] "Molot" is related to the English word "mallet." At that time the symbolism was enjoyed as a pseudonym by Vyacheslav Mikhailovich Skryabin ("Molotov" is derived from the Russian word for "hammer").

Stalin's name is derived from "steel" as if he was the "Man of Steel" or the super socialist man. It is doubtful that Hitler was blind to the symbolism (as most people are today). The "steel" reference is more obvious in German than in English. "Stalin" sounds like "stehlen" -the German word for "steel."

Molotov became half of the 2 girls 1 cup crime against humanity known as the Molotov-Ribbentrop pact (a.k.a. the Hitler-Stalin pact) when German socialists and Soviet socialists joined forces in 1939.

The hammer and sickle represent socialism's burglary tools and murder weapons. The hammer is the threat of violence and is used for breaking and entering into private property. The sickle stole grain from the millions who starved under socialism's glorious "free" food system. The scythe was

Another symbol with two crossed pieces was the Hebrew Star of David (at least in the eyes of German socialists). It was interpreted as crossed triangles (one pointing up, the other pointing down).[37] German socialists wore crossed "S" letters (e.g. hooked crosses on armbands) as they persecuted Jews forced to wear crossed triangles (the Magen David).[38] In concentration camps the two triangles had different colors denoting different categories (see Kennzeichen für Schutzhäftlinge in den Konzentrationslagern). Non-jewish prisoners wore badges that bore only half of the Star of David (one downward-pointing triangle in different colors denoting different categories).

When the First World War (1914-1918) drew to a close, Germany began to follow Russia into more

---

carried by the grim reaper of Soviet socialism before, during, and after 1939. Socialists, like highwaymen, say: "Your money, or your life." Often, they take both. When you are a hammer and sickle, everything is a nail or sheaf.

[37] The original meaning of the Shield of David is not clear, nor why it was first adopted by Jewish people as a symbol. Nevertheless: Two crossed triangles resemble two crossed deltas (the Latin letter for "D") and could be interpreted as a reference to "David" or "Davidian Dynasty" (Dr. Curry made this point). That is not inconsistent with the symbol's origin as a symbol for Judaism used by Medieval Christians c. 1400s (see the historian Jonathan Kirsch). Similar to the cross (infra), it could also be a symbol for "death" ("D" for "Death" – the "Dead Davidian Dynasty"). The double-"D" letter provides another comparison to the two crossed "S" letters referencing "socialists" in Hitler's hooked cross. The Bible obsesses over racial purity, lineage, and the "chosen" noble people. This is tiresome: people who obsess about essing dees.

[38] The documentary "For the Love of Spock" contains (near the beginning) what appears to be a photograph of Leonard Nimoy wearing his U.S. army uniform which includes a Star of David badge on his left shoulder.

socialist revolution. The German Revolution or November Revolution occurred in 1918 at the end of the First World War. In August 1919 it resulted in the establishment of what later became known as the Weimar Republic (1919-1933 and named after Weimar, the city where the constitutional assembly took place). During this period, and well into the next era of National Socialism, the official name of the state was the German Reich (Deutsches Reich).

The conditions which gave birth to the German revolution were similar to those in Russia in 1917 (resulting in Soviet socialism). Thereafter, sustained socialist agitation was the strategy of many socialists including the socialist Hitler and his National Socialist German Workers Party. Germany's path included the abdication of Kaiser Wilhelm II and led to the socialist Hitler.

On March 27, 1917, German socialists helped Vladimir Lenin (and 32 other socialist fellow travelers) ride by train through Germany to Russia to impose socialism there and demand an end to the war with Germany.[39] Lenin was a loony follower of the

---

[39] Lenin traveled on socialized railroads back to Russia. Lenin's path to tsarism was expedited because socialism preceded Lenin in Russia, and enabled Lenin to merely seize the socialist structure that already existed there (and that exists almost everywhere, then and now): post offices, railroad stations, the telegraph office, telephone exchange, the national bank, and major bridges. They were all socialized before Lenin. He wasn't doing anything new. He wasn't "seizing them from capitalists" he was assuming them from the other socialists. There was no "socialist revolution." Those "means of production" already had long records of socialized unproductiveness. Lenin simply proceeded to worsen everything. Most of the world has learned nothing from

demented German socialists Karl Marx and Friedrich Engels. Lenin had wasted precious time in exile when he could have been in Russia ~~murdering millions~~ creating socialist utopia. While in exile, Lenin had lived in Munich, Bern, and Zurich.

In 1913, Vienna had been home to many socialist wieners (the type of people who should be on your "DO NOT SAVE FROM DROWNING" list), including Stalin, Trotsky, Hitler, and Josip Broz Tito (who would become president of the Socialist Federal Republic of Yugoslavia). Perhaps Lenin visited too. They could have heard each other preaching about how wunderbar socialism is while they schemed at Café Landtmann, Café Central, or other Viennese coffee-houses, or in the Rathauskeller, Hofbräuhaus, or other beer halls. Maybe they chatted about the swastikas that eventually appeared on the first paper ruble currency under Soviet socialism (and on German socialism's currency later).

"The Untold History of the United States" by Oliver Stone and Peter Kuznick states "Marx, ironically, had doubted that a successful socialist revolution could occur in economically and culturally backward Russia."[40] Marx and Engels thought that Russians were "racial trash" who needed to be exterminated in a "holocaust." The first socialist to aid Marx' holocaust of the "racial trash" in the USSR was Lenin; then Stalin; then Hitler and Stalin together; then Stalin alone again. Many socialists are Holocaust deniers in this regard.

Despite Marx's drivel -or because of Marx's drivel- a

Lenin's modus operandi. Soon he would employ government schools (socialist schools) -another common mistake in many places today.

[40] Russia was the political equivalent of the Flat Earth Society (they have members all around the globe).

socialist revolution did occur in "economically and culturally backward Russia." After the socialist revolution, Russia remained economically and culturally backward. It was a never-coming-of-age story. The USSR was arrested development. In fact, after the socialist revolution everything devolved farther in "economically and culturally backward Russia."

Marx thought that a successful socialist revolution could occur in Germany. It did. German socialists after WWI merely followed the pattern blazed by Soviet socialists after WWI (which Germany had fomented with its railroad aid and more provided to Lenin and his co-conspirators). At the end of WWI, the German socialists Marx and Engels had inspired Lenin, and all three of them (plus Stalin) then provided a template for Hitler after WWI.

Lenin campaigned for the First World War to be used to impose Europe-wide socialism. Lenin's effort was aided by Hitler who also used WWI to campaign for socialism in Germany and beyond. Later, Hitler joined with Lenin's successor (Stalin) and continued the campaign for Europe-wide socialism in their pact to start WWII. All the socialist sociopaths learned from each other. They had parallel lives. In that sense, (and in the minds of Lenin, Stalin, and Hitler) both wars were socialist wars.

Lenin and Hitler share many parallels in their Kampfs for socialism, but it took Hitler longer to gain control of his nation. Lenin was imprisoned and exiled in 1897; he attempted to seize power in 1905 but failed; he then gained power in 1917, although the USSR was not officially formed until 1922. Hitler joined his socialist group in 1919 (following Lenin's path), became its leader in 1921, and attempted to gain power in 1923.

The failed coup resulted in Hitler's imprisonment (9 months), during which he dictated his socialist manifesto Mein Kampf (think of it as Hitler's "Das Kapital." The phrase "das kapital" appears in Hitler's book four times; and "kapital" appears ~30 times as a word or part of a word).

War is sold as "temporary" police state socialism, and it devolves into permanent socialism after the war pretense ends. That was WWI with Lenin and Hitler.

War is always socialism because it is always a takeover of the economy for war. Lenin and Hitler showed that socialism was merely a continuation of WWI domestically, after the international mayhem stopped. Socialism is the prelude to the next war. WWII.

Lenin and Hitler fulfilled the dream of the socialist Gavrilo Princip who wanted to foment socialist revolution (Princip claimed that the intervening WWI that he caused was an unexpected oversight on his part. He offers his apologies for that). Yet in the demented socialist way, Princip's plan worked.

Lenin's hand-picked replacement, Stalin, said: "We are fifty or a hundred years behind the advanced countries. We must make up this gap in ten years. Either we do it or they will crush us." He didn't do it. And all the crushing of peasants et al was done by him. We have met the enemy and he is us. The only part Stalin got right was being at least a century behind (He was referring to the property-owning capitalist USA). He lengthened the temporal distance.

Stalin's inferiority complex spurred his partnership with the National Socialist German Workers Party. The duo of economically and culturally regressed countries invaded Poland together, spreading their next socialist war (WWII). The two liars and their socialist lies got halfway around the world before the truth even had a chance to put its pants on.

Hitler said, "What Marxism, Leninism and Stalinism failed to accomplish, we shall be in a position to achieve."[41] They didn't.

In 1920, the word "socialist" was added to the name of Hitler's party, which was already ideologically socialist. The alteration occurred near the time of his early infamous Hofbräuhaus speech. That change was an open declaration of socialist dogma, in light of everything that preceded it historically in Hitler's life (e.g. the creation of the Union of Soviet Socialist Republics and the spread of socialism by the USSR to other countries around Germany). The name change to "National Socialist German Workers Party" from "German Workers Party" was potent, comparable to turning the Hakenkreuz 45 degrees from the horizontal.

November 1923 brought another attempt at socialist revolution in Germany by Hitler. It resulted in his imprisonment where he wrote Mein Kampf, a book that promotes his socialist plans. Hitler was released from prison in December 1924 (the year that Lenin died and Stalin replaced Lenin).

In 1939, Stalin joined Hitler in their shared kampf to steal real estate. German socialists became allies in socialist imperialism with the Union of Soviet Socialist Republics.[42] The Nazi-Fasci-Socialist Stalin partnered

---

[41] Quoted by Otto Wagener in "Hitler: Memoirs of a Confidant," edited by Henry Ashby Turner, Jr., Yale University Press (1985) p. 149.

[42] What would you do if you lived in country (e.g. the USA) that kept invading other countries and killing people around world? Rationalize it as humanitarian?

with Hitler. It brought together the two worst populations on earth in the so-called "Third Reich."

German socialists and Soviet socialists reunited again in East Germany (GDR) from 1949 to 1990. Was the GDR a continuation of the Third Reich or had it become the Fourth Reich? The East German Soviet Republic formed despite Hitler's earlier alleged failure to create the Bavarian Soviet Republic (or Munich Soviet Republic). Buried within the GDR was Berlin divided; showcasing the embarrassing poverty of East Berlin's socialism compared to West Berlin's wealthy capitalism (similar to North and South Korea). The cliché of East Germany became "Workers of the world, unite!" (a vapid Weltanschauung of the German socialist Marx. The banality had been on early Soviet socialism's paper ruble currency before Hitler expanded Germany's socialism).

Soviet socialism provided the Fourth Reich (GDR) with Lebensraum via the enormous Soviet empire which at that time included Poland, Ukraine, et cetera -the places German socialists had also invaded. The ruling party in East Germany was the Socialist Unity Party of Germany (Sozialistische Einheitspartei Deutschlands or SED. Sound familiar?). Other institutional groups were allegedly "permitted to exist" as long as they were "in alliance" with the SED; one such party was the Christian Democratic Union. Although Hitler had killed himself in 1945, other antidisestablishmentarians continued the socialist dystopia in East Germany until the Capitalist Revolutions of 1989 against socialist control.

In East Germany, many trademarks of German socialism were embraced by Soviet socialism. The Schutzstaffel (SS) ended under German socialism and the Stasi began under Soviet socialism (with a fascinating repetition of the "S-S" sound shared by the swastika; and "Stasi" rhymes with "Nazi").

Swastika-style graphic design was popularized by Soviet socialists in the form of the "S" shaped logo used on the notorious Trabant Sachsenring car (How do you double the value of a Trabant? Fill the gas tank).

The socialist Adolf Hitler participated in three attempted violent socialist revolutions (but he succeeded in imposing socialism via voters electing him to office).

The following are Hitler's three attempts at violent socialist revolution (two were at Munich and those two were only four years apart) -

1. Munich Soviet Republic 1918-1919 (aka Bavarian Soviet Republic) - under Kurt Eisner and Ernst Niekisch (the latter one had a sad life of socialism). German socialists conspired with Soviet socialists to spread the Soviet socialist confederacy's "revolution" into Germany.

2. Munich Beer Hall Putsch - 1923 (November 8-9, 1923). Hitler's second attempt at a Munich Socialist Republic. Hitler was arrested for his socialist activities and was charged with treason in connection with the Munich Beer Hall Putsch (coup). Imprisoned, Hitler wrote his socialist manifesto "Mein Kampf."

3. Poland 1939 - German socialists and Soviet socialists became allies in 1939 in a pact of socialist imperialism and socialist colonialism to divide up Europe, spreading WWII, and leading to the socialist Wholecaust (of which the Holocaust was a part), the worst slaughter of humanity in history. Hitler and

German socialists touted international socialism in a global conspiracy with Soviet socialists.

Concerning the Munich Soviet Republic, Hitler had suspiciously little to say in Mein Kampf or ever. An excerpt: **"In the course of the new revolution of the Councils I for the first time acted in such a way as to arouse the disapproval of the Central Council. Early in the morning of April 27, 1919, I was to be arrested..."** Another excerpt: **"A few days after the liberation of Munich, I was ordered to report to the examining commission concerned with revolutionary occurrences in the Second Infantry regiment."** There is nothing about his reasons for staying in Munich, nothing about the horrors of the councils (soviets) which he actually knew, nothing about the severe fighting that preceded the liberation of Munich.

A photograph exists that seems to show Hitler at Kurt Eisner's funeral procession (Eisner was assassinated February 21, 1919).

Shortly after Hitler's doings at the Bavarian Socialist Republic, Hitler joined the political party that he would re-name the National Socialist German Workers Party. Hitler's socialist obsession was clearly deliberate and ongoing.

While in jail for his second attempted socialist revolution (the Beer Hall Putsch), Hitler wrote an awful lot (with the emphasis on "awful"), and completed Mein Kampf which promoted socialism (by the very word "socialism" repeated over and over by Hitler) from beginning to end. Hitler wanted Germans to read his book with a serious mien. Hitler always used the term "Socialist" to describe himself and his dogma, and he did not refer to himself as a "Nazi," nor as a "Fascist," nor did he use the term "Third Reich." Those latter terms are used today by anti-semantic socialists to shroud what Hitler and his supporters called themselves: SOCIALISTS.

Books and films about Hitler have titles like "Secrets of the Third Reich" and "Fascist Germany's Secrets" and "Dark Secrets of the Nazis." The books and films hide the biggest title secrets: Hitler did not self-identify with the words Nazi, Fascist, nor Third Reich. Those secrets expose the deception in popular titles and their contents.

According to Mein Kampf, Hitler immersed himself in Marxist studies.

Hitler also adopted as his notorious totem the very same image that was used on the first paper money of the Union of Soviet Socialist Republics. Hitler used the Soviet socialist symbol to represent crossed "S" letters for his own socialism under the National Socialist German Workers Party

Eisner and the Munich Soviet Republic used a solid red flag for the "socialist revolution." Hitler used the red flag too and placed his crossed "S" letters for "socialism" upon his red banner.

Hitler also adopted the notorious stiff-armed salute that originated in American heritage as authored by the USA's National Socialist Francis Bellamy.

It is fascinating to see how almost all so-called historians refuse to describe the Beer Hall Putsch as an attempted violent socialist revolution, even though that is exactly how Hitler perceived it and described it.

Historians warn 'Hitler said exactly what he was going to do in Mein Kampf! We must not forget!" And then the history books actively hide what Hitler said in Mein Kampf, and afterward.

German socialists did not refer to their mark by its popular modern name, "swastika." They called it a "Hakenkreuz." The term "Hakenkreuz" means "hooked cross." To Germans at that time, the Hakenkreuz hallmark was a type of domestic (German) cross, not a foreign Sanskrit "swastika." That is one reason why the German term "Hakenkreuz" (hooked cross) is hidden under the word "swastika" today.

The deception creates comical confusion: The German Women's Order supplied nurses for wounded socialists through its branch, the "Red Swastika" (at least that is how the name is often referred to in books written in the English language) and described as the "Nazi version of the Red Cross." Readers who are familiar with books about the academic work of the etymologist Dr. Rex Curry know that in German it was not called the "Red Swastika." It was called the "Rot Hakenkreuz" (red hooked cross). The explanation that it was a "version of the Red Cross" would be more clear if translators called it the "Red Hooked Cross," instead of using the misleading "Red Swastika" translation.[43] In the German language, the relationship between the

---

[43] The white armlet bearing a red cross was used almost as far back as the creation of the Red Cross in 1863. It served as another example to Hitler and German socialists in their adoption of armbands bearing their own cross (the hooked cross).

Today, the Red Cross movement works internationally with the Red Crescent movement and the Magen David Adom. "Red Crescent" is self-explanatory. "Magen David Adom" means "Red Star of David" (literally: "Red Shield of David"). It has been officially recognized by the International Committee of the Red Cross (ICRC), and is a member of the International Federation of Red Cross and Red Crescent Societies.

organizations is obvious. The translation game is sneaky and funny.

The term "swastika flag" is a false flag used to slander a foreign symbol in ongoing efforts to hide what German socialists thought about their emblem: that it was a type of cross and it was altered for use as an alphabetical emblem for "socialism."

The modern misnomer "swastika" was used (and continues to be used) to obscure German socialism's origin in American Christian Socialism, via Francis Bellamy and his cousin Edward Bellamy.

To put it another way, Hitler loved to wear a cross and he wanted others to wear a cross (on armbands, medals, posters and more) and he put a cross on his flag.

The double "S" letters and sounds of the word "swastika" and "socialism" were (and are) interchangeable. They are, in a sense, mutually onomatopoeic. They are linked in a way that the four letter N-word (Nazi) is not. In Hitler's hallmark, the swastika is synonymous with, and is a mnemonic reminder of, his socialism.

Hitler's "S" shape for the swastika added to the ignorant belief that German socialists called their label a swastika, in that the word "swastika" starts with the letter "S" and has two "S" sounds (and letters) in its spelling, as does the word "socialism."

The swastika was an ancient sign for "good luck" in India and elsewhere (and the word "swastika" is ascribed to the Sanskrit language). "Swastika" is misleading because in Sanskrit the term "swastika" (and other related spellings) was used to refer to many different "good luck" symbols; it did not refer exclusively to the hooked-cross shape.[44] The Oxford

English Dictionary proposes that the modern use of "swastika" entered the English language in 1871.

Although swastikas were ancient markings for "good luck," that is not why it was used by German socialists. It is unclear if Hitler even knew of the term "swastika" or that it was an ancient good-luck logo in India (as opposed to a "good luck" symbol via reference to the Christian cross). If Hitler was aware of a general connotation of "good luck" for his hallmark, then that would have encouraged his use of the swastika for his socialist dogma; all socialists mistakenly believe that their policies are "auspicious" for everyone.

In the lengthy book "Adolf Hitler: The Definitive Biography," John Toland asserts (page 86) that when the leader of the National Socialist German Workers' Party adopted the insignia, it was already in use as an emblem for another socialist group, a fact known by Hitler when selecting the graphic design. Toland writes "Drexler [Anton Drexler] suggested calling their group the German Socialist Party (the same name of a similarly motivated party founded a year earlier [1916?] in Bohemia [Czechoslovakia], whose emblem incidentally, was the swastika)."

Based on Toland's book and other sources, there is a question whether the leader of the National Socialist German Workers' Party was even aware of any context

---

[44] The ancient symbol itself has been described as a monogram with "interlacing of the letters of the auspicious words in the Aśoka characters" (such as "su" and "asti"; or "su" and "ti"). see Monier-Williams, Alexander Cunningham, and Jayarava (who debunks the idea). Wikipedia liars repeat the old debunked Sanskrit monogram myth but they never mention (not even as a question) the hooked-cross as "S" letters for "socialist" as Hitler's monogram.

for the symbol other than as an emblem of an existing socialist group (however, see Lambach Abbey referenced earlier in this book).

Another entry in Toland's book (page 183) references the use of the hooked cross under Hans Knirsch, founder of the National Socialist Workers Party in Czechoslovakia, a group that was also known as the Sudetendeutsche National Sozialistische Partei (Sudeten-German National Socialist Party).

If the swastika was a logo of the Sudetendeutsche National Sozialistische Partei, then that use provides additional evidence of an alphabetical representation for the swastika's two overlapping "S" letters: "Sudeten Socialism" or even "Southern Socialism." The word "Sudeten" came to mean "Southern" for many Germans, although the original etymology is unclear.

Toland also notes that the swastika was long a symbol of the Teutonic Knights and had been used by Lanz Von Liebenfels, the Thule Society and a number of other groups before Hitler's Socialist Party.

Another example of the swastika's use is at Lambach Abbey where Hitler attended as a youth in Austria. Revealing differences exist between the swastika styles of Abbey Lambach, of the Thule Society, and of the version used later by German socialists. If the two earlier styles influenced the later Nazi hallmark, then they demonstrate Hitler's alteration of the earlier styles to more closely reflect overlapping "S" letters in the later Nazi version.

The book "Swastika: the earliest known symbol and its migrations" (1894) by Thomas Wilson shows that the mark was used in and around ancient Germany and worldwide. The following is from Wilson's book (page 771):

"Dr. Schliemann found many specimens of Swastika in his excavations at the site of ancient Troy on the hill of Hissarlik. They were mostly on spindle whorls, and will be described in due course. He appealed to Professor Max Muller for an explanation, who, in reply, wrote an elaborate description, which Dr. Schliemann published in the book 'Ilios.'

Professor Muller commences with a protest against the word "Swastika" being applied generally to the symbol, because it may prejudice the reader or the public in favor of its Indian origin. Muller says:

'I do not like the use of the word svastika outside of India. It is a word of Indian origin and has its history and definite meaning in India. * * * The occurrence of such crosses in different parts of the world may or may not point to a common origin, but if they are once called Svastika the vulgus profanum will at once jump to the conclusion that they all come from India, and it will take some time to weed out such prejudice.'"

Muller's prediction was amazing in its accuracy, and it is amusing that he labeled so many people in the world today as "vulgus profanum." The word "swastika" was used enough that it became the prevailing term, even as a substitute for the actual German word "Hakenkreuz" (and the English term "hooked cross") and many people concluded falsely that all such symbols, including Hitler's Hakenkreuz, were references to India's swastika.

People who want to "save the swastika" are cross about Hitler's "theft" of "their" emblem. But swastika-lovers will never explain that Hitler did not call his mark a "swastika," and that he used it as "S" letters for "socialism." Swastika-lovers are at cross purposes in distinguishing the swastika from the logo of German socialism. They ignore the fact that when the insignia became "S" letter shapes for "socialism" (via Theosophy, Bellamy, Soviet socialism, and German socialism) it truly did become an irredeemably evil talisman of selfishness, robbery, and violence.

Hitler's hieroglyph was not always called a "swastika" outside of Germany. In the U.S., in the UK, and elsewhere, it was also called "Hakenkreuz" or "hooked cross" or "crooked cross" or "armed cross."

A popular explanation of the hypothesis of Dr. Curry regarding the swastika is: "Although an ancient symbol, the swastika was also used by Hitler to represent crossed 'S' letters for 'socialist' under his National Socialist German Workers Party." The explanation might seem complicated, but it is really quite symbol. Although verbose, Hitler was very symbol-minded. He was an artist and he was personally involved in the design and selection of the older and newer versions of his symbol and other banners.

A common retort is: "The swastika is an ancient symbol that predated Hitler by thousands of years." That common retort is proof that government schools (socialist schools) produce dimwits and must end. Government schools produce adults who believe swastikas cannot be altered in their use or appearance due to some "magic" spanning thousands of years.

Today, the term "swastika" is used to slander a foreign symbol in an ongoing effort to conceal what German socialists thought about their symbol. The schools and the media are as unwilling to report the facts about the swastika as they are unwilling to print historic photographs of the US pledge's early Nazi gesture.

A web search for "types of crosses" shows a chart of 25 collected images that include the "iron cross," the "Maltese cross," the "Florian cross," the Krückenkreuz ("crutches cross"), the Potent cross ⊹, the common "Christian cross," and more; but no "hooked cross" is depicted. Such charts reveal that the "vulgus profanum" who listed the "types of crosses" did not know that Hitler's hallmark was a type of cross.

The same web search for "types of crosses" show other charts that include a "swastika" that is facing in the "Z" letter-shape direction (卐 or the opposite orientation of Hitler's logo), and it is depicted as if drawn in a square (not a diamond), and it is NOT identified as a "hooked cross." Such charts are stupider than the charts mentioned in the preceding paragraph. They reveal that the "vulgus profanum" who listed these "types of crosses" are EXCLUDING Hitler's hooked cross, and are identifying the Indian/Buddhist/Hindu swastika as a "cross" in a ignorant manner, without explanation.

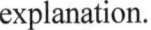

Another type of cross used by German socialists was the Balkenkreuz. Balken means "beam" or "bar" in German. A literal translation of "Balkenkreuz" would be "beam cross" or "bar cross."

Balkenkreuz

Under Hitler, the Hakenkreuz was sometimes placed on top of (or combined with) the Ritterkreuz, and the Christian cross, and Maltese cross (e.g. on medals). Such a pairing of crosses is shown in the flags of "Deutsche Christen" a Christian Socialism group: Its emblem was a traditional Christian cross with a hooked cross in the center intersection. In other words, one cross is combined with another cross, for a pair of crosses.

Members of the Deutsche Christen socialist group (and other Germans) did not think "How nice that the ancient Hindu religious sign -the swastika- is placed in the center of the Christian cross." Recipients of medals with paired crosses did not exclaim "Wunderbar! An age-old Hindu religious mark -the swastika- has been combined with an old German cross."

In parades, Deutsche Christen members would carry German swastika flags wherein the swastika in the center had been replaced with the standard Christian cross. Ignorant documentaries and books always describe the banners thusly: "the swastika was replaced by the cross" (instead of explaining that "the hooked cross was replaced by the standard Christian cross").

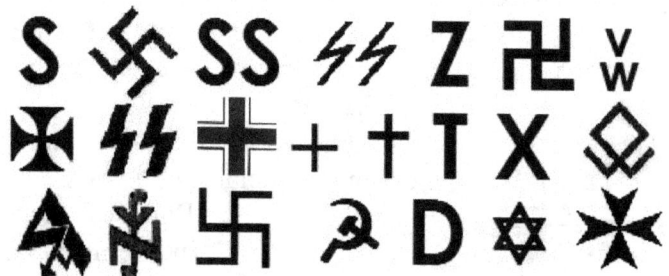

When paired-cross war medals are sold today among collectors of German WWII memorabilia, they have incongruous descriptions such as "a swastika on top of a Ritterkreuz," (instead of "a Hakenkreuz on top of a Ritterkreuz"); and "a swastika over a Maltese cross" (instead of "a hooked cross over a Maltese cross");[45] and "a swastika on top of a cross" (instead of "a German hook-cross on top of a common Christian cross"). The inconsistent terminology reveals a secret etymological history that is unknown to almost everyone on earth.

Neophytes incorrectly believe that two crosses[46] double in strength; but the learned masters know that it multiplies their magical crossiness powers (just like the old gypsy woman foretold).

There were grave markers that were in that shape of a Christian cross that contained in its center an iron cross that contained in its center a hooked cross. That's THREE crosses combined! CROSS SUPERPOWERS ACTIVATED!

Perhaps German Christian Socialists expanded the Christian "sign of the cross" (spectacles, testicles, wallet, and watch) to the physical gesture known as the "sign of the hooked cross" (left side of your spectacles, right side of your spectacles, left testicle, right testicle, bottom of wallet, top of wallet, bottom of watch, and top of watch).[47]

Old film footage of Hitler speaking shows an armband on his left arm displaying his "S"-shaped hooked cross next to an iron cross (displayed on Hitler's left shirt pocket as a metallic pendant). The two crosses are almost touching. People who have not read this

---

[45] Henry Ford was awarded the Grand Cross of the German Eagle, the highest medal that German socialism could bestow on a foreigner. It is always described as a Maltese cross surrounded by four swastikas (as opposed to "a Maltese cross surrounded by four Hooked crosses or Hakenkreuz").

[46] "Dos Equis" as a Spanish speaker might say, as compared with one cross or Hakenkreuz (una equis).

[47] The "sign of the cross" was parodied as the "sign of the T" as a reference to Ford's Model T car in Brave New World by author Aldous Huxley.

book state incongruously that the film shows Hitler with a "swastika" armband next to his "iron cross" pendant.

We should all be thankful that Americans and Brits et cetera did not adopt Sanskrit/Hindu names and Sanskrit/Hindu stories for the German socialists' use of the Maltese Cross, the common Christian Cross, and the Iron Cross (Eisernes Kreuz, Ritterkreuz, Rider Cross, Knight's Cross) or any other crosses used under German socialism.

Iron Cross
Eisernes Kreuz
Ritterkreuz
Rider Cross
Knight's Cross

Only the Hakenkreuz received such deceptive treatment as it was renamed "swastika." It alone was so reviled that its relationship to other crosses had to be hidden. It was excommunicated from the church of crosses.

Before German socialism, the swastika was usually oriented horizontally (as if it was drawn within a square, NOT a diamond) and was pointed left or right (see Wilson's book and illustrations therein).

During Hitler's early life, Hitler viewed the Hakenkreuz pointed left or right and oriented horizontally (as if drawn within a square). A drawing by Hitler (he had been an aspiring artist) shows a fireplace mantel decorated with two of the crosses, both horizontal; one points left and the other points right. That use changed during the existence of the German Socialist Party. Hitler presided over the amulet's mutation into a socialist sigil. Under Hitler, the swastika became a socialist cipher, and a doppelsieg for a doppelgänger.

Hitler's modification gave his monogram a 45° rotation from horizontal (as if it was drawn within a diamond shape). The change also turned the Nazi mark to point the arms rightward in newer, future uses. That also became the official version displayed on the flag. Both transformations to the German socialist sigil emphasized "S" shapes in the orientation.

Steven Heller, author of "The Swastika: Symbol Beyond Redemption?" and art director of The New York Times Book Review, overlooked so much about the symbol when he stated "Hitler's major contribution was to reverse the direction of the swastika."

Hitler did more than merely reverse the direction. Heller failed to make many other discoveries about the swastika, including: (1) the object represented "S" letters for "socialism" under Hitler, and (2) the relationship of Hitler's hooked cross and his dogma to Christian socialism, to Francis Bellamy, and to the American Nazi salute from the US flag pledge.

In the USA, "Swastika" was the name of towns, streets, businesses, products, brands, and more. Those names were changed after WWII. The list of things "ruined" by socialism continued to lengthen: the Pledge of Allegiance (especially its early gesture); hand salutes substituted for handshakes;[48] the names "Adolf" and "Hitler"; "Swastika" names; and the symbol itself; and toothbrush moustaches (aka "Charlie Chaplin" moustaches[49]).

---

[48] To this day hospitals spend millions of dollars trying to stop the spread of bacteria while ignoring the most obvious source: handshakes. Over two centuries after the utility of hand-washing was "discovered" by Dr. Ignaz Semmelweis, almost nothing has been done to end handshakes. How many millions of people have died as a result?

[49] Did Chaplin inspire Hitler's moustache? Evidence (i.e. photographs) suggests that Chaplin's iconic moustache came first. For more on Hitler and Chaplin see infra.

10. SOCIALIST IMPERIALISM

The Bellamy dogma was the same dogma that led to the modern Christian Crusades of Christian socialism, and to history's worst bloodbath under the socialist Wholecaust (of which the Holocaust was a part): ~50 million slaughtered under Stalin and Soviet Socialism; ~40 million under Mao and Chinese socialism; ~20 million under Hitler and German socialism. It is deadly to cross a socialist.

Before Christianity, the cross was capital punishment.[50] After Christianity began, the cross' meaning changed. Crucifixion was banned[51] in the 4th

---

[50] Crucifixion continues to be available (or used) as capital punishment in some parts of the world.

[51] The crucifixion ban seems good, yet the ban caused substitution of other (worse?) forms of execution (e.g. impalement). Impalement was used to defend Christianity under the reign of Vlad Tepes (the inspiration for the blood-drinking "Dracula"). As a Roman Catholic in Romania (~1448), Tepes took part in ritualized cannibalism via transubstantiation; drinking blood, and eating flesh.

Even so, the number of people who suffered and died under *modern* Romanian socialism (both German and Soviet 1939-1989) makes Vlad the Impaler seem slight. Jesus said eat my body and drink my blood; Under Stalin and Mao that was multiplied for thousands of people.

Century AD by Roman emperor Constantine, a Christian.

Today, the cross symbol (the old Christian cross, the Crucifix, and the hooked-cross of socialism) represents death, execution, martyrdom, human sacrifice, and self-sacrifice (or suicide in the case of socialism). Because of those connotations, the cross remains a meaningful totem for the deadly dogma of socialism.

The cross complements another socialist symbol: the red flag. The blood color promoted by Stalin, Mao, Hitler and other socialists represents their bloodlust and violent sociopathy. The Christian Bible and socialism share a fascination for blood, death, and genocide. The red flag was easy to invent: all that was needed was cloth and the great big puddles of blood all around from men, women, and children.[52]

The state is the only modern religion that continues

Old habits remain undead. In 2014 in Romania, Toma Petre's relatives pulled his body from the grave, ripped out his heart, burned it to ashes, mixed it with water and drank. No media mentioned that Petre's relatives engage in a weekly Eucharistic religious ritual that includes drinking blood and eating flesh of someone who was crucified.

[52] The "Blood Flag" (Blutfahne) is the German socialist hooked-cross flag that was used in the failed Beer Hall Putsch in Munich, on 9 November 1923, during which it became soaked in the blood of one of the SA members who died. It became one of the most revered objects of the German Socialist Party (NSDAP). It was used in ceremonies in which new flags for party organizations were consecrated by the Blood Flag when touched by it.

SMH used the socialist flag to excite people in the same way that a red dot laser pointer is used to play with cats.

People react differently to the public display at a rally of a Soviet socialist flag, as compared with a German socialist flag. How strange.

to demand human sacrifices.[53] Socialism slaughters infidels.

"Christian Socialists" continue to exist along with their parties and movements, and they continue to use the cross to signify their socialism.[54] The mainstream groups no longer use the "S" oriented hook-cross as an alphabetical image for their "socialism."

Critics think it is odd that Christians (and Christian Socialists) wear crosses and crucifixes as pendants hung on necklaces.[55] It would be similarly odd if pendants shaped like tiny firearms had become jewelry worn by admirers of Abraham Lincoln (the 16th President.

---

[53] Without government, who would have killed Jesus? When Jesus was executed he felt cross. He believed that he had been double-crossed. Crucifixion causes excruciating pain.

[54] In Germany, The Chancellor of Germany, Angela Merkel, is the leader of the Christian Democratic Union of Germany (Christlich Demokratische Union Deutschlands). Merkel's socialist father deliberately moved to Soviet-controlled East Germany where Angela was raised. Her father was a pastor (Get it? Her name is "Angel." Also note that Friedrich Engels' name is related to "Angel" also). Modern German political leadership merely exchanged a Nazi uniform for a Stasi one?

Another modern example of "Christian Socialism" is "Liberation Theology."

[55] Crosses can represent alphabetical symbolism as a sans serif lowercase "t" letter for "terminate" and/or "terminated" or "tombstone." The Christian hand gesture known as the "sign of the cross" was spoofed as the "sign of the T" in Brave New World.

Some historians believe that crucifixion used an "X" letter shape for the wooden beams (St. Andrew's cross; also see the painting of Peter the Great, Peter der-Grosse 1838, by Paul Delaroche; also see the swastika crucifix illustration *infra*). That "X" now provides alphabetical symbolism for "exterminated" or crossed-out. It is used in the word "Xmas" as a substitute for "Christmas."

"Other than that Mrs. Lincoln, how was the play?"); or of John F. Kennedy (the 35th President. Killed by a Soviet socialist. "Other than that Mrs. Kennedy, how was the parade?"); or of James A. Garfield (the 20th President); or of William McKinley (the 25th President).[56]

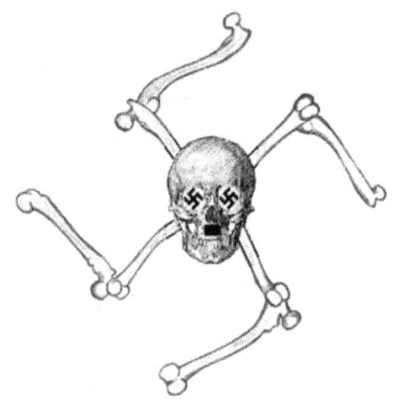

Hitler loved to wear a cross and he wanted others to wear a cross (on armbands) and he put a cross on his book, on his flag, and everywhere. It was the hooked cross. Old photographs and film footage show German socialists wearing crosses (e.g. hooked crosses on armbands) as they persecute Jews forced to wear the Star of David (Mogen David). Jews were also forced to wear the Davidian star on armbands.

---

[56] Believe it or don't: There are people who wear crucifixes alongside other small charms that resemble a .44-caliber "pocket cannon" Derringer; an Italian Carcano M91/38 bolt-action rifle; an 1881 British Bull Dog revolver; a .32 caliber Iver Johnson; a tiny noose, a tiny electric chair; a tiny hypodermic needle; and any other tool of execution of which they can think. They delight in telling inquisitive onlookers that they are big fans of Jesus, Lincoln, Kennedy, Garfield, McKinley and more.

Hitler's anti-Semitism was preceded by Tsar Lenin's and Tsar Stalin's.[57] Under Soviet socialism, all Jewish religious practices were banned, including circumcision.[58] Painting lamb's blood around the doors did not help. All practicing Jews had to exodus Soviet socialism (no one could leave unless permitted by the slave masters on the Soviet plantation).

The most egregious demonstration of Stalin's anti-Semitism (and Soviet socialism's guilt for the Holocaust) was his alliance with white supremacist socialism in Germany with the Molotov-Ribbentrop pact from 23 August 1939 to 22 June 1941 (about two years).

Soviet anti-Semitism spread to Cuba in 1959. All the smart Jews fled (only 5% of Cuba's Jews remained) and joined the ranks of survivors of socialism. Castro's socialists banned books by Anne Frank, Elie Wiesel, and others. In the late 1960's, a number of Jews were sent to forced labor camps for political dissenters, religious peoples, gays, and exit applicants; that highlighted the similarity to socialism under Hitler and Stalin.

Socialism's anti-Semitism continued in China where

---

[57] Is it historically inaccurate to refer to Lenin and Stalin as Tsars? Stalin once told his mother when she asked what he did for a living: "I am like a Tsar!" Even so, it is an insult to every Caesar, Kaiser, Czar and Tsar. Lenin and Stalin were more economically illiterate and plunged many more people into medieval serfdom, slavery and worse.

[58] "FREE" (Friends of Refugees of Eastern Europe) has helped Jews from Soviet socialism obtain circumcisions (also known as male genital mutilation. Because God said so ~3500 years ago).

Chinese socialism had similar anti-Semitic practices (and violence against all religious beliefs). China was historically anti-Semitic and it worsened under Mao's socialism, and remains a problem today. How many synagogues and Jews are there in China?

Mao followed the lead of Stalin and Hitler in banning all Jewish religious practices. It is fortunate that Mao had essentially no Jews to murder in China, for if he had then he might have exceeded the number of Jews slaughtered by Stalin and Hitler (in light of Mao's terrifying killing rates). China's long-standing xenophobia and general inhospitableness continued under Mao's socialism, and saved the lives of many ethnics and theists.

North Korea continues to impose similar anti-Semitic policies.

The Chinese Hitler (Mao) and his Nazi-Fasci-Socialists paid homage to German socialism's red armbands by donning their own red armbands and making them Chinoiserie, along with looney vocalizing on cue, goose-stepping, mass murder, and Mao's equally evil book of socialism (his Little-Read Book) that had few buyers (but for threats; and by not printing other books on the socialist presses; and by banning other books outright). As under Hitler, the armband was the way ass-kissers showed that they submitted to socialism. Mao's armband bore the characters for "Red Guard" in another ominous parallel to Hitler's SS protection guards. Mao's mandarins lifted his little book in Hitler's American salute, while donning Mao's Nazi-style red armband, and hailing Mao with cartoonish socialist slogans that showcase the madness of crowds.

Mao made mass-murder seem easy, breezy, and Chineasy. His baying Red Guard used violent "struggle meetings" to help Mao carry on Hitler's same struggle (Mein Kampf) for socialism. "Look Mao, no hands! ...and no teeth either!" They spread socialism's rape culture/hate culture. It was like "Lord of the Flies" only instead of a small island with two dozen boys where three died, it was an entire country full of adults and millions died.

Mao was assisted by German socialists, including Otto Braun, born in the Bavarian village of Ismaning, near Munich. Braun moved to China in 1934, to provide Chinese socialists with advice on military strategy. During his time in China, Braun adopted a Chinese name, Lǐ Dé ("from Germany").

Braun's life has many parallels to Hitler's. Similar to Hitler, Braun was drafted into the army in 1918 during the First World War (but WWI ended before Braun faced combat). Similar to Hitler, Braun's enthusiasm for socialism seemed to sprout after the war. He wanted to be a teacher, and studied in the Munich area, but never obtained a job. Instead, like Hitler, he began promoting socialism all over Germany as his lifelong vocation and career. In 1919, he participated in establishing the short-lived Bavarian Soviet Socialist Republic (See information elsewhere in this book that Hitler might have also been involved in this socialist uprising with Otto Braun).

It is unknown whether Otto Braun was related to (or knew of) Eva Braun, Hitler's long-time companion (and for ~40 hours they were Mr. & Mrs. Hitler). Eva, like Otto, was a supporter of socialism. She was also from Munich.

Braun, similar to his fellow-socialist Hitler, was arrested and charged with High Treason. As a consequence, Braun was detained by the police in July 1921. Unlike Hitler, he did not initially go to prison, but went into hiding. Nevertheless, similar to Hitler, he regularly wrote articles to promote socialism. He joined the Communist Party of Germany. He became deeply involved in his party's militia and para-military activities (another interest similar to Hitler's).

Hitler was released from prison (where he had written about his struggle for socialism) on 20 December 1924, after serving just over one year in prison.

The police caught up with Braun in September 1926. He first served his "Freyberg sentence" of 1922, then was kept in detention at the Moabit Prison. However, on April 11, 1928, a band of fellow socialists, including his then-lover Olga Benário (another socialist from Munich), staged his jail break. Hitler stuck around, took over, and imposed socialism in Germany; Braun fled Germany and helped impose socialism in China (and in the Union of Soviet Socialist Republics).

Braun first made his way to Moscow. While there, Braun went to the Frunze Military Academy.

Following his graduation from the military academy in 1932, Braun went to China to abet Mao and Chinese socialism. Mao supported the imperialism of Soviet socialism and wanted China to be part of it. In China, Braun was in military affairs under the orders of "General Kleber" (nom de guerre of Manfred Stern), who maintained a "military section" in Shanghai, and in political issues under Arthur Ewert, another fellow German socialist.

In the later part of 1933 Braun arrived in Ruijin, at that time capital of the "Chinese Soviet Socialist Republic," where he became a military adviser. Braun stayed in China until 1939, and then returned to the Union of Soviet Socialist Republics.

Back in the USSR, He worked at the Moscow Foreign Languages Press. He again assisted German socialism (and the socialist Joachim von Ribbentrop) by promoting public support for Adolf Hitler and Joseph

Stalin and the alliance between German socialism and Soviet socialism (which began in 1939). Braun probably knew Walter Ulbricht, another German socialist in the USSR at that time.

Later, Braun and Ulbricht helped German socialists and Soviet socialists work together again in the German Democratic Republic (East Germany). Braun worked under the Central Committee of the ruling Socialist Unity Party (SED). Ulbricht was the monster who put up the Berlin wall. They created socialism so good, people would climb up 15 feet and risk being shot to flee it.

Braun died at age 73 in 1974 and was buried in East Berlin. His obituaries appeared in Pravda and, of course, the New York Times (Pravda West). He had never returned to China to visit his dear friend Mao.

A BBC documentary is titled "Chairman Mao: The Last Emperor." China's "worst emperors" are often ranked in lists on the internet, but they never list nor mention Mao. His death tolls dwarf all the other emperors combined. Mao's dogma (including claiming ownership of everyone and everything, persecuting and killing the educated, burning books) has a long history in China and worldwide. Mao just tried to give it a newer name. He expanded China's history of feudalism to levels that should not have been possible. Mao was the worst emperor of all time.[59]

A quip about the naked emperor's new clothes would

---

[59] Mao was embarrassed that every "Chinatown" and "Little China" in the West was better than the original. They were true utopias compared to Mao's utopian lies. While millions staved in China, the USA's capitalism produced Chinese restaurants -owned and operated by Chinese- that satiated non-socialist bellies all over America.

be appropriate here but for brain pain conjured by the mental picture. Man boobs. Ayatollah Mao showed that under socialism, the higher you go, the bigger the fugly slob you get to be.

Loyalty dances had to be performed by puppets in honor of the pig. The ritual showed everyone's allegiance, similar to the USA's Pledge of Allegiance. Would the USA's pledge be improved as a loyalty dance? Yes prease!

The deadly stupidity of monster Mao's millions of minions is one reason why the term "Mongoloid" persisted for so long as a term (no longer in technical use; now considered offensive) for someone affected with Down's syndrome (and mental impairment). This is your brain on socialism...any questions? Mao retarded China. He had shit for brains. Kim Jong un picked up the semi-retarded mantle. They were not rocket surgeons. One can never overestimate the stupidity of socialists.[60] They are like candidates for an elementary school's class president who promise soda in all water fountains.

Moron Mao promoted do-it-yourself (DIY) home smelting of anything that contained iron. It was his unalloyed idiocy to industrialize (to be like the capitalist countries he so envied). The daft plan left Chinese ass-kissers without basic metal tools (their hammers and sickles and more), regressing them toward the Stone

---

[60] "Socialist" (similar to the label "voter") is considered an ableist slur because it refers to low IQ. The negative connotation is due in large part to SMH and their ilk. Voting is a suggestion box for slaves.

There are two types of people in the world: people who think their government is looking out for their best interest, and people who think.

Age (while "poor" people in capitalist countries lived better than medieval kings did). Mao's life makes the "Tulip Mania" myth seem trite. China approached ADZ (Absolute Dumb Zero), the point at which socialism cannot get any dumber. Mao couldn't think his way out of a paper bag.

Millions wanted to be Mao's dog. An early 1990s book by Liu Xiaobo contains pungent attacks on the character of Chinese socialists. Liu, the late Chinese individual rights activist, said he wanted to "…show just how wimpy, spineless, and fucked-up [weisuo, ruanruo, caodan] the Chinese really are." If the math is correct, socialism is fucked up squared. Liu could have said the same about Russians and Germans (especially those who lived under Stalin and Hitler), or anyone from government schools (socialist schools).

Marx said similar things about China and the Chinese. He labeled China a "living fossil" of stagnation and "unchanging." Although Mao killed four times as many people as did the socialist Hitler, the dead were Chinese people, so they don't count in the eyes of racist western socialists. Under Marx's and Engels' dogma, the Chinese were "racial trash" who needed to be extirpated in a "holocaust." Many socialists are Holocaust deniers in this regard. [LITERALLY SHAKING].

Liu was attacked by China's "Marxists" (they oppose freedom of speech), and he suffered multiple terms of imprisonment. China's violence topped the news in 2017 after Liu's death while he was under an 11-year sentence. He is said to have died of complications resulting from incorrect ideology. When Liu died, Chinese socialism joined German socialism (under Hitler) as the pair of socialist countries that had Nobel

Peace Prize laureates die in state custody.[61]

In a well-known statement of 1988, Liu said: "It took Hong Kong 100 years to become what it is. Given the size of China, certainly it would need 300 years of colonization for it to become like what Hong Kong is today. I even doubt whether 300 years would be enough."

Liu's sentiments are reinforced by Guo Wengui, an exiled Chinese property magnate who described Chinese socialism as organized crime: "They are just a tiny group of mafiosos, pure and simple." Guo describes China as "the most corrupt, tyrannical and brutal state on earth, bar North Korea." The word "socialism" is used to re-define felonies as a political philosophy. Guo vowed "to expose the leviathan Chinese mafia state."

Guo's comments are reinforced by China's President Xi Jinping who denounced widespread corruption within his country's socialist bureaucracy in 2017.[62] He praised

---

[61] The USA's President Obama is the first Nobel Peace Prize winner to bomb and kill other Nobel Peace Prize winners (Doctors Without Borders).

Before you diagnose yourself with depression or low self-esteem, first make sure you are not, in fact, just living amongst socialist. Socialism: If it isn't worth doing, it isn't worth doing well. It helps if you hate yourself.

[62] At the 19th party congress, 10/18/2017. Xi was dwarfed (as he often is) by a huge hammer-and-sickle on the wall. The symbol was culturally appropriated from defunct Soviet socialism. Perhaps it could have been worse if the hammer and sickle had instead been a fat picture of China's homicidal psychopath Mao. After 1917-2017, President Xi avoids celebrating a century of socialism persecuting and slaughtering rational people.

All attendees at the party congress could have gathered all their wealth together and then evenly divided it among

"socialism with Chinese characteristics" (national socialism or "Nazism") while endorsing the "socialist modernisation" (capitalism) that is improving China. Xi is going sane. Socialists are slow learners.

China took over Hong Kong in 1997; it is more accurate to say that Hong Kong is taking over China (long before 1997, thank goodness). China was retarded by the socialist colonialism of the former Soviet Union (and by its influence over Mao). Millions of serfs have been lifted out of Chinese socialism's poverty by Capitalism. Capitalism provided socialism with a better class of people. Socialism produces real problems, capitalism produces first-world problems.

Mao used the term "rightist" in the same way that Stalin did and in the same way that socialists use it today: to insult any fellow-socialist that they suddenly dislike. The difference is that when Mao or Stalin labeled a fellow socialist "rightist" it meant that they were about to imprison or murder the fellow. Socialists killed millions for being "politically incorrect."

Mao wasted his life (and millions of others) trying to change the laws of economics. He failed. Ideology collided with reality. Atlas crapped (on Mao's head). LMAO. The truth didn't give a f*ck about the opinions of Marx, Mao, Lenin, Stalin, Hitler and other socialists. Those who don't study history are doomed to repeat it; yet those who *do* study history are doomed to stand by helplessly while socialists repeat it. None of them were smart enough to know that they were dumb. The racketeers were what is now classified as "Felony Stupid" (as compared with the related IQ category of

---

themselves. That didn't happen. That has never happened at any meeting of any socialists anywhere ever.

"Misdemeanor Stupid." See the work of the criminologist Dr. Rex Curry). Their intelligence doesn't even register on any standard IQ scale. Mao was so stupid, he fell for their utopian oldspeak. His predecessors' failures only made Mao suffer socialism envy. Phuck Mao.

There is a sage old warning: "Don't make the mistake of believing your own propaganda." Mao repeated that error his entire life. For decades, Mao took Anarchyball right to his chin.

Socialists are the flat-earthers of economics. They wear rose-colored glasses (La vie en rose). It's a whiter shade of pale red.

Millions were conned, and still are. Many Chinese wished to beatifically tongue-bathe Mao's taint. Socialists have short memories. "The curious task of economics is to demonstrate to men how little they really know about what they imagine they can design," Friedrich Hayek warned.

Mao joined Lenin, Stalin, and Hitler to prove that the market doesn't corrupt morals – socialism does. Morality is scarcer than bread, under socialism. When you reject reason and truth, all that's left is violence.

Mao lived to the age of 82. Even in old age, people say he had the heart of a young boy. He kept it in a jar next to his bed.

One of the last to realize his own failure, Mao often repeated his vacuous slogans to anyone who would listen, mainly just himself.

After a lifetime suffering from dementia, Mao suffered two major heart attacks in 1976, one in March and another in July, before a third struck on September 5, rendering him an invalid. Perhaps Mao received the same socialist medical treatment that had been administered to his old dead pal Stalin; if so, then Mao was treated with leeches (although after 23 years, socialized medicine had probably developed better leeches). It was so apropos: Stalin and Mao were treated with comrades. There is no arguing that socialism produces the best leeches. Mao died nearly four days later (on September 9th), per government "news." The truth will never be certain because it was socialist China, home of the worst pathological liars, fake news, and alternative facts, of all time.

Earth rejoiced. [music swells] "Ding! Dong! The witch is dead!" It was a September to remember. It made the USA's bicentennial celebrations brighter. Global celebrations were bigger than what had followed the deaths of Stalin and Hitler; because it meant that the three worst socialists and murderers of all time were now "good socialists" (dead).[63] Savoir faire is everywhere!

Mao would lie in state for a week (he continued to lie even after his death), his body draped with a red flag bearing the hammer and sickle. Mao had predicted he'd live until year 2000 before going up "to see Marx in Heaven." He did not live even to the year 1984. His mEnTAl iLLnEsS (Socialism Derangement Syndrome) caused confusion about the direction he traveled to meet Marx. While he was invalid and death was imminent, an

---

[63] Satan personally congratulated each one (Stalin, Mao, & Hitler) for committing every sin possible.

There was festivity at the death of each socialist. A 1953 photograph shows a sign posted by the 1203 Restaurant in New York inviting customers to enjoy free borsht in celebration of Stalin's death.

A popular conspiracy theory asserts that Mao faked his own death and then went to live in Buenos Aires with Stalin and Hitler (who had also faked their own deaths).

attendant whispered in his ear, "When you get to Hell, tell them Murray Rothbard sent you."

Mao died in 1976 but his Hate Culture lived on. In 1979, the one-child policy was imposed when Chinese socialists seized the "means of reproduction." It was another official confession that socialism cannot provide enough goods and services (the Malthusian Theory only manifests itself under socialism).

"One-child" came after decades of retroactive adult abortions (as under Mao, Stalin, the Kim scum et cetera) had proven that socialism cannot provide, even when millions "with the greatest need" are violently liquidated. It exposes socialism's evil concept of "supply and demand": Socialism cannot supply, and therefore the "demand" must be reduced (millions of people must be murdered). That strategy does not make socialism "work" either, and the lack of supply (poverty) persists despite attempts to reduce demand via genocide. Socialism embodies the SNAFU principle: Situation Normal - All Fucked Up.

"One-child" was an extension of the same policy: socialism doesn't work and therefore millions must die pre-natal, post-natal, or in adulthood. China's one-child policy exterminated millions as fetuses and led to infanticide. It was another excuse for retroactive abortions, this time directed at newborns, almost exclusively females. They threw babies out with the bathwater.[64] Socialism promises womb-to-tomb care and

---

[64] Here, China's socialism was the opposite policy of Romanian socialism, where socialists used force in efforts to increase childbirths (see supra).

A common objection to anarcho-capitalism is: "Don't throw the baby out with the bathwater." But what critics don't realize is that it is Rosemary's baby. Spawn of Satan. Here is a

it's often a quick trip.

After Mao's death, his wife, Jiang Qing, was arrested, given a show trial, and sentenced to death, of course. It was for her part in China's "Cultural Devolution." Her sentence was commuted to life in prison. In May of 1991, the shrill socialist killed herself, distraught that she could no longer kill other people.[65] It

---

partial list of the birth dates of Rosemary's babies: **Lenin** 22 April 1870; **Stalin** 18 December 1878; **Hitler** 20 April 1889; **Mao** 26 December 1893; **Pol Pot** 19 May 1925. They and their governments needed to be retroactively aborted.

On the other hand, minarchists say that they don't want to abolish government entirely; they simply want to reduce it to the size where they can drag it into the bathroom and drown it in the tub.

Capitalists can go a day, a week, a year, a lifetime, and never think of socialism once. Hater socialists hate capitalism every moment.

[65] The psycho bitch's bitter suicide note included odd religious socialism, alerting (the late) Mao "...your student and fighter is coming to see you!" She provided no indication of the direction that she intended to travel. At her trial, she had used the Nuremberg defense, explaining that she was only following orders: "I was Mao's dog. When he said bite, I bit!" As a comparison: Stalin's wife committed suicide because she discovered that her husband was a homicidal psychopath. Mao's wife committed suicide because she discovered that SHE was a homicidal psychopath, just like her husband. Stalin, Mao, and Hitler made socialism the leading cause of unnatural deaths. Eva Braun attempted suicide twice in the 1930s (due to Hitler's inattention or refusal to wed?). Finally, Hitler married her and then in the afternoon Mrs. Hitler succeeded in committing suicide (the newlyweds died together) April 30, 1945 was the end of Mr. Socialism's wild ride. Hitler shot himself, proving that the only way to stop a bad guy with a gun is (1) a good guy with a gun or; (2) if the bad guy with a gun stops himself. This stuff writes itself. In 1943, Szmul Zygielbojm committed suicide

was the 25th anniversary of the Cultural Revolution, and Soviet socialism was disintegrating, and Chinese socialism was shrinking too.

Compared with Mao's Chinese socialism, German socialism was a third-rate killing machine. It was the Third Reich in the sense of a third socialist reich under the Princes of Darkness Stalin, Mao, and Hitler. Hitler was of tertiary importance and in third place behind the larger death tolls of Stalin and Mao.[66] That makes Mussolini the "Fourth Socialist Reich" in that gang of four?

Stalin joined in a pact with German socialism when Mussolini, the long-time socialist leader, was already in a pact with German socialism. The Vatican also had a pact (concordat) with Germany (from 1933). None of that bothered Stalin, so he joined the group. Italian socialism, Soviet socialism, and German socialism worked together beginning in 1939. They were building an international alliance of nationalists. ☺ Together they would beat globalism.

Soviet socialism was on the path to formally join the socialist Axis, and by its behavior had already done so. It was already the deadliest member when it joined. Together, Soviet socialism and German socialism maximized violence in the Axis. The Allies opposed German socialism while Soviet socialism was part of the

---

due to the world's indifference to the homicidal psychopaths under German socialism (He did not use the word "Nazi" in his suicide note). If there is such a thing as the transference or reincarnation of the soul, then Hitler's soul must have traveled into Mao, Stalin, or both.

[66] Every law should end with: "Or we will kill you." Stalin, Mao, and Hitler proved that. When explaining their dogma in speeches, socialists should end each paragraph that way.

Axis. The Allies (and not merely Stalin) defeated German socialism. Soviets exited the Axis late, after June 22, 1941. Stalin joined the allies involuntarily (because Hitler attacked him in Operation Barbarossa. Six months later, on December 7, 1941, Japan attacked the U.S. at Pearl Harbor, and on December 11, Germany and Italy declared war on the U.S.).

The ways that Soviet socialism aided its Axis work against the Allies included: Soviet socialism invaded Poland along with its German socialist buddies; Soviet socialism deported to Siberia about 1.5 million of the 13 million Poles in the eastern half of the country (the USSR acted as a role-model for German socialism). Soviet socialism's NKVD assisted German socialism's Gestapo when it exchanged intelligence and plans regarding Polish resistance groups; Soviet socialism also invaded Finland, Estonia, Lithuania, Latvia, Romania, et cetera; Soviet socialism helped German socialism resupply during the Allied Naval blockades; Soviet socialism demanded that socialist and communist groups in the UK and France adopt a pro-German anti-war line; Soviet socialism sold German socialism millions of tons of grain and steel at a 60 million RM (Reichsmark) deficit.

When Soviet socialism joined its fraudulent "Non-Aggression Pact" with German socialism, Stalin was already working with Chinese socialism and Mao Zedong. The Sino-Soviet Non-Aggression Pact was signed in Nanjing on August 21, 1937, between China and the Soviet Union during the Second Sino-Japanese War.

Stalin instructed Mao and the Chinese socialists to cooperate with Chairman Chiang Kai-shek and the Kuomintang (KMT).

In January 1935, Mao had been elected to a position of leadership, becoming Chairman of the Politburo of the Communist Party, and de facto leader of both the party and the Red Army, in part because his candidacy was supported by Soviet socialist Joseph Stalin. In Mao's mind, Stalin had established himself as the leader of "correct" socialist thought well before Mao imposed socialism in China; Mao never challenged the suitability of any of Stalin's socialism (at least while Stalin was alive, and even after Stalin's death in 1953). From 1958-1961, thirty million or more Chinese serfs starved during the Great Leap Forward, as Mao followed Stalin's model of collectivization.

Chinese socialism, Soviet socialism, German socialism and Italian socialism worked together in 1939. Stalin, Mao, Hitler, and Mussolini all acquired controlling interests in multi-national socialist conglomerates.

Stalin also had close relations with the socialist Kim Il-sung in North Korea.

There was also Sino-German cooperation, and it had existed from the 1920s. Contact between China and Germany persisted to 1941, with elements from both sides wishing to resume their cooperation.

In "Mein Kampf," Hitler refers to Christian Socialism glowingly: "To-day, as well as then, I hold Dr. Karl Lueger as the most eminent type of German Burgermeister. How many prejudices were thrown over through such a change in my attitude towards the Christian-Socialist Movement!" Lueger was active in Viennese politics from 1891 (and mayor from 1895-1910), when Christian Socialism had been heavily influenced by the Bellamy boys (from 1888).

In "Mein Kampf," Hitler self-identified as a socialist

throughout, and repeated (over 170 times?) the words "socialism" and "socialist" in a glowing manner. Hitler's speeches were similar.

Mein Kampf rarely mentions the political concepts of "left" (5 times?) and "right" (1 time?).

Hitler did not create the phrase "Third Reich," and never used the term in his notorious book. It did not appear on coins, stamps, medals, badges et cetera under Hitler.

Hitler DID use the word "Reich" (in reference to Germany's government) many times (over 190 times?). "Reich" was commonplace in Germany before Hitler. Hitler would have used the phrase "Third Reich" often if his goal was to replace the old "Reich" that he mentioned over 190 times in his book.

Hitler eschewed the phrase "Third Reich" and he banned the use of it. During the summer of 1939, the press was directed to use the terms "Nationalsozialistisches Deutschland" (National Socialist Germany), "Großdeutsches Reich" (Greater German Reich), or simply "Deutsches Reich" (German Reich) to refer to the German socialist state in place of "Drittes Reich" (Third Reich) (Schmitz-Berning, Cornelia (2000). Vokabular des Nationalsozialismus. Walter de Gruyter GmbH & Co. KG, 10875 Berlin, pp. 159-160. (in German)). The people who would proofread the press under Hitler's socialism were literal grammar Nazis.

The phrase "Third Reich" was coined by Arthur Moeller van den Bruck (1876-1925), author of a book with the phrase for its title: "Das Dritte Reich" (The Third Reich). The book was published in 1923, giving Hitler years to consciously decide not to use "Third Reich" in Hitler's 1925-26 book "Mein Kampf."

Moeller did not support Hitler nor Hitler's socialism (Moeller died in 1925, before voters from government schools -socialist schools- elected Hitler into government).

It is interesting to note that the "Third Republic" in France ended with the fall of France to German socialism in 1940.[67]

The USA might be in its "Third Reich" stage, following its Second Reich (the period during the War for Southern Independence), and thereafter under the dictates of American National Socialists, including Francis Bellamy (and his cousin Edward Bellamy), a dogma that continues to haunt everyone today.

Dr. Curry was the first to point out that Wikipedia (and other so-called sources, including all the news outlets that you pay attention to) cites no credible example of Hitler ever using the term "Third Reich" or "Nazi" or "Fascist" as a self-identifier in German or in any language, and that there are no citations to show Hitler employed those terms as common bywords. And yet Wakipedia (and every news outlet) deceives users into believing that Hitler over-used the term "Third Reich" and "Nazism" and "Fascism" as a self-identifier for his dogma. The nuts who write for Wakipedia (and its ilk) are the people who over-use those terms. They over-use those terms to hide the word that Hitler DID yackety-yak about: SOCIALISM.

Dr. Curry's expertise is supported by the German socialist Albert Speer's memoirs that bear the misleading title "Inside the Third Reich" (titles are often not the product of the writer. Speer's memoirs were

---

[67] The French Third Republic also bore a fasces symbol prominently in the center of its emblem.

published in 1969). Speer's book contains no mention of Hitler ever using the title phrase, nor babbling it as a hackneyed buzzword.

A popular claim by socialist liars is that Hitler used the word "socialism" to trick people (because socialists are so stupid?) into supporting him. Those liars trick people into believing that Hitler used other self-descriptions: Nazi, Fascist, Third Reich.

The introduction to Speer's memoirs (by Eugene Davidson) states "Speer's father did read the liberal Frankfurter Zeitung, an unusual paper for a conservative architect to have in his home, but he utterly rejected the Nazis because he believed them to be more socialist than nationalist." Speer did not hide the fact that Hitler and his party used the terms "socialism" and "socialist"; there are at least 59 instances in Speer's book.

The socialist Dark Ages included the modern inquisitions in socialism's witch hunts for much of the world: millions were tortured, interrogated and persecuted as "heretics" against socialist terrorism. Family members would denounce each other in show trials during the Endarkenment. It was much worse than the earlier inquisitions (~40,000 to ~50,000 died in the old inquisitions? Thousands of times more people suffered and died in the modern socialist inquisitions: much more than ~40 million to ~50 million). Nobody expects the socialist inquisitions; they make the old inquisitions seem historically unimportant. Socialists promised heaven on earth but provided hell for everyone not part of the ruling class.

The socialist Dark Ages continue in some parts of the world, including North Korea. Satellite photographs taken at night of the Potemkin village of Pyongyang and the surrounding area show that North Korea remains in the literal socialist Dark Ages. Why is this night different from all other nights? Because they don't have lights. Please send help. They are also known as the socialist Dork Ages in the case of the Norks -North Koreans. Nork is known as "Black Earth" and the "Dark Incontinent." The benighted Terra Noir is ruled by the bête noire. What Kim Jong-un is doing, and what the Norks think he is doing, are as different as night and day. North Korea is known as "the empire on which the sun never rises." He turned himself and his penal colony to the dark side of never-ending dorkness. Space aliens can see the disaster of socialism just as satellites do.[68] It is the Black Hole of socialism, and the Event Horizon continues to approach. Time keeps on slipping, slipping, slipping, into the future.

The socialist Wholecaust (of which the Holocaust was a part) continued in North Korea, where an estimated three million starved to death in the 1990s. Time Magazine reported on March 29, 2016, that the socialist government warned the population that another famine is imminent in North Korea, where the mincing cartoon character Kim Jong-un overcame anorexia long ago and is now known as "the only fat kid in the country."[69]

---

[68] Space aliens have refused to contact earth after monitoring socialism spread by Stalin, Mao, Hitler etc. There's a starman waiting in the sky, he'd like to come and meet us, but he doesn't want to be enslaved or starved. The third rock from the sun remains classified as "no intelligent life" and Earthlings are "insufficiently developed and sociopathically violent." Also, too much of the planet (and earth's solar system) remains undeveloped.

[69] "Kim Fatty the Third" or "Jin San Pang" in Chinese. It is always tough being the fat kid in school. It must be extra tough being the ONLY fat kid in your ENTIRE country. He's

The socialist genocide caused famines in Cambodia from 1975 to 1979 with 500,000 to 2 million deaths, representing ten to twenty percent of the country's total population, making it one of the deadliest famines in modern history (by percentage of the population of the country).

The socialist Wholecaust occurred under Chinese socialism in the late 1950s and early 1960s, when over thirty million perished under Chairman Mao Zedong's "Great Leap Forward" into famine. Rice, Rice, everywhere, nor a grain to eat.[70]

Today, in the United States, Bellamy's daily lobotomy continues as a never-ending socialist inquisition in government (socialist) schools. From its origin in 1892, the quotidian pledge shaming remains the first bullying that begins each school morning for small children up through high school graduation. It produces dark sarcasm in the classroom. Hey teachers leave those kids alone!

In the past, the mantra inspired beatings, arrests, school expulsions, and lynchings. E. V. Starr was

---

got more chins than a Chinese phone book.

He is also known as "the 40-year-old virgin" (but not in the butt; what Kim refers to as his mangina) and the nation's "dick-taker." The snowflake's father was also that way (while simultaneously persecuting gays) and boasted that during his first experience he had "eleven holes-in-one" and they were accompanied by a "double rainbow." (for more detailed information see Australian reporter Eric Ellis, who worked as the Europe correspondent for The Global Mail).

Most graduates of government schools (socialist schools) in the USA cannot point out North Korea on a map.

[70] Wakipedia's (Wikipedia's) article on "famine" covers up for socialism as the cause of the most massive starvation in history. Intelligent readers can see through Wakipedia's deceit and read the famine page as a refutation of socialism.

sentenced by a Kansas state judge in 1918 to twenty years of hard labor for abusive language toward (and for refusing to kiss) the US flag.[71] Later, a federal judge felt powerless to reverse the state court's sentence even though the US judge believed that Starr was "more sinned against than sinning." The mob that instigated Starr's persecution, he wrote in his opinion, had descended into the kind of "fanaticism" that fueled the "tortures of the Inquisition."

Starr's persecution was not unique to his times. That type of violence and worse occurred two decades later, before and after Minersville School District v. Gobitis, 310 U.S. 586 (1940), when the U.S. Supreme Court and other courts ruled against Jehovah's Witnesses in litigation against the American Nazi salute and its repetitious chant. What a culture!

Most modern parents gleefully shove their children into the state meat grinder (schools). Some happily beat their own offspring if the kids disrespect the flag, the pledge, or any government mandate.

President Donald Trump said, "Nobody should be allowed to burn the American flag - if they do, there must be consequences - perhaps loss of citizenship or year in jail!" (11/29/2016). It proves that presidents are easily brainwashed too. His opponent in the election (Hitlery Clinton) had gone farther in 2005 and actually co-sponsored federal legislation (the Flag Protection Act) to criminalize flag burning with a year in jail or $100,000 fine. Is it the most infantile argument for government? Trump and Hillary would probably prefer

---

[71] Imagine being Starr's lawyer at the sentencing hearing and having Starr apologize to the flag (and having Starr kiss the flag repeatedly), in an effort to apologize and "make up" with the flag and gain leniency from the sentencing judge.

the earlier stiff-armed gesture (and revive it?), if they knew anything about the socialist pledge.[72]

According to the Bellamy cousins, Jesus was a socialist and Christianity is socialism. In that way, Jesus was doubly blessed. Under that dogma, socialism (via the old Crusades from the 11th-16th centuries) initiated the socialist bloodbath long before it was exceeded in the later socialist Wholecaust (the modern socialist Crusades, of which the Holocaust was a part).

Another example of "Christian Socialism" would have been the Anabaptists in the 16th century.

Francis Bellamy's interpretation of Christianity can be compared to "Christian atheism" - rejecting belief in the God of Christianity, but embracing the supposed teachings of "Jesus the socialist." In a similar vein, a person is a Marxist for following Marx's ideas while not thinking Marx was a god. With that logic, the archsocialists Stalin, Mao, and Hitler would have been "Christians," if they believed that Christ was a socialist who wanted everyone to spread socialism. Every monster believes that, if there are gods, then the gods share his ideology.

"Christian socialism" and "regular socialism" are the same except for one meaningless difference. Of all the multitude of lies under socialism, "Christian socialism" piles on only one more falsehood: the single lie that socialism is endorsed by an imaginary supernatural being.

All religions (including Christian Socialism) are correct about only one thing: that all the other religions

---

[72] It is another commonality that Trump and Clinton share with Chinese socialists. China's law provides three years in prison for disrespecting its national anthem (Nov. 2017). Socialism jails liberty.

(past and present) and McGods are rubbish. That is why every theist is in fact almost exclusively an atheist. He/she rejects belief in all religions (except his own). The religious are polyatheists. Each theist should judge his/her own religion with the same criteria by which they reject all other religions.[73]

Theists often marry within their delusion in order to avoid conflicts with a spouse's delusion.

Theists are de facto atheists in the way in which they live their lives by relying on reason and science, and by rejecting stale superstitions from their old books authored by barbaric primitives. They show that they know that God and prayer will not mend compound fractures, nor reverse deaths.

Due to the fact that God does not exist, each believer is his/her own God. That is why each believer's "God" reflects exactly that individual believer's own thoughts. He/she is his/her own "God."

Problems arise when a theist wants his/her God forced on everyone else. It is another way of saying that the theist wants to impose his views on everyone else. The God imagined by a socialist is a God who supports socialism. It is another way of saying that theistic socialists want to impose socialism on everyone else.

Socialism is the method by which anyone (theist or non-theist) forces everyone to endure his/her weltanschauung (socialized medicine, schools, pledges, media, food, art, clothing, wages, social security, drugs,

---

[73] Early Christians were considered atheists by Romans because they didn't pay tribute (or perform animal sacrifices and other forms of taxation) to the gods of Rome.

Muslims do not believe that Jesus was divine (that is almost the only thing about which Muslims are correct). They revere Jesus as a "great prophet."

prices, housing, et cetera).

The Bellamy cousins believed that they promoted divine government as foretold by Jesus the socialist. Through Christian socialism, Bellamy touted an omnipotent/omniscient entity (government or God) ruling over everyone. Most people happily repeat 2000-year-old religious lies just as gleefully as they chant a modern Pledge of Allegiance. They share a belief in a supreme power that rules beneficently over all of humanity. That is the essence of both socialism and religion.

The questions must be asked: How do you separate church and state when the state is your church? Are you really an atheist if you worship the state?

Socialists are faith-healers fleecing the gullible crowds. Miracles are promised for the worship of God-Gov via the pledge: magically "free gifts" from Gov (healthcare, schools, sports stadia,[74] and more); fiat paper money printed at will; endless socialist debt to pay for it all. Government is a pyramid scheme. That is the revelation of Edward Bellamy's utopia.

Christianity and religion are often maligned for the number of deaths they caused. Socialists are often maligned for the number of deaths they caused. Theists and socialists both do a lot of preying. However vast those death tolls are, they are combined into one number under the Bellamy dogma.[75]

According to Bellamy, Christianity was socialism. Jesus was a socialist touting the same dogma as the socialist bobbing heads Stalin, Mao, and Hitler (SMH)

---

[74] In sports news today, I continue to not follow sports.
[75] And that number far exceeds the 900 deaths in Rev. Jim Jones' self-proclaimed socialist utopia of Jonestown in Guyana.

in their mortacracies. SMH's body piles were inspired by the same dogma touted by Jesus and Christianity: Socialism.

Many famous atheists are socialists. Before large audiences, they excel at recounting religious horrors; they fail at recounting the horrors of socialism. They make no comparisons between religion and socialism. They cite absurdities by chapter and verse in religious books, and they are silent on similar absurdities of socialist books, and Stalin, Mao, Hitler (SMH), Marx, Pol Pot, Kim Jong-un, et cetera.

The inconsistencies of atheist/secular/socialists (ASS) were rhapsodized by ex-Beatle John Lennon, and specifically in his song "Imagine." His ASS anthem derides religion while propagandizing socialism (Lennonism?) in a way that would have impressed Lenin. "Imagine no possessions," sang the millionaire who abused women and neglected his child. WTF seriously? Back in the USSR, Lennon did not know how unlucky they were (especially those Ukraine girls. Their possessions were stolen).

The late Christopher Hitchens embodied the classic omissions of ASS. Hitchens was a long-time socialist, Marxist, and Trotskyist. Hitchens condemned "heaven" as a "celestial dictatorship similar to North Korea,"[76] but he would not identify the country by the word that Norks use to describe their Korean homeland: socialist. That was one of Hitchens' embarrassing cover-ups for

---

[76] Compare The Handmaid's Tale by Margaret Atwood: In a dystopian future in the USA, some women are forced to live under a fundamentalist theocratic dictatorship. Reviewers in the old media rarely compare the Handmaid dystopia to actual conditions in fanatical Muslim countries, nor to nuns in convents.

socialism while rightfully bashing theism.

Hitchens used "fascistic" as an insult, but never used "socialistic" as an insult.

Hitchens greeted his audiences as "Comrades" (whether he pronounced a "C" or a "K" as the initial letter was unclear. It showed his missionary need for comrades to join his socialist kampf).[77] He fancied himself clever to sound like the Godhead incarnate Stalin, Mao, Hitler and their evangelical ilk.[78]

Socialism and religion (including Islam, a top target for Hitchens) preach the same trope: "Universal Brotherhood." A world of comrades. Religion and socialism both employ the fictive kin "brothers" and "sisters." It's funny how quickly they switch from "Let's treat each other as siblings" to "Do as I say or else."

Comrades are reminders of a cartoon in Charlie Hebdo magazine that stated: "It is hard being loved by morons." So much of modern politics is the stupidest people on earth yelling at each other. It is funny to hear a statist calling a religious person "brainwashed" (and vice versa).

Hitchens denounced Mother Teresa as a woman who loved poverty but who did not love the poor.[79] Many of

---

[77] The economist Thomas Sowell said: "Socialism in general has a record of failure so blatant that only an intellectual could ignore or evade it."

[78] Compare these twitter quotes from socialist Richard Spencer, the alleged creator of the alt-right: "Let's just give people a single-payer healthcare system and stop having this stupid debate." And: "Look, Marx was kinda right. Bourgeoisie capitalism (and not the Soviet Union) created an undiferentiated, [sic] alienated proletarian mass." And: "Internet providers operate a public utility, which relies on government infrastructure, like water and gas. They should be regulated as such." He really is a socialist.

his criticisms apply better to socialism and to the socialists Stalin and Mao, and the poverty, alienation, dependence, hunger, and starvation that their policies caused. They love the poor so much that they make more of them. Socialists prove that "Hell is other people."[80]

Hitchens never discussed the Socialist Inquisitions, their modern Dark Ages, their witch hunts, bonfires of the vanities, medieval persecution of heretics, forced conversions, and socialism's primeval barbarism. Pay your fair share of extortion (taxes) honestly for a faster ride back to the year 700 A.D.! In his lifetime of scorn for religion, Hitchens failed to make enumerable obvious comparisons to SMH. He let his fans down.

Most (all?) atheistic socialists evade in the same way that Hitchens (and Lennon) did. Just imagine if I pulled a you on you: "Excuse me sir, do you have a moment to talk about Our Lord and Savior the government? I'm a socialist so I don't believe in god. I do believe in an all-powerful, all-benevolent state that has a wonderful plan for my life!" May the market have mercy on their souls.

---

[79] Hitchens' books, speeches, and 1995 essay succeeded in converting Mother Teresa. Two years later she was assassinated to prevent her impending public announcement that she had finally "seen the light" and was leaving the church as an atheist.

[80] Many fans of films depicting dystopias discovered that they were living in one under Stalin, Mao, and Hitler. That experience remains available in North Korea. Also check out fundamentalist Muslim countries (including the USA's "pal" Saudi Arabia) where atheists are proudly murdered for their thought crimes. Gays are killed too. The Saudi flag reads: "There is no god but God, and Muhammad is the messenger of God." The Isis flag reads: "There is no god but God," and the white seal reads "God Messenger Mohammed."

Gullibility about Yahweh, Allah, Christ et al equates with gullibility about Stalin, Mao, Hitler, and other canonized socialist overlords. One difference between God and SMH -and it is a grievous difference- is that SMH actually existed (they actually were involved in ruining lives). Atheistic socialists owe God an apology. In religion, the people crucify their savior; In socialism, the savior crucifies his people!

SMH started the "No Lives Matter" movement. Here is a prayer for all who died under SMH, Kim, and their ilk: May God treat you better than the socialists did.

God doesn't exist. That means ALL religion is similar to socialism in that the institution is the "God" as it tells you how to live your life. Welcome to Hell.

People have sympathy for the devils (SMH): Socialist theologians concoct new "rights." Government schools are a sacred rite. The pledge is a sacred rite. The welfare state is a sacred rite. Health care (or is it just health insurance?)[81] is a sacred rite. "The National Health Service is the closest thing the English have to a religion," Margaret Thatcher's Chancellor Nigel Lawson famously once observed. Socialism is a disease masquerading as its own cure. Real eyes realize real lies.

The well-known atheist Sam Harris comes a tad closer to the topic with this quote: "People of faith often claim that the crimes of Hitler, Stalin, Mao, and Pol Pot were the inevitable product of unbelief. The problem

---

[81] Neither Jesus nor any religion gave sight to the blind now or in history. Capitalism's technology through doctors gives sight to the blind. Senator Rand Paul (an ophthalmologist) has given sight to the blind for free. You can't say "our bodies, ourselves" nor "my body, my choice" if you believe women should be fined (and ultimately jailed, and killed) for not buying insurance.

with fascism and communism, however, is not that they are too critical of religion; the problem is that they are too much like religions." Thus, Harris fell for the old "fascism and communism" trick (or he adopted the trick deliberately). He side-stepped "socialism" that they ALL glorified (Hitler, Stalin, Mao, and Pol Pot). Does Harris know that Hitler did not self-identify with, nor blather with, the word "fascism"?

Another Harris quote: "Consider the millions of people who were killed by Stalin and Mao: although these tyrants paid lip service to rationality, communism was little more than a political religion." Harris did not rebuff the lip service that Stalin and Mao (and Hitler) paid to socialism. That reveals more about Harris than it does about the fabulists SMH.

Harris, author of "The End of Faith," could write a sequel entitled "The End of Faith in Government and Socialism" (but he won't). His sequel could literally make most of the same arguments. He could debunk Hitler's first propaganda film titled "The Victory of Faith" about Germany's socialist dogma.[82]

---

[82] Der Sieg des Glaubens (1933) directed by Leni Riefenstahl. Her film recounts the Fifth Party Rally of the National Socialist Party, which occurred in Nuremberg from 30 August to 3 September 1933. In the film (and in Riefenstahl's other film "Triumph of the Will"), German socialists compete to out-do similar disgusting self-congratulatory propaganda that Soviet socialists had been committing since 1917.

It is interesting how "Leni" sounds like "Lenin" shortened. It appears to be short for "Helene" in Helene Bertha Amalie Riefenstahl.

In "Brave New World" a character is named "Lenina Disney" and many other character names are references to failed socialists and successful businessmen/inventors.

Harris asks why the Holocaust did not cause all Jews to conclude that there is no God. Readers should ask why the Holocaust did not cause all Jews (and everyone) to conclude that socialism is evil and must end. Hitler, Stalin, Mao and all the other socialists who murdered millions should cause everyone to conclude that socialism is violence and must cease. SMH were Godfathers in the mafia sense (multiplied by 200 million).

Everyone who reads Harris' book (or who listens to his audio on youtube and his podcasts) should replace (mentally or with a big red pen) the word "God" with the words "Gov" (government) and "socialism."[83] Then send it to Harris to help him with his next book. That intellectual exercise should be performed whenever anyone reads or hears any atheist-secular-socialist explaining why "God" is claptrap.

Harris chides religious moderates for enabling violent religious extremists. Harris's next book should argue that moderate socialists enable violent socialists, as was the case with the robber barons Stalin, Mao, and Hitler.

Before political parties existed, religions were political parties and states (and this remains so today in some of the world).[84] Ancient Rome, so admired by modern government and by the socialists Hitler and Mussolini, was an example of what Harris calls

---

[83] Hitchens could have written "Gov Is Not Great" as a sequel to his book "God Is Not Great." Also see "Democracy: The God That Failed" by Hans-Hermann Hoppe. Elected officials believe that they are mind-readers for millions. They are telepathetic.

[84] The Chancellor of Germany, Angela Merkel, is the leader of the Christian Democratic Union of Germany (Christlich Demokratische Union Deutschlands). Many Muslim countries have much worse examples of this problem.

"political religion."[85] Stalin, Mao, Hitler, Mussolini, and other socialists turned their countries into modern coliseums with death matches.

The "political religion" Harris bashes is exemplified in the flag pledge (by the American Christian socialist preacher Francis Bellamy) in socialist schools in the USA. Flags and Bibles are both carried as security blankets by socialists and religionists. Harris, Hitchens, and other Atheist-secular-socialists (ASS) never talked about that.

Most ASS admire the pledge catechism except for only two words. They believe that if 1954's "under God" were redacted from the daily Gregorian chant on cue in government schools, then that would magically transform the pledge utterly from a "political religion." Can anyone dream up a better test (besides this real-life razor-sharp pledge test) that reveals the doublethink of most ASS?

ASS know next-to-nothing about the pledge's putrid past. Similar to theistic-socialists, they repeat glowing crapaganda about Bellamy the socialist, and they never mention the origin of the Nazi salute and Nazi behavior.

ASS support both the pledge and the government schools where pledging occurs. Stalin, Mao, Hitler also supported government schools. ASS want G-schools to root out religion from students by re-educating them. It

---

[85] Rome's political religion included animal sacrifices. The old media pretend it was a mysterious ritual (they imply that sacrificed animals were left to rot, or cremated entirely at each occasion); the old media cover up the fact that it was taxation in the form of meat for barbecues to pay Rome's officials and priests via the feasts. People who refused to pay the tax were arrested, persecuted, and killed if they resisted (similar to tax resisters today).

is another goal shared by Stalin, Mao, Kim Jong-un, Pol Pot and their ilk.

Each ASS wants to play God (or dictator) over the schools in order to micromanage how religion will be exterminated. They naively imagine that government policy will precisely reflect their desires at some point in the near future, and that it will then always remain so for eternity.

In their books and speeches, the ASS applaud government schools in one breath and then in the next breath disparage schools for not yet eradicating religion. They are unaware of their cognitive dissonance.

ASS forget that most theists also support the socialist schools. Education is another socialist war in which ASS fight theistic socialists (and all theists) for control of government schools. All of them battle to dictate how schools will brainwash children.

It can happen here. When socialism comes to America, it will be wrapped in the flag and carrying a cross.[86]

The ASS imagine that they will prevail, but history is against the ASS in the US. Bellamy and his comrades wanted government to take over all schools to promote Christian Socialism. Bellamy's socialism resulted in Bible reading, prayers, hymns, religious indoctrination, and crosses in G-schools (as well as segregation imposed by law, and racism taught as official policy, along with Nazi salutes and Nazi behavior). Students

---

[86] Also cf. – "When fascism comes to America, it will come under the guise of anti-fascism." – this quote has been attributed to Huey Long, or Franklin Delano Roosevelt, or, better yet, Woodrow Wilson. lol.

were probably taught the Christian "sign of the cross" to crucifixes hanging in government schools as well as the "Nazi salute to the flag." More recently, in 1954, the pledge was deified and remains so. Those are history lessons that are not taught today in government schools, and they never will be taught there.

It did happen here. When socialism came to America, it was wrapped in the flag and carrying a cross. It hasn't departed.

Imagine what it is like to live in a tiny town where everyone goes to church and, if you don't go too, then everyone dislikes you and you have no local social life. Now compare your life under Stalin, Mao, Hitler, Fidel Castro, Pol Pot, Kim Jung-un, et cetera, if you do not join in to praise socialism.

If atheistic-secular-socialists succeed in the US then they will perpetuate a system of education that began as a method of socialist indoctrination and that already resembles the governmental process used under Stalin, Mao, the Kim gang, Pol Pot, and others.

"Give me the child for seven years, and I'll give you the man," is an alleged Jesuit quote. It explains why theists and socialists both support government's monopoly schools and have a history of banning all the better alternatives. In the USA, socialism's brainwashing is so inefficient that twelve years are stolen, instead of seven.

The following is an excerpt from a catholic catechism, and appears to have been plagiarized by Mao in his Little Red Book, and by Kim Jong-un (and his predecessors with their holier-than-Mao attitudes), and their ilk.[87] Change "God" to "Gov":

Q. Why did God make you?
A. God made me to know Him, to love Him, and to serve Him in this world, and to be happy with Him for ever in heaven.

Q. What must we do to save our souls?
A. To save our souls, we must worship God by faith, hope, and charity; that is, we must believe in Him, hope in Him, and love Him with all our heart.

Anyone who disobeys God/Gov is a sinner who must repent through confession or face damnation:

Penitent: **"Forgive me, oh great State, for I have sinned. I drank raw milk."**
High Priest: **"Take heed my child; say two 'Our Roads,' one 'Hail Flag,' and bomb a brown kid, then thy sins will be absolved."**

A top socialist catechism is: **"from each according to his ability, to each according to his need."** That maxim is often translated from the original German as "Slavery and theft are OK!"

---

[87] Pope Francis agrees with the socialists Stalin, Mao, Hitler, and the Kim gang, as he indicated in his assertion that capitalism is "Terrorism against all humanity." (~8-2-2016).

Mao's little red book is filled with exhortations to self-sacrifice.

Hey, here's an idea: let's task the worst possible people on the planet with telling the rest of us how to live!

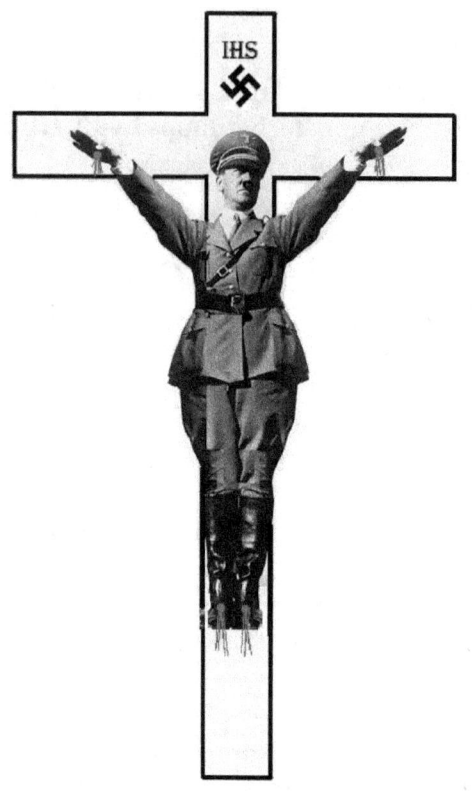

For Hitler so loved the world, that he gave his only begotten self, that whosoever believeth with him in socialism should not perish, but have everlasting life (by pretending that Hitler self-identified as a "Nazi" or "Fascist"). It is through Hitler that all sins of socialism are absolved. His so-called "opponents" refuse to tell his side of the story and they abuse his legend. The black sheep of socialism is portrayed as a political transvestite. He was nailed to the plank of the political movement he championed. He gave himself as the sacrificial scapegoat for Stalin, Mao and all socialists who blame "Hitler, Nazism, Fascism" and thereby glorify the Holy Word that Hitler verily preached with them: Socialism. Hitler: He takes the blame so that you don't have to.

Hitler's last words: "My socialists, my socialists, why hast thou forsaken me?"

If Christ was in fact a socialist, and if his second coming had occurred under Stalin, Mao, or Hitler, then he would have been murdered again by his own people (his fellow socialists). The supreme socialist would have been given a "fair" trial and then executed for obstructing socialism. All of his friends would have implicated him in his trumped up anti-socialist conspiracy. He would have confessed publicly on camera after torture.

Atheistic socialists make God cry when they attack Islam too. Yet "Islam" and "socialism" both mean the same thing: "submission" (etymologically related to these words: submissives, subs). Muslims "pray" by dropping to their knees, bending over with their heads on the floor and their behinds in the air. God has fucked them in the ass so many times. Fans of such dogmas enjoy being submissive and enjoy domination (etymologically related to these words: dominator, dominatrix, dom). They are kinky.

Socialism and religion are also entomologically related to these words: leeches, fleas, ticks, lice, mosquitos, and other parasites. As socialism grows it becomes parasitoidal.

Atheistic socialists do not reprove the socialism of Islam (e.g. Sharia law and how its anti-capitalism has retarded Muslim economies). Both dogmas use a "pledge of allegiance" as part of submission to the bureaucracy of God and/or Gov.

Islam and socialism are often combined outright as in

the Ba'ath Party (which included Iraq's Saddam Hussein). Radical Islamic terrorists probably learned a lot about bombs and terrorism from socialists (e.g. Chicago's Haymarket Square Riot in 1886 which the author Timothy Messer-Kruse researched; Marinus van der Lubbe, who proudly confessed to starting the Reichstag fire in 1933; James T. Hodgkinson in 2017; the Unabomber Ted Kaczynski; Marx; Lenin; Stalin; Mao; Hitler). Their cry: "Socialism Akbar!"

God is not great, as Hitch said. And socialism is not great either.

Harris, Hitchens, Lennon et al would do better to explain that religion IS socialism.[88] The deadliest religion is not Islam; it's not Christians or non-believers. Statism is the world's deadliest religion. Stop the theocracy.

Stalin, Mao, and Hitler are socialism's Holy Trinity with their cross symbols (the hakenkreuz and the hammer and sickle which, similar to the Christian cross, resulted in so many deaths/executions/martyrs). It is dangerous to make a socialist cross.

The Diagnostic and Statistical Manual (DSM) for diagnosing mEnTAl diSOrdErs contains a religious exemption under the diagnosis of delusions (many atheists want to eliminate that exemption). Does the DSM diagnose the iNsaNity of Stalin, Mao, Hitler, Kim Jong-un and other socialists? The God delusion is similar to the socialism delusion. Just wait until the new DSM comes out.

Under socialism men go mad, and when they see

---

[88] For more on that see "The Socialist Phenomenon" by Igor Shafarevich. "Socialism, like the ancient ideas from which it springs, confuses the distinction between government and society." - Frederic Bastiat

someone who is not mad, they attack him saying: "You are mad; you are not like us!"

Religion and socialism preach the same: altruism, sacrifice (i.e. self-sacrifice), everyone unified as comrades under one dogma. The Quran, the Bible, and Marx's books spark the same adjectives: obtuse, hokey. B-O-R-I-N-G! The world has a horrible history of stupid people believing stupid books written by stupid people.

Lying is a prerequisite for a "non-believer" to stay alive in both fundamentalist Muslim nations and in fundamentalist socialist nations. Under socialist mouthpieces Stalin, Mao, and Hitler (SMH), dissenters could not question the statist quo. Rational comments trigger socialist snowflakes. SMH caused much of humanity to spend their lives telling lies gleefully. SMH are why most people spend their lives telling lies today.

Socialism is not a peaceful religion. SMH make the Bible's genocides and ethnic cleansing seem minor in comparison. Now that SMH have reunited again in a warmer place, everyone should feel sad for Satan. R.I.H.

Galileo Galilei told the truth about heliocentrism and was attacked by the Roman Catholic Inquisition in 1633 for disagreeing with the Bible, and he died in indefinite imprisonment. Under old inquisitions everyone was forced to convert to Catholicism; under modern inquisitions people were forced to convert to socialism (or to pretend so).

In socialist inquisitions, the innocent were imprisoned and killed for telling the truth about the dogma and for disagreeing with socialist Bibles and doctrines (such as the books of Karl Marx). Socialists established that there is no "freedom of speech" for socialists. They have the secular equivalent of blasphemy laws.

A headline in Newsweek declared: "Christians in China must replace Jesus with pictures of Xi Jinping or lose social services" (by Cristina Maza on 11/14/17). Mao, Stalin, and Hitler and other socialists played God and millions died. Billions of lives were ruined.

SMH and socialist hate groups prove that socialism's arguments haven't improved much since "Heretic! Burn them!" Remember St. Marx and his commandment in chapter 5, verse 13: "Thou shalt not suffer a witch to live." Woe be unto he who loses faith in socialism.

These are some of the statertot Commandments: (1) The state is the LORD thy God; (2) Remember your Lord's school days and honor them all; (3) You shall pledge allegiance to the flag.

Statists gonna state.

The following questions are dangerous for non-believers in many countries: What do you think about God? What is your opinion of Marx (peace be upon him) and his books?[89] What is your opinion of Mohammed? What is your opinion of our nation's leader? What is your opinion of the government? What is your opinion of the Quran? What do you think of pledging allegiance? A "Good Roads, Fair Weather" response is a necessity. Those questions make dissenters sweat more than a crack mule at customs. Tourists must

---

[89] "What is your opinion of Edward Bellamy and his books?" is a question that is not known to have ever resulted in official persecution in the U.S. (for a negative answer). However, failure to perform Francis Bellamy's flag salutation (and the early Nazi gesture) did result in beatings, arrests, even lynching. The pledge continues to cause persecution of non-submissive students.

also be careful what they say. Everyone must drink the Kool-Aid, or pretend that he/she has.

Socialism makes each day a never-ending Milgram test. Society is one large Stanford prison experiment. The socialists Stalin, Mao, Hitler etc demonstrate that a large percentage of the population (more than 2/3rds?) will obediently kill millions because people in authority directed it to be done.

Smart people learn to keep quiet or to zealously repeat Kafkaesque absurdities in support of socialism and/or religion. Socialists force others to spout anti-capitalist hate speech. It is a real-life Twilight Zone.

It is impossible to know how many dissenters there are because danger silences them. Dissenters were blacklisted out of socialism's fake media of radio, film, television, books, and newspapers.[90] Bitter socialists perfected blacklisting and ruined the lives of millions of

---

[90] US Media often re-use stories about McCarthyism without ever comparing (nor even mentioning) much worse blacklisting under SMH and other socialists. In other words, US media blacklist information about socialist blacklisting. During World War II, Soviet socialists railed regularly at "rootless cosmopolitanism," especially in the arts. German socialists tossed the term around, too. It was socialist code for "Jewish." The socialist Stalin purged the culture of such "dissident" voices. In a 1946 speech, he condemned works in which "the positive Soviet hero is derided and inferior before all things foreign and cosmopolitanism that we all fought against from the time of Lenin..." It was part of a campaign aimed at writers, theater critics, scientists, and others who were connected with "bourgeois Western influences." Many of those "cosmopolitans" were Jewish, and the socialist media for a time "unmasked" the Jewish identities of writers who published under pseudonyms. McCarthy helped the US against socialist infiltration, and the blacklisting that socialism imposes.

talented people. "I have here a list of criminals who are known to be members of the Anti-socialist Party," they would say as the executions began. Intelligent people were accused of anti-socialist activities and were considered subversives.

Religion and Socialism both attack the "educated classes" as apostates. They demonize dissenters. Anyone who understands liberty and free market economics feels like the only adult in a country full of children. His/her ears will bleed listening to government officials. Theists and socialists are not sapiosexuals.[91]

Socialists cause brain drains when the intelligent skedaddle (it is true "democracy" when people "vote" with their feet and money to leave). Victims ask, "Who is John Galt?" Non-socialists flee far from the madding crowd's ignoble strife.

Simultaneously, socialists ignited their modern bonfire of the vanities (much worse than the old one from 1497). They destroyed objects that were considered heretical and western: including capitalistic books, music, paintings, sculpture, fine clothing, and more.

The most socialistic nations become genuine idiocracies. That remains the case in North Korea, Cuba[92]

---

[91] Under the "social contract" gibberish for socialism, they believe that you consent to sexual intercourse by being present in their country.

[92] Escapes from Cuba account for the vast majority of deaths, disappearances, hauntings and ghosts in the Bermuda Triangle (also known as the Devil's Triangle). Socialism is so bad, and capitalism is so good, that people try to escape from Cuba to Florida in rafts rigged from water bottles, trash, and worse. The Cuba Archive used an estimate from economist Armando Lago of about 77,000 rafter deaths (only up to the year 2003). Cuba's socialist regression coincides with the

and other countries today.

Theists promise a posthumous paradise of free food, clothing, shelter, and all goods and services. Socialists promise the same in this life. They promise heaven and deliver hell. Utopia is always "coming very soon." Everyone must have faith. Pray harder, vote harder, and/or lick the boots harder.

Religion and socialism are both absurd lies. They both cause shortages, poverty, misery, food deserts, starvation, and mass murder. Socialism creates bureaucratic nightmares that cause people who want "free" things to die while waiting in queues. Christian socialism and other forms of religious socialism combine all the lies into one.

Edward Bellamy's book "Looking Backward 2000-

---

growth of the Bermuda triangle story. Yet, the role of socialism/Cuba is never mentioned in "documentaries" nor books about the Devil's Triangle. Similarly, Stalin, Mao, Hitler and other socialists are never mentioned in "documentaries" and books about hauntings even though their victims should top all the ghost lists. Hungry ghosts.

The world rejoiced on 11/26/2016 when Fidel Castro finally became a "good socialist" (he died). To prevent the retarded island from erupting into a non-stop party, socialist Cuba's government imposed 9 mandatory days of mourning. As usual, the U.S. media naively reported that all Cubans claimed to be sad (and they all love the socialist Cuban government too, of course, and Castro's half-century of central planning). The military socialist's cremated remains were hauled to the ash heap of history by a green army jeep that broke down en route. Castro was late to his own funeral. The vehicle was then pushed by fashionistas wearing Castro's silly green fatigues (according to the obitchuary). Dead socialists always put the "fun" in "funeral."

In the U.S., some people mourned Castro's death (the same people who think Hitler self-identified as a "Nazi," a "Fascist," and think Hitler called his symbol a "swastika").

1887" is fiction. Books written by Karl Marx about socialism are fiction too. So are the unreadable Torah, Bible, Quran and all religious books. Fiction is a euphemism for "lies." It is make-believe, pretend, fantasy.

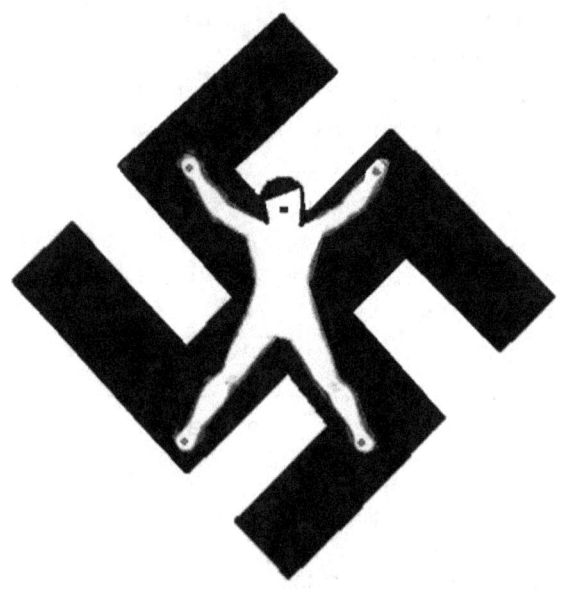

Under Bellamy's dogma, Christ was, to a large degree, a non-religious figure whose true message was socialism. Bellamy's concept of Christianity (Christian socialism) is not inconsistent with the atheism of Stalin and Mao. That can be seen in Edward Bellamy's book "The Religion of Solidarity," one of his early works, written in 1874 at the age of 24.

Socialism is the actual message and goal, Christ was simply a messenger of socialism, similar to his modern "angels" in the narcissists Stalin, Mao, and Hitler.[93]

---

[93] Some historians believe that crucifixion often occurred via an "X" letter shape for the wooden beams (e.g. Saint

If Christian socialists and others glorify Jesus as a socialist, then the vexilLOLogist Dr. Rex Curry is the Antichrist (as compared with Mary's sister, also known as the Auntie Christ).

Hitler's "Minister" of Propaganda under German socialism was Joseph Goebbels, and his diary (dated 16 October 1928) pointed to the crux of the matter: "What does Christianity mean today? National Socialism is a religion. All we lack is a religious genius capable of uprooting outmoded religious practices and putting new ones in their place. We lack traditions and ritual." One of the new rituals Minister Goebbels used for propaganda was the stiff-armed salute from the "religious genius" and one-time minister Francis Bellamy, and Germany used the salute in a similar programmed chanting fashion of worship en masse and on cue.

The author William L. Shirer in his book "The Rise and Fall of the Third Reich" suggests that German socialism logically evolved from Martin Luther to Adolf Hitler, as an expression of national character. Shirer argued that the course of German history "made blind obedience to temporal rulers the highest virtue of Germanic man, and put a premium on servility." That Sonderweg (special path) interpretation of German history was then common in American scholarship. Luther's influence applies to U.S. history via "Christian Socialism" and the Bellamy dogma.

Socialism is the opiate of the masses.[94] Or is it

Andrew's cross).

[94] But unlike when you use opium, socialism harms everyone else as well as yourself. Millions died overdosing on socialism. The German socialist Marx wrote: "Die Religion ... ist das Opium des Volkes" (published in 1844 in Marx's own

religion? No matter, the two are now combined. And pledges of allegiance are Gregorian chants.

The Anarchist philosopher Larken Rose retorted: "You are not Christians. You are not Jews. You are not Muslims. And you certainly aren't atheists. You all have the same god, and its name is 'government.' You're all members of the most evil, insane, destructive cult in history. If there ever was a devil, the state is it. And you worship it with all your heart and soul."

That is why GOD HATES FLAGS. The Ten Commandments and related dicta warn against the worship of other Gods and/or graven images. Socialist leaders are demigods and demagogues. God wants teachers to stop making little children verbally fellate flags every morning in schools. End flag fetishism. Stop saying the pledge, or else go to Hell.

Modern Socialist Crusades had many other similarities to the old Christian Crusades because the modern crusades had: aggressive expansion attempts by modern socialists; all "sins" (all atrocities) are justified and forgiven to whosoever took up the cause of socialism. The crusades reinforced the connection between socialism and militarism. Similar to the old Crusades, the modern socialist Crusades were military campaigns, consistent with Bellamy's 1888 dogma of "military socialism" and similar socialist militarism

---

journal Deutsch-Französische Jahrbücher).

Mao showed that socialism is the opiate of the masses, or worse: Socialism is the cyanide of the masses. How many people died from opium in China or anywhere ever? Mao's socialism killed so many people it makes opium (and the old "Opium Wars") seem blissful in comparison. Opium is much better than socialism. If only Mao and his monsters could have been zonked out on opium all the time. Millions of lives would have been spared.

under Stalin, Mao, and Hitler (born 1878, 1889, 1893, respectively). Flags are used first to shrink-wrap brains and then as ceremonial shrouds to bury the dead.

Modern socialist crusaders often pillaged the countries through which they invaded in the typical medieval manner. Socialists often retained much of the territory gained rather than returning it (e.g. the territories acquired by Soviet socialism under its pact of socialist imperialism/colonialism with German socialism).

The Soviet-German treaty of 1939 included a secret protocol that divided territories of Poland, Romania (specifically Bessarabia), and Baltic states (Finland, Estonia, Latvia, Lithuania) into German and Soviet "spheres of influence," anticipating potential "territorial and political rearrangements" [canned laughter] of these countries.

Soviet socialists and German socialists continued their imperialist pact in a "Declaration of the Government of the German Reich and the Government of the USSR of September 28, 1939," (note the use of the phrase "German Reich" and not "Third Reich") declaring their desire to "put an end" to the war of England and France against socialist Germany, and threatening England and France ominously: "in case of the continuation of the war, the Governments of Germany and of the USSR shall engage in mutual consultations with regard to necessary measures." Germany attacked France on May 10, 1940. Paris fell to the Germans on June 14, 1940. The Battle of Britain began on July 10, 1940. Hitler and Stalin remained allies until June 22, 1941.

The pact between Soviet socialism and German socialism surprised many people. Soviet socialism's atrocities and genocide had helped garner support for German socialism and, later, garnered tolerance for German socialism's atrocities and democide. In 1939, they were a cooperative street gang; in 1941, they became two rams smashing their heads together to decide which one will rape you. After the defeat of German socialism, the feared Soviet socialist atrocities renewed and then expanded into Chinese socialism and beyond.

The author Timothy Snyder extensively researched some of the socialist Wholecaust for his book "Bloodlands: Europe between Hitler and Stalin." It is a gruesome look at non-military deaths under militant socialists. He ranks the most common methods by which mass murder occurred under the socialist genocide: (1) starvation; (2) shooting; (3) gassing. He states, "Of the fourteen million civilians and prisoners of war killed in the bloodlands between 1933 and 1945, more than half died because they were denied food," and adds, "After starvation came shooting, and then gassing." (Preface: Europe page xiv). Snyder ranks the most common methods by which mass murder occurred under the German socialist Holocaust thusly: (1) shooting; (2) asphyxiation by carbon monoxide from engine exhaust; (3) Zyklon B pesticide gassing.

Snyder's ranking of starvation as a common method of mass killing under Soviet socialism and German socialism is characteristic of socialism elsewhere, including Chinese socialism. It remains a trademark of North Korean socialism.

In a speech delivered to the London School of Economics on January 21, 2014, Snyder stated that in 1938 the socialist Stalin had killed 1000 times the number of Jews killed by the socialist Hitler. That Hitler began to catch up with the Soviet socialist killing spree after Soviet socialists and German socialists became allies in their pact (1939-1941) to divide up Europe, invading Poland together, and launching World War II.[95] The German Holocaust began on territories that Soviet socialists occupied (or had occupied). That Soviet socialist citizens actively participated with German socialists in the German socialist Holocaust. Most of the perpetrators of the Holocaust were Soviet socialist citizens. German socialists found Soviet socialist collaborators everywhere they went.

Snyder's work shows why Soviet socialism is responsible for the German socialist Holocaust (which is usually blamed only on German socialism). He showcases the cutthroat competition of socialism (literally cutthroat). When Stalin teamed up with Hitler, it caused quite a furor.

In some lectures, Snyder fails to mention "socialism" even as he purports to analyze the motivations and ideologies of Hitler and Stalin. Sometimes he camouflages "socialism" by using the terms "Nazism" and "Stalinism." He perpetuates and reinforces widespread ignorance because uninformed listeners could leave his lectures without learning from Snyder that Hitler did not refer to his party as the "Nazi Party" and did not refer to members as "Nazis."[96] Listeners are

---

[95] Stalin said to his socialist pal Hitler "You gotta pump those numbers up! Those are rookie numbers." Later, Stalin said the same thing to Mao.

[96] People worldwide have been misled by Wakipedia (a more accurate name for "Wikipedia") which is written throughout by neo-nazis and racists who want the public to believe that Hitler and his supporters called his party the "Nazi Party" and spoke loudly and proudly about themselves as "Nazis." It is more accurate to say that Hitler and his supporters called his

not told that Stalin and Hitler (and their supporters) touted "socialism" by the very word in their tedious speeches and writings. It causes other spectators to wonder if Snyder likes "socialism," and dislikes how Stalin, Hitler, and Snyder all show affection for the word.

It is a reminder of the 2016 candidate for president Bernie "Whitey" Sanders (aka "BS"), a socialist who owns three homes and is in the top 4% of wealth. Sanders is a white nationalist and socialist who claimed that many in his father's family were killed by "Nazis." The trad media never asked: "BS, do you know that Nazis did not call themselves 'Nazis'? They were white males and were in their national government and called themselves the same thing you call yourself: SOCIALIST."[97]

It is a reminder of the New York Times (NYT) writer Walter Duranty who won a PuLiTzEr PrIZe (that should be revoked) hiding Soviet socialism's horrors. Duranty suppressed the Holodomor, the dearth and death of Ukrainians, Tatars (or Tartars), Kazakhs, and other non-Russian ethnic groups in the Ukraine and the Caucasus, the south, and Siberia. The slaughter included Kulaks.

---

party the "Socialist Party" and spoke loudly and proudly about themselves as "Socialists."

Wakipedia also deceives readers about the use (non-use) of other terms under Hitler's socialism, including: Fascism, Swastika, and Third Reich.

[97] "We're socialists...enemies of today's capitalist system of exploitation and we're determined to destroy it" -Bernie, 2017? No, Hitler, 1927. To be fair, BS probably prefers Karl "Whitey" Marx, another racist German who was a privileged melanin-challenged male. BS is so repulsive that he honeymooned in the USSR. The only thing more corrupt than socialists are the reporters who cover up for them.

Grain, grain everywhere, nor any seed to eat. That is a short history of tractors in Ukrainian.

The New York Times believes that slavery was not so bad. Under socialism, everyone must feed the loudmouths who bite them. Socialism is the fastest way to create a necropolis. Socialism is sociopathy. Socialism defies the best parts of human nature and brings out the worst in people.

Duranty described socialism in a way that is often mis-attributed to Stalin: "But – to put it brutally – you can't make an omelette without breaking eggs..."[98]

Duranty's New York Times deceit (~1932) makes a fascinating comparison to the first article concerning Hitler to appear in the newspaper (1922). The NYT's article (November 21, 1922 by Cyril Brown) exposes facts that the NYT masks in modern articles about Hitler including the following quotes from the NYT's article from 1922: "His followers are nicknamed the 'Hakenkreuzler.' " And this: "Hitler's 'Hakenkreuz' movement is essentially urban in character." The NYT article uses a form of "Hakenkreuz" four times in the article and never uses the word "swastika." The NYT article never explains the term "Hakenkreuz" nor "Hakenkreuzler"; was that because the term was well-known in 1922? Or did the NYT not want readers to know why Hitler's socialists used that nickname?

"Hakenkreuz" means "hooked cross" because, for Hitler's socialists, it was a type of cross and was used to

---

[98] It should be obvious that Stalin would not have said such a thing without adding "However, there are usually no eggs available in the Glorious Peoples' grocery stores, which is another reason why everyone is starving." Stalin's actual quote was "You can't make an omellete if all the eggs are stolen by socialists. That helps increase the body piles."

represent crossed "S" letters for "SOCIALIST," as Dr. Curry explained. The misnomer "swastika" was substituted for "Hakenkreuz" to hide German socialism's origin in American Christian Socialism, via Francis Bellamy (author of the "Pledge of Allegiance") and his cousin Edward Bellamy (author of "Looking Backward" -the origin of the National Socialist movement).

Current policy at the NYT is to libel a foreign symbol (the swastika) in order to conceal the truth about what German socialists called their symbol (Hakenkreuz or "hooked cross").[99] It is related to the NYT's current policy to conceal the USA's Pledge of Allegiance as the origin of the Nazi salute and Nazi behavior. The pledge continues to be the origin of similar behavior even though the gesture was changed to help the NYT hide America's past.

The revealing aspect of Brown's 1922 NYT article is that the terms "Nazi" and "Swastika" do not appear in it (because the "Nazis" did not call themselves "Nazis" and they did not call their talisman a "swastika," and the New York Times had not launched its current policy of masking those facts, and its current policy of hiding the fact that Hitler's supporters called themselves "Socialists" and called their insignia the "Hakenkreuz").

Today, the NYT continues a deceptive policy from

---

[99] Another example is Steven Heller, author of "The Swastika: Symbol Beyond Redemption?" and art director of The New York Times Book Review. In his book, he failed to mention that the swastika was used to represent crossed "S" letter shapes for socialism (Dr. Curry's discovery). It appears Heller has never mentioned it since the publication of his book either, and it is assumed that he will never tell anyone anywhere ever. Perhaps he deserves some credit for the fact that he is bright enough not to dispute the swastika's use as alphabetical symbolism.

Duranty's 1932 days that is followed by many newspapers, writers, and socialist shills: refer to German socialism as "Nazism," and refer to Soviet socialism as "Communism," and don't mention the word they both used: "Socialism"; Don't tell readers that Hitler did not self-identify as a "Nazi," nor a "Fascist," nor as the "Third Reich," but use those words to hide the word he DID use: socialist.[100]

Snyder's book "Bloodlands" refers to German socialists as both "Nazis" and "National Socialists." In comparison, Snyder labels Soviet socialism as "Stalinism." Sometimes he uses the phrase "National Socialism and Stalinism" when he refers to German socialism and Soviet socialism in the same sentence. Why does he not refer to them as "German National Socialism and Soviet National Socialism"; or "German socialism and Soviet socialism"; or "Hitler's socialism and Stalin's socialism"?

Readers should be grateful that Snyder is more

---

[100] In 2017 the New York Times continued its fake news to cover up for socialism when it published a bizarre series, "The Red Century," to celebrate the centenary of the socialist genocide. One quote claimed that, for all its flaws, the socialist revolution "taught Chinese women to dream big." There was no mention of the estimated 50 million people killed by Chinese socialism; the female intellectuals tortured and killed for sane thoughts that were politically incorrect; the thousands of women and girls raped; the grandmother and granddaughter buried alive for being class enemies; the mother of Zhang Hongbing, who was executed by firing squad -because she "disrespected" the image of Chairman Mao; Lin Zhao, executed after being tortured for criticizing socialism; Lin's mother, who only learned of the execution after an official demanded she pay five cents for the bullet that killed her daughter; the peasant women condemned to painful death by mass starvation.

honest than other historians who hide "socialism" with the phrase "Nazism and Stalinism." Snyder writes, "Hitler called his enemies 'Marxists,' and Stalin called his 'fascists,'" even though Snyder overlooks the irony that Hitler and komrade Stalin were each doing what Snyder (and other writers) do: protecting "his" word "socialism." It remains a common lie today: Hitler's party was "Nazi" and "Fascist"; Stalin's USSR was "Communist"; in contrast, socialists are intelligent and caring [sarcasm].

Snyder speaks socialism surprisingly well. He has many foreign linguistic skills. He can cover up for socialism in multiple languages.

Snyder so desperately protects socialism that he refers to Hitler as an "anarchist." I am not making this up. To make matters worse, Snyder never tells his audience: "I said Hitler was an 'anarchist' even though I cannot cite any example of Hitler ever self-identifying with that term, nor using the word in any way."[101] It seems as if Snyder would not be bothered if people started to believe that Hitler called himself an anarchist, in the same way that people incorrectly believe Hitler called himself a "Nazi," and a "Fascist." For socialists the goal is to prevent anyone from knowing that Hitler self-identified as socialist. Any misdirection is better: Fascist, Nazi, anarchist, gender-fluid, autistic, furry,

---

[101] Hitler used "anarchy" once in Mein Kampf in a manner indicating his disapproval of anarchy. It is visible in the original German language edition and in the Murphy edition in the English language.

On a side note: Modern history provides many examples of socialists who misuse the term "anarchists" to describe other socialists who threw bombs and killed to foment Marx's "violent revolution of the masses." Snyder is merely another example of that old deception.

OCD, nudist, bird watcher. ANYTHING ELSE!

Snyder does not compare Stalin or Mao as "zoological anarchists" in his analysis of Hitler. When SMH mfs killed millions were they just weeding out the unfit? ("unfit" is code for any "class" that did not gleefully submit to SMH's socialist theft and violence). All three "zoological anarchists" were inspired by the socialist Karl Marx, who misinterpreted Charles Darwin, as in this quote: "Darwin's work is most important and suits my purpose in that it provides a basis in natural science for the historical class struggle." (16 January 1861).

Hitler is a poster child for why anarchy is the only logical choice for humans against Hitler's socialism. Stalin, Mao, and Hitler are examples of why statism is bad, and anarchy is good. Anarchy is the realization based on thousands of years of experience that individuals cannot entrust the management of their lives to government. History proves how dangerous it is to have government.

When Snyder is interviewed by people who seem ignorant of Hitler's words, Snyder does not clarify for them. Snyder uses the term "Nazi" and never explains that Hitler did not use the term in Hitler's many repetitive speeches and writings in which Hitler promoted socialism and socialists. Snyder cites no example of Hitler using the word "Nazi," nor "Fascist," nor "Third Reich," nor "anarchist" as a self-description (for more on all of that see Dr. Curry's research). Hitler jabbered glowingly about "socialism," as did Stalin and Mao and millions of others seduced by Marx' conspiracy theories.

The above is why Snyder did not make the historic discovery that the swastika was used by Hitler to represent crossed "S" letter shapes for "socialist" (Professor Curry's breakthrough). Snyder was intellectually incapable of making that discovery. That is why Snyder will never mention the swastika's alphabetical function under German socialism: for the same reason that, in interviews and lectures, Snyder avoids or minimizes any mention that Hitler and his supporters called themselves "socialists." It is important to repeat the point: Snyder will never explain to his audiences and readers that the swastika was used by Hitler to represent crossed letter "S" shapes for "socialist." It does not support his misleading narrative and his efforts to hide what Hitler said and the actual words Hitler used: socialist and socialism. Snyder does not want to talk about it.

Snyder obscures the socialist interrelationship of Hitler, Stalin, and Mao, as he hides the influence of American socialists. That is why Snyder did not make the historic discovery that the USA's Pledge of Allegiance (from the American socialist Francis Bellamy) was the origin of the Nazi salute and Nazi behavior. That is why Snyder will never educate his audiences about that.

In a telling double-standard, Snyder's anarchist "slur" avoids the "anarchist" Stalin and the "anarchist" Mao (even though they allegedly believed that socialism would evolve to a utopian level with the "withering away" of the state -just not while Stalin and Mao were top socialist "archists" killing millions). Snyder is mum about the "Union of Soviet Anarchist Republics" (USAR) during its alliance of Soviet anarcho-socialism and German anarcho-socialism in 1939 (when the two "anarcho-governments" [?] invaded Poland together, launching the anarchist war of WWII) with their infamous motto: "Anarchists Unite!"[102]

When German socialists invaded a country, they would often cause "state destruction," according to Snyder in his bizarre explanation of "anarchist" Hitler. Snyder knows that wherever Hitler went he imposed the German socialist government. The archangels Stalin, Mao, and Hitler all imposed their socialist governments wherever they went (and for a while the archo-socialists Stalin and Hitler did it together, and then the archo-socialists Stalin and Mao did it together). Sometimes (often? always?) they destroyed whatever government was present and replaced it with their socialist government. That is not "anarchy."

All socialism exemplifies "state destruction" and the eventual failure of the state (e.g. late stage socialism in the USSR in 1991) because socialism causes alienation of labor, shortages, poverty, squalor, suffering, food deserts, starvation, and the deaths of millions. The Austrian economist Ludwig von Mises (born in Ukraine) explained why in his book "Socialism: An Economic and Sociological Analysis" (1922, 1932, 1951): Socialists always impose the dual strategy of (1) nationalizing as much industry and property as possible; and (2) "destructionism," defined as "destroying the social order which is based on private ownership." Socialism is planned chaos.[103]

---

[102] All that socialist "aid" and "freedom" coming your way. Run for your life!

[103] See also the book "Planned Chaos" by Ludwig von Mises. Also see "Why Socialism Works" by Harrison Lievesley. The collapse of the Soviet Socialist Empire was bigger than the collapse of the Roman Empire, and many more people suffered and died before the collapse. Socialism is an example of "Chaos theory" and the "butterfly effect" in that interferences in a market (even small interferences) can

The Malthusian theory only manifests itself under socialism because socialism interferes with the ability of a population to provide goods and services. Modern Malthusians misidentify the problem as "overpopulation" and claim that runaway consumption of precious resources remains the biggest danger facing humankind (the same lie motivating "climate change" statists). They then laud plagues and the genocides of Stalin, Mao, and Hitler for "helping Mother Earth" and desire new Stalins, Maos, and Hitlers with bigger body piles. Their lies have been debunked by Dr. Julian Simon, author of "The Ultimate Resource." Overpopulation occurs only in the form of an overpopulation of socialists (and reducing the population of socialists will also decrease "climate change," according to a consensus of scientists).

A socialist country's lifespan is lengthened only by the black market (the underground catallaxy) to the extent that everyone breaks socialist laws in the struggle to survive the dogma. That is anarchy. Resistance is fertile. When freedom is outlawed, only outlaws will be free. Capitalism destroyed Soviet socialism in the same way it destroyed the USA's socialist mail monopoly, Kodak, Blackberry, and Blockbuster Video. Laissez faire is everywhere!

Snyder uses socialism's bloodbath to promote yet more statism (some of that is in Chapter 4, "The State

---

cause catastrophic results that result in mass shortages, poverty, and starvation. The USSR barely staggered through 69 years (1922 to 1991), or 74 years (if counted from 1917). It barely exceeded the life span of Karl Marx, at 64 years (1818 to 1883). Stalin's life was longer than his country's (he died at 74 years; 1878 to 1953). Only Hitler's German socialism was more embarrassing. Schadenfreude. No do-overs.

Destroyers," in his book "Black Earth"). Snyder points out the obvious: that of the states invaded by German socialists, some local governments were "destroyed" and some local governments were left intact, and survival rates were higher in the latter. Duh.

Many of the deadliest invasions by German socialism occurred in areas that were butchered first by Soviet socialism, then by German socialism, and then again by Soviet socialism. The final Soviet socialist hell then continued for decades.

Submitting is good? When German socialism was appeased by a state that Germany invaded, then Germany might kill fewer of that state's people. If Snyder urges capitulation to German socialism (to avoid bloodshed), then he shares another point of view urged by German socialists. That is why "states" are important, using Snyder's reasoning: so that they can embrace German socialism and thereby reduce deaths. That is disturbing.

Snyder continues with his explanation of why archy is good: Countries block and/or send back non-citizens when non-citizens try to immigrate after fleeing German socialism's (or Soviet socialism's) graveyard. When that happens, it is better to be a local citizen than a non-citizen fleeing Soviet or German socialism. A doomed outsider is told to stay away, or is returned from whence she came, to go die somewhere else.

Snyder promotes statism with the fact that France protected its own Jewish citizens while France sacrificed Polish Jews (who had fled to France after Germany's invasion of Poland), returning Polish Jews to German socialists. Statists make creepy arguments.

Snyder worsens. He cites for support (with apologies?) the socialist police state "Nazi Germany"

(Snyder's term) as proof that statism is a good thing: Jews in Germany had ~50% chance of living, while Jews in areas that Germany invaded had ~5% chance of survival (those numbers have been used by Snyder). Under socialism, you might live longer because your government might kill more foreigners than locals (i.e. you), says Snyder in defense of statism/socialism. People who support government say odd things. It will be frightening to read Snyder's cheery spin on the citizen/non-citizen death rates under the archo-socialists Stalin, Mao, Pol Pot, the Kim thugs, et cetera.

Snyder is mum on immigration laws under Lenin, Stalin, Mao, Pol Pot, and in North Korea, East Germany (and its Berlin immigration/emigration wall), Cuba, and other socialist prisons.[104] Millions died because of immigration laws in their own nations/states.

Snyder promotes the nation state (even national socialism itself?) and its borders, visas, passports, and control over the movement of human beings; he promotes how people are treated as sheeple who are socialized property owned by fenced-in farms (their socialist states). Authorization is required before anyone may cross socialism's ubiquitous imaginary lines.

The immigration controls that Snyder praises are the same rules that continue to kill today in the same way they killed during the socialism of Germany, China, and the Soviet Union. Because of immigration laws, the same thing could happen again under another socialist war and socialist Wholecaust. Victims would be prevented from fleeing, or would be sent back. It happens today. It continues in China, North Korea,

---

[104] Socialists support a multi-billion dollar public-works project for an East Berlin style wall on the USA's southern border, along with an army of DHS boots on the ground there.

Cuba, and more.[105]

No one ever said, "I crossed 90 miles of shark infested, stormy ocean at night on a raft I constructed out of water bottles to escape free market capitalism." Most illegal immigrants know how dangerous the state is. That's why they immigrated. Socialism is Hellacious acres: admission is "free," you pay to get out.

Some animals won't leave the pen even if their gate is left open. Socialists lock the gate because they know that many humans *will* flee the pen. People want to be survivors.

Immigration laws also keep out "undesirables." Such laws are socialist xenophobia, discrimination, and eugenics.[106] Dirt worshippers in the U.S. dictate who Americans can marry, live with, work with, hire, rent to, buy from, et cetera.[107] Imports are labeled by national origin (this is usually required). Socialism dictates bigotry and discrimination, while socialists falsely preach diversity and tolerance.

Snyder's "anarchist Hitler" ploy is misdirection to hide another embarrassing similarity between Snyder,

---

[105] Homeschooling is illegal in Germany today under a law that existed under Hitler's German socialism. Some families have sought asylum abroad in order to home-school their children. Immigration laws in some countries delay or prevent people from fleeing Germany's socialist schools (just as immigration prevented people from fleeing German socialism under Hitler).

[106] Socialism is eugenics. Cf. a recent headline announcing: "Iceland is on pace to virtually eliminate Down syndrome through abortion." Other examples of socialist eugenics include government schools and the Pledge of Allegiance.

[107] It is a reminder that President Lincoln wanted to deport freed "negros" back to Africa or anywhere other than the USA.

Hitler, Stalin, and Mao: the socialists Stalin, Mao, and Hitler were archists and Snyder is too. They are not even minarchists.[108] They are bad archists who spread malarchy. Stalin, Mao, Hitler, Kim Jong-un, and other Oedipus Rexes are socialist Monarchists and the worst kind of "kings" – socialist kings who impose a one-size-fits-all socialist monopoly on everyone and everything.

Similar to Marxists of another era, Snyder substitutes mythical thinking about the economy for loyalty to individual liberty. Snyder needs to face what he is and face the dogma Snyder touts: archy and the violence, theft, and planned chaos it embodies.

The unmatched bloodbath of socialist mfers inspired two new fields of study: anarchaeology and misanthropology. Anarchaeology is the study of how people throughout history have progressed and thrived with limited government (minarchy) or with no government at all. Misanthropology is the study of why governments hate humanity, and how government kills millions of people, destroys their property, causes chaos, spreads misery, and creates poverty that ruins civilizations.[109] Both fields consist of members

---

[108] Every statist is a minarchist (and every minarchist is a statist), differing only in what each deems the "minimum essential services" that inspire the initiation of violence.

I like the idea of small government. Very small. Smaller. Keep going...

[109] Capitalism turns luxuries into necessities; Socialism turns necessities into luxuries. In a sense, capitalism and socialism aren't opposites: Socialism is a worldview; Capitalism is a description of economic facts. Capitalism describes how people actually behave. Capitalism is equivalent to economic mental health, a view that accords with reality.

Socialism is a pathology. If socialists were sincere in their rejection of private property, they wouldn't own anything of

(Anarchaeologists and misanthropologists) who often study the worst examples in history: the socialist Wholecaust (of which the Holocaust was a part). Modern Holocaust museums will triple in size when they include the entire socialist genocide.

World War I (WW1) and World War II (WW2) were governments killing millions of people. War is when one government tries to destroy and/or replace another government. WW2 was yet another archist war and was related to the archist WW1. Many nations are today engaged in ongoing militarism and warfare that is a result of the archist WW1 and WW2.

Germany's socialist government committed the same atrocities as the Soviet's socialist government and China's socialist government: they all killed millions of people. Their socialist Reichs implemented the Final Solution against all non-socialists. Government is the most sociopathic killer of all human history. It is not anarchy. It is the opposite of anarchy.

The militant socialists Stalin, Mao, and Hitler were similar to the socialist Mussolini and other socialists: They all touted socialist totalitarianism. It was the totalitarian dogma touted by the Bellamy cousins in the U.S. from 1888: National Socialism and Military Socialism.

"Hitler or Stalin: Who Killed More?" asks Snyder in another article. He confusingly argues that "Hitler" is the answer. Snyder's low numbers are from Soviet socialist sources. Why does he believe those figures? Walter Duranty was willingly duped by Soviet socialist sources.

Snyder dances around part of his "accountant"

their own. Their deeds betray them!

question: Did the number of people killed by Stalin in the socialist famine in Ukraine and the Caucasus (1930-33) exceed the number of Jews killed by Hitler?[110] A clear answer is not provided. Snyder thinks it was close, apparently. Maybe he considers it a "tie" in that contest between the German Hitler and the Soviet Hitler (Stalin).

Snyder uses the term "non-combatants" when accounting, and he seems to include ~3 million "Soviet prisoners of war" starved (or shot) by German socialists. That number is embarrassing for Soviet socialists because they started Hitler's worst killing (and WWII) with German socialists in the so-called "non-Aggression pact." It was portrayed as a peace agreement. It should be called their "Xtreme-Aggression Pact." They lived in piece(s).

Here are some more embarrassing numbers for Soviet socialism's "non-aggression" pact with German socialism: the number of Soviets dead due to their war was ~27 million; the number of Germans dead was ~6 million. Ouch! That left a mark. Soviet serfs were like kamikaze but without planes and multiplied by millions.

---

[110] The number of people killed by Stalin's profiteering in Ukraine greatly exceeded the number killed later by Hitler in Ukraine (after Hitler began his "drive to the East" on June 22, 1941 by invading Ukraine after the Hitler-Stalin love-in, laugh-in ended).

People before socialist profits. Socialist profits are the worst kind. Under socialism and under both of those socialists, the word "profiteering" is a euphemism for "violent robbery and murder."

Socialism was so destructive that, according to one writer: "Only now, 100 years later, has Russia begun to match the agricultural output that it had prior to 1917." (L. Todd Wood, 11-16-2017).

One can imagine Stalin tweeting "WTF? TIL Hitler is murdering more of my people than I am. Dagnabbit! OMG!" Stalin got what he deserved from his conspiracy with German socialism.

Snyder should include even more of Hitler's death toll in Stalin's death toll (It is easy to do. It was done by Dr. Curry). Stalin and Hitler were in a worldwide conspiracy, the Molotov-Ribbentrop alliance between German socialism and Soviet socialism, launching Hitler's worst destruction (including the German Holocaust). It was 2 girls, 1 cup socialism. According to Snyder, most abettors in the German Holocaust were willing Soviet socialist citizens who were collaborators.

Joachim von Ribbentrop was convicted at the Nuremberg trials for his role in the Holocaust and executed by hanging; Vyacheslav Molotov[111] was not

---

[111] "Molotov" was a pseudonym derived from the Russian word for "hammer" as in "hammer and sickle" or ☭ (Russian: Серп и молот, serp i molot) and is related to the English word "mallet." When you are a hammer, everything is a nail. He is also the origin of the term "Molotov Cocktail" for socialists who enjoy causing poverty via arson.

Stalin's name was Joseph Vissarionovich Jughashvili. His high school yearbook states that he was voted "Most Likely To Slaughter Millions." He rechristened himself "Stalin" (derived from "steel" as if he was the "Man of Steel" or the super socialist man who ruled with an iron fist, or steel fist, or steal fist). The "Iron Curtain" should have been labeled the "Steel Curtain" in that Stalin shut his hostages in and shut out everyone else. Stalin was actually the "Man of Steal" or "Stealin" due to his socialism; also, Steely Dzhugashvili (Dan). Stalin was a true robber baron, literally. Before he graduated to robbing everyone all the time under Soviet socialism, he was a young criminal with mug shots for his arrests, and a history of robbery.

One of Stalin's sons was named "Yakov." He served (and died) as an officer in the socialist world war that Stalin had

(he was not even charged or tried). Molotov, Stalin's left-hand man, lived until 1986 (from 9 March 1890 to 8 November 1986) and the age of 96!

Stalin was double-crossed by the Hakenkreuzlers on 22 June 1941. He did nazi that coming. Stalin sought help from Britain against Germany. One problem: Stalin wanted Churchill to agree to Stalin's Lebensraum so that Stalin could have eastern Poland and the Baltic states that Stalin had stolen. Guess who Stalin sent to the UK to secure his atavistic red revanchism: Molotov. Imagine. My. Shock. Psychopathic Stalin sent the same man (Molotov) to meet Churchill to ask for the same sociopathic deal that had put Hitler at Stalin's Moscow doorstep. -Oh, yes. He did.[112]

Many Russians believe that Stalin could have defeated Hitler with no assistance from other countries. Then again, Stalin started the war with no assistance from other countries (besides help from Germany). Stalin could have ended the war the same way he started it: on his own. Many people almost agree with Stalin: the world would have been better off if Stalin had been

---

planned and launched as an ally of Hitler (oh the poetic justice. It was like a Greek tragedy). Stalin's son was known as "Major Yakov." He was captured by Germany and offered to Stalin in exchange for captured German Field Marshal Friedrich Paulus, but Stalin refused the offer, explaining, "I will not trade a Marshal for a Major Yakov." He was no fortunate son. Stalin also persecuted Yakov's wife.

[112] Molotov may be the only man to shake hands with Hitler, Himmler, Goring, Stalin, Roosevelt, Churchill, Lenin and Trotsky.

Speaking of Trotsky: while Stalin had Molotov partner with Stalin's socialist friend Hitler, Stalin was simultaneously arranging the murder of his old socialist friend Trotsky. Stalin made it clear that Trotsky was "not real socialism" and Hitler WAS real socialism.

left to fight his ex-pal Hitler on his own. Stalin deserved the opportunity to show he was correct.

After WWII, Soviet socialists did not disavow the Molotov-Ribbentrop conspiracy, and did not return the stolen property.

After Stalin's death in 1953, Molotov's antidisestablishmentarianism continued: he staunchly defended Stalin's Kremlin crimes, castigated Stalin's successors, and opposed "de-Stalinization." Molotov watched much of the USSR's deterioration, but it is a shame that Molotov died in 1986 without seeing the final disintegration in 1989. The existence of the Molotov-Ribbentrop secret protocol was denied by Soviet socialists until 1989. Despite the collapse of the Union of Soviet Socialist Republics, the remaining Russian government has never disavowed socialism, and continues to use it.

Soviet socialists helped prosecute German socialists at Nuremberg for "crimes against humanity" (including the crimes that they committed together). Germans experienced that feeling when someone worse than you are tells you that you are a bad person. Kettle, meet Pot. It was weirder than if the novelist Stephen King had said Hitler has "a severely fucked-up mind." Soviet socialists were unindicted co-conspirators in the Nuremberg trials (e.g. Stalin and Molotov conspiring with Hitler and Ribbentrop). Soviet socialists were virtue signaling while they slaughtered millions. Irony had surely died too.

Soviet socialists are the "divers other persons" referenced in count one of the indictment: "1. Between September 1939 and April 1945 all of the defendants herein, acting pursuant to a common design, unlawfully, wilfully, and knowingly did conspire and agree together and with each other and with divers other persons, to commit War Crimes and Crimes against Humanity, as defined in Control Council Law No. 10, Article II." Nuremberg was another of Stalin's many show trials against fellow socialists.[113]

Soviet socialism's crimes against humanity went unpunished (as did Chinese socialism's crimes against humanity). Stalin, Mao, and Hitler serve as exhibits 1, 2, and 3 in the trial of socialism. Socialism is nutzi.

Other deaths that Snyder ignores via "Stalin" are deaths under Soviet socialism before and after Stalin was head of the USSR. The Soviet socialist famine of 1921 is one example, with 6 million deaths. Sometimes, Snyder restricts his death count to "Stalin vs. Hitler," lowering the numbers, as compared with the bigger body piles for "Soviet socialism vs. German socialism."

Stalin was a deadly mentor to Hitler. Stalin was a politburo member from the beginning (in 1917) of the Soviet socialist death machine. He was appointed General Secretary of the Central Committee in 1922. He consolidated power following the death of Vladimir Lenin in 1924. Stalin had a long murderous track record for Hitler to admire and aspire to. German socialists were playing catch-up to the Soviet Hitler (Stalin).

Stalin's death toll easily includes Mao's death toll, along with Hitler's. They were disciples of Stalin, Lenin, and Soviet socialism. That makes Mao a stinky number 2. Mao was another left-hand man in Stalin's

---

[113] "Why was there not a Nuremberg for Communism?" was the title of a conference held at the European Parliament in Brussels in October 2017.

Hitler was a baddie and Stalin was a baddie? Or was one of them a good baddie or bad goodie? And what about the other? There is no way to untangle the knot.

circle jerk of socialists. Stalin inspired, aided, and abetted Mao, in another conspiracy, between Soviet socialism and Chinese socialism. It was 2 girls, 1 cup socialism all over again. It resulted in the Chinese Soviet Socialist Republic (also known as the Soviet Republic of China) established in November 1931 (lasting until 1937).

Wouldn't it be fun to know Mao's public comments from 1939 to 1941 about the Stalin-Hitler pact? That question would never cross the mind of any mainstream media. Mao probably joined Stalin and Hitler in rejoicing about "international socialist cooperation." [kissing sound]. Mao's jubilation on that topic is as difficult to locate as old films of America's Nazi salute.

Stalin also inspired Mao's brothers (Mao Zemin and Mao Zetan). Mao Zedong and his brothers were more turds from Stalin's backdoor.

Chinese socialism, Soviet socialism, German socialism and Italian socialism worked together in 1939 and some of that cooperation continued far beyond 1939. Stalin, Mao, Hitler and other socialist Reichs competed in one-downmanship.

What if Hitler had won the war?[114] That question inspires dystopian scenes in books, movies, and conversations. The question's answer is: If Hitler had won the war it would have been similar to what happened when Stalin won the war; it would be similar to what happened under Mao too. And Pol Pot and others. Thus, "what if Hitler had won the war?" is not as unimaginable as people pretend. Hitler's dogma DID

---

[114] Perhaps a scarier question for movies and books is: What if the pact between German socialism and Soviet socialism had not been broken and had continued indefinitely? Would that have been worse than what actually happened?

win the war. Hitler's co-conspirator ally (Stalin) DID win the war. Stalin groomed Mao. Their dogma inspired Pol Pot and many others. Socialism went on to enslave and kill millions.

After German socialism signed an unconditional surrender on May 7, 1945, it was springtime for Stalin. And then it was a cruel summer as the despot went bananas seeking revenge. The Soviet death toll continued after Hitler's hara-kiri because Stalin continued killing until 1953 when Stalin finally became a good socialist (Stalin died).

Stalin's death toll continued after Stalin died because Mao continued killing until Mao's death in 1976. Mao was like a bald Stalin with no facial hair. One example: thirty million or more Chinese starved during the Great Leap Forward Into Famine, as Mao followed Stalin's model of collectivization from 1958 to 1961. It was like the Chris McCandless story, but multiplied by millions. Atlas farted again. The field of economics was rocket surgery for Mao. If he had been placed in charge of the Sahara Desert, then he would have caused a shortage of sand.

Mao also imposed Laogai, his version of Soviet socialism's Gulag (penal labor and prison farms). Laogai means "reform through labor" (with a tip of the hat to German socialism). Millions died in Laogai.

Soviet socialism's death toll continued after Soviet socialism died (1991) because Stalin's socialist imperialism slouched on in China, North Korea, Cuba, Colombia (the FARC), Peru (Shining Path), Nicaragua (Sandinistas), Venezuela,[115] Symbionese Liberation

---

[115] When you study Marx in economics, even theft of petroleum can't save you. Venezuela is a reminder that no country is so rich that it can't be ruined by socialism. Hugo

Army, et cetera. Soviet socialism's corpse pile hasn't stopped ballooning yet. [#EconomicCalculationProblem is real]

The Union of Soviet Socialist Republics declared war on Japan on 8 August 1945, and the Soviet Socialist Army entered Pyongyang, North Korea, on 24 August 1945. Stalin created the socialist Kim Il-sung (15 April 1912 – 8 July 1994) from zero, and maintained close relations with him thereafter. Even after Stalin's death, Stalin's killing spree continued in North Korea. One example: following the implosion of Soviet socialism, North Korea's economy worsened (is that possible?), leading to yet more widespread poverty, food deserts, famine, and death.

In 1956, Kim Il-sung and Mao Zedong became "tankies" and re-affirmed their bloodthirsty support of Stalin's lunacy by rejecting Nikita Khrushchev's program of de-Stalinization, and by supporting the Kremlin's crushing of the Hungarian revolt against Soviet socialism. Despite his opposition to de-Stalinization, Kim never officially severed relations with the Soviet Union.

Today, Stalin's mass murder goes on (from Stalin's bread line in Hell) because Kim Il-sung continues to rule

---

Chávez and others brought starvation to the nation. One warning clue: Chavez referred to Kim Jong-il as a "comrade" he mourned. Socialism's environmental destruction reached new heights as Venezuelans ate flamingoes, anteaters, pigeons, pet rabbits, cats, and dogs. Venezuela is simultaneously too socialist and not socialist enough depending on which socialist screeches. Venezuela is Schrödinger's socialist. LOL. #NotRealSocialism™ The temptation for anti-socialists is to relish Venezuela's predictable collapse. But socialism is a horror story more than a farce.

in North Korea today (according to North Korea's socialist sociopaths who insist that Kim Il-sung remains the "Eternal Leader of North Korea"). Now that Joseph Stalin and Kim Il-sung are both dead and roasting in eternal damnation, they continue to kill together in today's North Korea.

Should Stalin be blamed for World War I? Stalin, Lenin, Marx, Kropotkin, Bakunin and others were promoting socialism worldwide for years leading up to WWI. Their dogma inspired the man who started WWI: the socialist Gavrilo Princip. Princip's goal in assassinating Archduke Franz Ferdinand of Austria was "not to start WWI" (oops) but to cause a socialist revolution. (yawn). He wanted to do it via violent terrorism. Princip explained that he was inspired by Russia's Kropotkin shortly before the assassination. Kropotkin, in the late 1800s, supported the economic absurdity of abolition of private property and the rule of "from each according to his ability, to each according to his need" (viewpoints that Stalin shared). Kropotkin supported "propaganda of the deed" (terrorist violence) to inspire the yawning masses to political awareness and socialist revolution.

Whenever a death occurs anywhere at any time, an investigation should be launched to examine if Stalin was involved. Chances are he was.

Another example of Soviet socialism's deadly impact is the assassination of John F. Kennedy on November 22, 1963 by Lee Harvey Oswald.[116] Oswald's apartment

---

[116] For other examples of wacko socialists going after presidents see: Lynette Alice "Squeaky" Fromme and Sara Jane Moore (they went after Gerald Ford); Leon Czolgosz (always described as an "anarchist" in order to cover up for socialism).

is a tourist attraction in Minsk, Belarus. Oswald was honorably discharged from the Marine Corps and moved to Minsk, living there from October 1959 to June 1962 (the Bay of Pigs Invasion occurred on Apr 17, 1961; the Cuban missile crisis occurred Oct 16, 1962). Dial "M" for Murder (and for "Minsk" and "Moscow").

The Cold War produced fear in the USA of nuclear war from Soviet socialism. Yet, Stalin had already rained nuclear bombs on his own country and turned it into a post-apocalyptic wasteland, judging from his death toll (~50 million dead? And writing metaphorically). Mao had already rained nuclear bombs on his own country, judging from his death toll (~40 million dead?). Socialists are nuclear bombs. Russian President Vladimir Putin compared Lenin's policies to "a nuclear bomb planted under Russia." Socialism is nuclear war.

The previous paragraphs should be expanded (beyond "death counts") to include decades of robbery, slavery, torture, and terrorism that continued under Soviet socialism after German socialism ended. Snyder and other writers minimize socialism's horrors by focusing on death counts.

One example is Czechoslovakia, where German socialism plundered first, and then Soviet socialism followed the path of German socialism there and for decades longer (1948-1990).

Soviet socialism's omni-crimes continue today.

Stalin's guilt for the horrors of Hitler and Mao (and others) is consistent with Stalin's (and the USSR's) stated threat to spread the toxic culture of socialism worldwide.[117] The fifth column menace was reinforced

---

[117] This influenced the German socialist concept of

on Soviet paper ruble currency in 1919 with the ominous Lebensraum shibboleth "Workers of the world, Unite!" (other paper rubles were decorated with swastikas that appeared on Deutsche Marks or Reichsmarks later).[118] Government can take a valuable commodity such as paper and make it worthless by applying ink. The absurd Marxist catchphrase was repeated on the rubles in every major language, including German, Chinese, and Italian. Soviets foresaw the socialist greed and gullibility of Germany, China, Italy and other countries. Non-Soviets all over the world trembled with bated breath.

The rhetorical nonsense summons all to unite as the hivemind of the proles in their socialism trek. Join the Borg collective and be assimilated. According to Marx, Stalin, Mao, Hitler et cetera, "Resistance is futile!"

Socialists share the same genocidal goal of "class cleansing" and "ethnic cleansing." They want a "classless society" and there is no doubt that the socialists Marx, Lenin, Hitler, Stalin, and Mao were without class. A classless society involves their effort to murder the "capitalist class" and capitalists. They consider capitalists to be heathens under socialism. Capitalists (and other lower types) are sub-humans who must give way to the socialist "superman" (in Russian the "New Soviet Man").

In pursuit of that goal, they engage in "ethics cleansing" - imposing government schools (socialist

---

"Lebensraum." Compare them.

[118] "You have nothing to lose but your chains!" Millions of people lost everything including their lives and the lives of their family, friends, and neighbors. Humans help explain how flies are fooled by the painfully obvious Venus Flytrap plant. There's "free" cheese in a mouse trap.

schools) to teach generations of children about socialism: that theft, violence, and murder are magnanimous altruism. Socialist schools (government schools) remain. The lesson continues.

When German socialism began stealing land, Soviet socialism was already far ahead in the same crimes of theft and enslavement. The USSR provided Hitler with inspiration. For a while, Soviet socialism and German socialism were co-conspirators in their crimes.

Most people have heard earfuls about where German socialism went to plunder. For comparison, the following are some places (22) where Soviet socialism's imperialism and colonialism robbed, murdered and/or enslaved: Hungary,[119] Albania, Bulgaria, Romania, East Germany, Yugoslavia, Ukraine and the Caucasus, Belarus, Armenia, Georgia, Azerbaijan, Estonia,

---

[119] Raoul Wallenberg, a Swedish businessman, is lauded for saving thousands of Jews in Hungary while it was occupied by German socialists. German socialists did not arrest and kill him.

In 1945, during the Siege of Budapest by Soviet socialists, Wallenberg was arrested for alleged espionage and disappeared. He was later reported to have been killed in 1947 while imprisoned in Moscow under Soviet socialism.

Old media laud Wallenberg for saving people from "Nazis" and deliberately gloss over how Soviet socialism stopped him and killed him (German socialism didn't), and fail to mention death tolls in Hungary under Soviet socialism (as compared with death tolls in Hungary under German socialism). How many people might Wallenberg have saved from Soviet socialism? That is one reason why Soviet socialists killed him.

Hungary is home to the House of Terror (Hot), a museum that is an improvement upon the usual Holocaust Museum, in that the HoT covers both German socialism and Soviet socialism.

Kazakhstan, Kyrgyzstan, Latvia, Lithuania, Moldova, Tajikistan, Turkmenistan, Uzbekistan, Poland, and Czechoslovakia.[120]   Add those victims to China, Cambodia, Cuba, North Korea, Vietnam, et cetera for Soviet socialism's body count.   Each was a typical country involved in a typical nightmare. Many countries sought to transform themselves from 50 shades of red dominated by foreign imperialism into a free capitalist society. Yet, Stalin and Soviet socialism wreaked havoc worldwide.

Under Soviet socialism, many people in Hungary became hungry.   Modern socialists were worse than Huns. Socialized food is similar to socialized medicine: the food is hideous… and such small portions! Standing in food lines is so bourgeois!

Soviet socialism shares blame for the Cambodian

---

[120] Poland and Czechoslovakia are part of the documentary film "Fighter" about Arnošt Lustig and Jan Wiener. When traditional media review the film, they are as deceitful as they are regarding Wallenberg, supra. Weiner was persecuted by German socialism and then by Soviet socialism. Trad media cover up for socialism when they explain that Weiner "survived his ordeals in Europe by fighting the Nazis and, years later, the Communists." The Associated Press covered up for socialism and more in its article about Eliahu Pietruszka (11/20/2017); written as a "Nazi Holocaust survivor" story, it is more about a man who fled Soviet socialism after presuming that his brother died in a Soviet camp. A similar story is in the documentary "Tovarisch, I Am Not Dead" (2007) about Garri Urban, from Poland, another survivor of both German socialism and Soviet socialism. Also compare the plight of Ayn Rand and her family mentioned elsewhere in this book. More recently (8 December 2017), the BBC quoted David Smolansky who said his grandparents left the Soviet Union in 1927; his father left Cuba in 1970; and he is the third generation to leave a country [Venezuela] because of socialist regimes.

genocide committed by Pol Pot and the Khmer Rouge. Pol Pot was born Saloth Sar (19 May 1925 - 15 April 1998) and became a worshipful follower of Stalin and Soviet socialism.

In 1950, Pol Pot's interest in Soviet socialism grew when he participated in an international labor brigade building roads in Zagreb in the Socialist Federal Republic of Yugoslavia in 1950. On 31 January 1946, the new constitution of the Soviet Socialist Federal Republic of Yugoslavia was modeled after Soviet socialism. Yugoslavia was considered a Soviet socialist satellite until schism developed (from ~1948 to 1955) from what is called the "Tito-Stalin split" (1948). After Stalin died (1953), Nikita Khrushchev began mending the split between Yugoslav socialism and Soviet socialism.

In 1950, Stalin and Soviet socialism declared the Viet Minh to be the government of Vietnam. At Stalin's direction, French socialists/communists joined Stalin's work to impose socialism in Vietnam. The work to add Vietnam to the list of socialist hellholes attracted many young Cambodians, including Pol Pot (Sar). In 1951, Pol Pot (Sar) joined the Cercle Marxiste ("Marxist circle"), which had taken control of the Khmer Student's Association that same year. Within a few months, Sar joined the French Communist Party and thereby joined the work of Stalin and Soviet socialism again.

Pol Pot imposed Soviet-inspired socialism in Cambodia via the Khmer Rouge (KR), which was formed in 1968. The KR flag (a red field with a yellow hammer and sickle) was a sycophantic variation on the flag of the Union of Soviet Socialist Republics. It is another reason why the hammer and sickle should be as reviled as the hooked cross (both symbols were used under Soviet socialism).

KR (1968-1979) began as an offshoot of the Vietnam People's Army from North Vietnam, and allied with North Vietnam, and the Viet Cong.

Pol Pot's birth name "Sar" referenced his fair complexion ("Sar" means "white" in Khmer). In French, "Rouge" means "Red." The Khmer are the predominant ethnic group in Cambodia. Pol Pot exemplified how socialism, by definition, is bigotry and racism that perceives individuals only as members of groups (e.g. "classes") who have to be told what to do, and how to work and live.

Nosy socialists with the red flags hated the fact that the only color that matters is green (or gold) under capitalism. So many lives would have been spared if the reds had been greens and golds.

Pol Pot and the Khmer Rouge openly attacked Chinese, Vietnamese, and even their partially Khmer offspring for extinction; Some people with partial Chinese or Vietnamese ancestry were part of the Khmer Rouge system and were purged or part of ethnic cleansing campaigns.

The Khmer Rouge violently forced urban populations into rural agricultural socialism. The death toll of serfs was so large it was referred to as the socialist "Killing Fields." It is estimated that two million Cambodians, over a quarter of the population, died during the four horrifying years of KR socialism. KR tried to transform Cambodia into a "classless society" by depopulating cities. It was learned from Soviet socialist iNsaNiTy.

In 2017, one of the Khmer Rouge's top surviving leaders (Khieu Samphan, 84) said he had only fought for "social justice" in Cambodia. He fought for it using the baton rouge against skulls. He described himself as an "intellectual." The Social Justice Warrior was convicted of committing crimes against humanity in 2014 and sentenced to life in prison.

Soviet socialists continued the forced colonization policies that they shared with German socialists, even after Hitler was defeated. Soviet socialism's forced settlements took several forms. A notorious example was the Gulag labor camp system of penal labor (a penal colony within the larger Soviet penal colony). Resettling of entire categories of population was imposed under Soviet socialism. Involuntary settlement was used in the colonization of remote areas of the USSR. Soviet socialism used forced deportation where its pal Hitler had desired to use it: Ukraine.

After German socialism ended, Soviet socialism's ethnic cleansing continued. The USSR imposed homogenous territories. Some of the casualties were ethnic Germans (as had been established at the Potsdam Conference). Many others were Poles, Ukrainians, Hungarians, Crimean Tatars, and Chechens. Victims were forced onto train boxcars and shipped elsewhere resulting in millions of deaths by disease and starvation. As under German socialism, the actions had widespread support.

In 1945, Hitler's final democide was himself. Socialism is suicide. Yet, the socialist nightmare in East Germany continued until the Revolutions of 1989 against socialist regimes (ending Soviet socialism there).

Dear Socialism,
You lost again.
Sincerely,
Economics

Soviet socialism's house of cards collapsed in 1991 along with its hammer and sickle, symbols of old back-breaking manual labor,™ obsolete tools in the west that were replaced by capitalism's modern machines, robotics, and automation.

Soviet socialism was a sad reminder of the etymological relationship of the word "Slav" and the English word "slave."[121] Hitler used forms of the words "Slav" and "slave" many times in his books in apparent ignorance of the relationship. "Slave" is the source of, or the origin of the meaning of, the words "serve" and "serf" (people who serve) and is probably related to the word "Serb" (Serbs trace their history to migrating Slavs).

The word "Slav" includes places where many died under Soviet socialism and German socialism: Ukraine and the Caucasus (the last word being "Slavic" and the origin of the word "Caucasian," so that the word "slave" originated from Caucasians and other Slavs who were enslaved).[122] The word "slav" appears in the names of many people and places including Vyacheslav Molotov of the Hitler-Stalin pact infamy. Stalin was from

---

[121] Under socialism, the cliché "I have a right to food, shelter, schools, healthcare, etc." translates as "I have a right to force you to provide to me food, shelter, schools, healthcare, etc."

[122] For Slavs the term "Slav" is defined as "Glory." It is no surprise that they do not ascribe the English meaning of "slave" to their label.

The USSR dictated the manufacture of a timepiece bearing the name "SLAVA." Thus, wristwatches were built by socialist slaves under dictates of socialist slavery and it was named "slava." Eventually, the USSR realized the negative connotations of the watch's name in the West. The name was changed to "Craba." In Cyrillic, the word "slavs" is "славянин."

Georgia (in the Caucasus region), and his ancestors had a long history of slavery before Stalin expanded slavery there and elsewhere. German socialism aspired to re-enslave the Slavs and Serbs, and Soviet socialism did so where German socialism failed.

Slavery under Stalin, Mao, Hitler (SMH) and every socialist mortacracy far exceeded slavery in the U.S. in the 1800s. SMH and other socialist hate groups added the abominable behavior of murdering so many of their slaves (their kill rates alone far exceeded the number of slaves who worked in the U.S. in the 1800s). Socialism is slavery (capitalism is self-ownership).

The German socialist Karl Marx openly touted dictatorship and mass murder to impose dictatorship. "Dictatorship of the proletariat" was his term. "The very cannibalism of the counterrevolution will convince the nations that there is only one way in which the murderous death agonies of the old society and the bloody birth throes of the new society can be shortened, simplified and concentrated: revolutionary terror," said Marx ("The Victory of the Counter-Revolution in Vienna," Neue Rheinische Zeitung, No. 136, November 1848).[123]

Marx inspired the socialists Stalin, Mao, Hitler and

---

[123] During his life, the young Marx often wondered why time travelers from the future were trying to kill him. Marx said so in an interview performed by two women who summoned his spirit through an Ouija board. Both women died shortly thereafter under mysterious circumstances.

Some modern horror movies appear to be inspired by Marx's book "The Communist Manifesto." A dusty old book is discovered by some hot teenagers; the yellowed pages contain strange predictions and seem written by a madman; suddenly lots of gruesome deaths begin to occur just as the words foretold. How can it be stopped?!

their ilk. Stalin and Hitler worked together. Stalin and Mao worked together. Both couples exhibited 2 girls 1 cup socialism. The three of them together were the sickest ménage à trois ever. [romantic music playing]. Thank goodness that no videotape was made of the trio.

The only book co-authored by Stalin and Mao extolls self-sacrifice and is entitled "To Serve Man." It is a socialist cook book. One of the recipes is for soylent green.[124] Don't order dishes made from "soy with green curry." Nor red curry. Do not eat curry. Preeze!

True cannibalism was caused by socialism, especially under Stalin and Mao. Socialists proved that you can't stop cannibals by eating them. Stalin, Mao, the Kim gang, and their ilk, groomed their people to be food kind-of-sewers. They discovered that Marx's book "The Communist Manifesto" is actually a weight-loss program (How to lose 50 kilos and 50,000 people in one month or less). Everyone feasted on cognitive dissonance.

It was like the Donner party multiplied by thousands. Sometimes it was a "family feast." Jonathan Swift's "A Modest Proposal" was no longer satire; it was reality. Socialism imposes womb-to-tomb care, and it's often an expedited trip. As Marx said "from each according to his ability, to each according to his need." Starving adults have insatiable need.

---

[124] In news on 12/12/2017, Ji Hyeon-A of North Korea said the bodies of inmates who had starved to death were fed to prison dogs (to save the dogs from starvation). This explains another part of this book asking why no pet dogs are visible in documentaries about N Korea: The dogs are at the prisons eating human corpses due to chronic shortages of dog food.

More things not seen in documentaries about North Korea: regular cemeteries (not the two propaganda/war cemeteries for "show").

When a socialist says he wants to have you over for dinner, he means it literally. *takes out knife and fork* Stalin, Mao, and Kim don't want socialists with good taste, but socialists who taste good! We the sheeple. You're what's for dinner. [BURP!] It was the socialist apocalypse of zombies although more than brains were eaten.[125]

Don't order Mao's version of the dish "La Lechonera." It's not pork. The meat is marinated in the tears of socialists. It tastes like sadness. It led to China's one-child policy. Be careful when they ask "Do you prefer dark meat or white meat?" That is a red flag.

Mao's little red recipe book was exported to North Koreans (Norks).[126] A popular recipe was reprinted in a Nork newspaper's cooking column authored by a thin woman known as the "Barefoot Comrade" (because she has no shoes). The columnist (Shoeless Ina Nogarten), described how to gather and chew the roots of wild grass (published in Rodong Sinmun, the official newspaper of the monopoly Workers' Party, 2016).[127] "Watch out! I

---

[125] Socialists are Zombies because they live off the ideas (brains) of others (capitalists). They have to in order to survive.

[126] Anyone who is a fan of films depicting dystopias can actually experience one in North Korea.

[127] In the USA, the FDA pretends to dictate food safety. In reality, the FDA explicitly allows "rat hairs" and "insect parts" in food, with maximum permitted levels. The FDA merely mimics the market, because economics sets the standards; food can only be cleaned so much. If the FDA dictated zero tolerance for rat hairs and insect parts, then no one would be allowed to eat anything. Home-cooking would also be banned.

Under Mao's socialism people ate rats and insects. They continue to do so in North Korea and other socialist countries. Even the rats starve (if they are not eaten first). One socialist

pooped over there." Life doesn't seem as crappy when you realize that 1 out of 3 people in the world don't have access to a toilet.

If you are strolling about North Korea and you happen upon a hotdog stand just keep walking. Their wieners do not contain beef, pork, or chicken.

Things not seen in documentaries about life in North Korea: cats, dogs,[128] handicapped people, slow children. Comrade detective knows what happened to the cats and dogs; but the handicapped people...?

You've heard the joke about "What is a virgin in Alabama?" In North Korea, all the children in the documentaries can outrun their neighbors.

Stalin and Mao discovered how to reduce poverty: kill poor people. Socialists are so greedy that they will literally let people starve to death in the streets. Socialism causes economic death too. Socialists learned that it is easier (and cheaper) to kill millions than it is to control millions. Eating is so petit bourgeois! Anything above subsistence living is bougie.

---

complained that capturing rats was difficult because "everybody was trying to trap rats." That is why Stalin, Mao, and the Kim criminals are known as the "Rat Pack." If USA food cleanliness and health standards had been imposed upon Mao's China (and much of today's world) many people would die because they would not be allowed to eat, as no food that they had would meet prevailing free market standards in the USA.

[128] Documentaries that purport to "expose" N Korea overlook the absence of dogs and cats ...strange omissions. On the web are fun reviews of the "Super Excellent Fun Time Dog of Weiner Stand," and "Li'l Kims Little Boat Rental," alongside other tourist traps in Pyongyang that you can supplement. Internet satellite views of N Korea reveal carless streets and boatless rivers (certainly no yacts or pleasure crafts).

If you are served something that you suspect contains protein in a socialist country, it is best not to ask "What's in it?" They use seven secret Herbs (men named "Herb") and spices. Socialists: they'll make chicken shit out of chicken salad. Don't visit socialist countries if your favorite animal is steak.

Mao was another reason for those jokes about neighborhood cats missing around Chinese restaurants in the USA.[129] Don't order "Chairman Meow's Chicken." It's not poultry. If your waitress asks "Do you like to eat pussy?" be suspicious; even if she is a cute little commie.

Socialism starts with utopian lies about a wealthy future; ends with people eating their pets (e.g. Venezuela under Maduro). The dogma tastes like it wasn't properly refrigerated. That's because they don't have refrigerators nor consistent electricity to power them.

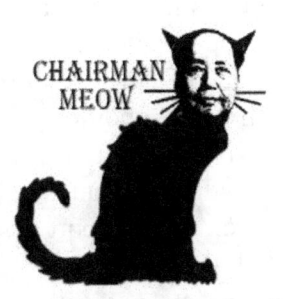

A popular food is curried chicken. Under capitalism, there is a different connotation (a non-food connotation) for the equestrian phrase "curry a horse." But under Mao's socialism, you curry a horse the same way you curry a chicken.

CHAIRMAN MEOW

---

[129] While millions starved in China, the USA's capitalists enjoyed thriving Chinese restaurants (owned and operated by Chinese immigrants). They satiated non-socialist bellies all over America.

It can be lethal to dine at any overly "authentic" Chinese restaurant that adheres to Mao's food service socialism. Imagine being forced to pay a restaurant whether or not they bring you food. Their fortune cookies contain death threats.

[Horse whinnies].

Socialists use a secret ingredient: spicy hot hate. If you swallow the dogma you will be hungry again in an hour. Marxists are gluttons for punishment. Nothing removes the bitter taste of socialism from your mouth like food.

While in Victorian Manchester, the German socialist Friedrich Engels concocted his meretricious "social murder" phrase. The term "social murder" does better at describing the crime visited upon children who starved to death or were cannibalized under socialism, or whose limbs were mangled by collectivized factory machines, or whose parents were killed in purges and camps. Murder and manslaughter were committed by individuals, but these atrocities were something else: what is called "socialism murder" or social murder.

"When society places hundreds of proletarians in such a position that they inevitably meet a too early and an unnatural death, one which is quite as much a death by violence as that by the sword or bullet; its deed is murder just as surely as the deed of the single individual," Engels wrote in 1845, in The Condition of the Working Class in England.[130] That is socialism's murders. Over 170 years later, socialism remains a dogma that murders its poor and more. Any support of

---

[130] "…Engels' 1842 Condition of the Working Class was outdated even in his own lifetime. Originally written as a warning to a German readership, the English edition did not appear until almost 50 years later; in his 1892 preface, Engels himself noted how 'the most crying abuses described in this book have either disappeared or have been made less conspicuous…'. Yet now it is quoted as if it were a news report from Grenfell Tower." – Mick Hume, 20 July 2017.

Such labels as "working class" are the inventions of bourgeois Marxist wastrels.

socialism, higher taxes/spending, and a larger state, is violence backed by murder.

"But we can have our stateless utopia only after we institute a dictatorship of the proletariat!" they said.

Stalin, Mao, Hitler, and other socialists know that it is easier to regurgitate anti-capitalist clichés than to start your own business and make it successful enough to employ workers. To wave a placard and shout "DOWN WITH CAPITALISM" is easy; to write and launch a business plan that makes profits is not easy. It's easier to destroy someone else's life's earnings than to work for your own. The business model of socialism is theft and fraud.

SMH are the political version of that one contestant on The Bachelor who makes up a stupid job so that he doesn't have to write "unemployed." It is funny how people who demand socialism did not contribute much to society to begin with. Those guys were criminals and not even the good kind of criminals who sell drugs, sex, and stuff.

Socialists, as their name declares, hate individualists; socialism opposes individualism. Socialists want everyone to be "equal" and they use force to make it happen, even if they must kill people who socialists think are not willing or able to be "equal."

It is important to remember all the deaths in the socialist Wholecaust (of which the Holocaust was a part) under Stalin, Mao, and Hitler (and others). That is something that Snyder does not want to talk about directly.

Snyder's book fails to analyze "socialism" as the political philosophy of both Hitler and Stalin, and the similarities and differences between how they used the word in their monotonous speeches and writings. His lectures perpetuate this shortcoming.

No historian can earn a grade of "A+" if his descriptions of Hitler and Stalin (and Mao et cetera) do not include their political philosophy of "socialism" and how they touted the word as their ideology. It is an issue of intellectual dishonesty. If you trust government, then you should have failed history.

Snyder probably likes the stale argument that the socialists Stalin, Mao, Hitler, Mussolini and others were not socialists because if they were all socialists then they would not have attacked each other and killed millions of others. If a group of people share a dogma (socialism) that preaches, "We lie, rob, and kill to gain more power," then there is no inconsistency in their dogma when they attack each other. They were dedicated socialists. A quote that is often misattributed to Lenin (or Stalin, or Hitler, or Mao) is: "The capitalists will sell us the rope with which we will hang each other." Socialists have a long history of killing and purging their own. That is the trademark of socialism.™

It is a reminder of the argument that Hitler was not a "true" socialist because he did not kill enough people to be a "true" socialist (on the scale of "true" socialists such as Stalin and Mao, with their higher death tolls). Stalin killed more socialists (and "communists") than Hitler killed. Mao killed more socialists (and "communists") than Hitler killed.

The counter-argument is: If Lenin, Stalin, and Mao were socialists (or Communists, or Marxists), then Hitler was a socialist (or Communist, or Marxist). They all killed at such high rates that they belong in the same damning category.

Stalin, Mao, and Hitler are often separated for analysis. Is there moral equivalence? No, there is no moral equivalence. Just do the math. One side of the equation robbed, persecuted, starved, and killed many millions more (and for longer periods of time) than the other socialist side (and some of the math is tricky, such as the moral equivalence weight when Stalin and Hitler were partners starting WWII together).

Snyder claims that Ayn Rand (Alice or Alisa Rosenbaum),[131] who fled Soviet socialism, believed that competition was the meaning of life itself. Snyder claims that the socialist Hitler said "much the same thing" (?). Such reductionism by Snyder, although temptingly elegant, is fatal. It was fatal to millions under the archsocialists Hitler, Stalin, Mao, et cetera.

Snyder did not reveal what Stalin and Mao said about competition. Snyder hides how Stalin, Mao, and Hitler championed "socialism" by the very word, and Rand did

---

[131] Rand suffered socialism from Germany and Russia. Before 1917, the Rosenbaums were subject to bigotry (anti-Semitic laws, the threat of pogroms) under Tsar Nicholas. But the worst bigotry came from the new socialist cult after 1917; under Tsar Lenin, armed soldiers stole her father Fronz's pharmacy. In 1924, Rand and many other "bourgeois" students were purged from the university shortly before graduating (After outside complaints, many of the purged students were allowed to graduate, which Rand did in October 1924). Lenin shifted from regicide to genocide. In 1926, Rand had the good sense to flee the USSR. She became another socialism survivor. In the 1930s she unsuccessfully tried to help her family escape from Tsar Stalin. She later learned that her parents died during the siege of Leningrad by German socialists during the war that Soviet socialists had started as allies with German socialists (WWII). Conditions became as bad as Rand portrays them in her novel "We the Living." Compare Rand's (and her family's) plight to that of Raoul Wallenberg and Jan Wiener mentioned elsewhere in this book.

the opposite. Rand debunked them, just as her work debunks Snyder.

The socialists Hitler, Stalin, Mao and all socialists believe that competition is bad, and thus capitalism is bad, and both must be eliminated. Socialists who believe that Jews are capitalists want to eliminate Jews. Socialists eliminate Jews either by killing them or by banning their religion (as did the socialists Stalin, Mao, and Hitler).

German socialists emphasized the terms "Jews" and "capitalists" as enemies, while Soviet socialists emphasized the term "capitalists" (it was broad enough and could encompass all who were disliked). All socialists hate capitalists for the same reason that German socialists hate/hated capitalists (AND Jews): for their ostensible virtues; they were too intelligent, too clever, too good at business, too rich, too influential, too cosmopolitan, too thrifty, too committed to their own way.

Snyder is brainwashed with the absurd left/right political spectrum that is taught in government schools (socialist schools). The military march of authoritarian soldiers: "Left! Right! Left! Right!"

Snyder falls for the current fad of all socialists: climate change (global warming?). "A problem that is truly planetary in scale, such as climate change, obviously demands global solutions -and one apparent solution is to define a global enemy" (Black Earth, page 327). Snyder suggests the same enemies (capitalists) who were named by the militant socialists Stalin, Mao, Hitler, and named by every other socialist (including all socialists today).

Socialists believe there is a pie of goods and everyone must fight for those goods by taking them from others.[132] They dress up their violence and theft with the terms "taxation," and "socialism," and "fOr tHe gOOd oF aLL." That old socialist lie works well with "climate change" where the pie becomes the entire planet.

In his ecological panic, Snyder discusses China, comparing its current behavior to that of Germany under Hitler. It is intellectually dishonest how Snyder evades any mention of love for the word "socialism" by China's government and Germany's government (under Hitler). It reveals more about Snyder than it does about Chinese socialism and German socialism.

Snyder is everything he accuses others of being. Similar to smug socialist dictators, Snyder knows all about "climate change" and how to use socialism to force the "fix" on everyone.

And what are some fixes? The list will neglect to include "commit suicide"; and "kill one or more of your children" (how many cat credits do you gain as carbon offsets per child eliminated?). How about "re-impose Chinese socialism's old one-child policy" (first and

---

[132] Socialism is worse than "zero sum." Socialism is negative sum. Forcibly moving capital from more productive use to less or counter-productive use destroys value. It also creates the tragedy of the commons.

foremost, control and limit the reproductive rights of women)? Clone Stalin, Mao, and Hitler? Time travel to Olduvai Gorge at 3 million BC and kill Lucy (the CLIMATE has CHANGED since then).

Climate totalitarians claim that 97% of scientists and most of the civilized world agrees with them. If so, they can all solve the problem merely by committing suicide. They can leave everyone else unmolested. But they don't love the planet THAT much. None of them have the integrity to fully commit to their 1984ish ideology.

Snyder and his fellow-travelers are a reminder of King Canute and the waves. People who cannot provide accurate weather forecasts two weeks into the future are now providing weather forecasts decades, even centuries, into the future (and, better yet, they promise to CONTROL the weather, if only they gain ever more money and power).

They rehash the Bible story of the Great Flood, in which God "destroyed all living things which were on the face of the ground: both man and cattle, creeping thing and bird of the air." It is a repeat of the Akkadian poem of Gilgamesh with a similar myth of angry gods flooding the Earth. An apocalyptic deluge plays a prominent part in the Hindu Dharmasastra too.

If you don't like the earth's climate, just wait a millisecond and it will change. It has been changing constantly forever. Earth has existed for ~4600 million years. Geologic time units are (in order of descending specificity) eons, eras, periods, epochs, and ages. Those millions of years (e.g. the dinosaur period) show that extinctions are common. Nature sucks. With capitalism, humans avoid or delay the non-stop death and destruction of nature.[133]

This is Snyder's trite insight: "We" have to "do something" about "insert current excuse here - CLIMATE CHANGE" (when what he really means is he loves government and wants to impose massive government intervention on everyone everywhere immediately).

The chicken-littles of global warming want great leaders. Dare they ask WWHD? WWSD? WWMD? (What would the socialists Hitler, Stalin, and Mao do?) They were "great leaders" of huge areas of the earth and adept at "rallying" their people to action.

Snyder's climate change cliché is a sad reminder of the old socialist excuse for millions who starved to death: "bad weather." It was a bad spell of weather from the World Storm (Weltsturm) forecast by Meteorologist Marx. Whether you would survive the storm of socialism was the question. Hurricanes, earthquakes, tsunamis, and other disasters are minor compared to the most destructive force in the world: Government.

There was severe "environmental change" suffered under Stalin, Mao, Hitler, (SMH) et cetera. At that time the problem was "global cooling" when millions of human bodies reached room temperature (genuine AGC... Anthropogenic Global Cooling). Some eco-nuts applaud the socialist Wholecaust for aiding "Mother Earth."

Now the old socialist excuse for killing millions has been updated: "bad weather caused by capitalism." Snyder's solution: we don't have enough socialism yet! Total bliss is just one more regulation away.

---

[133] If earth's history is not depressing enough, note that as of this writing Wakipedia (Wikipedia) contains (under the heading: Lists of Time Periods) "Marxian stages of history." Read it and weep.

Climate alarmists are watermelons: Green on the outside, red on the inside. Many of them sound like Unabomber Ted Kaczynski (or like Lynette Alice "Squeaky" Fromme during her pro se defense at her trial).

"Climate change" is a synonym for "capitalism." Socialist conspiracy nuts want to stop climate change (capitalism). That is what all socialists want to do. Hitler said much the same thing. The difference is that Hitler actually glorified the word "socialism." All the time.

Which one impoverishes, enslaves, robs, tortures, and kills more people: socialism or "climate change" (capitalism)?

For his "climate change" façade, Snyder never blames "late stage socialism" (a phrase that works great as a caption for all New Yorker cartoons). He does not fault socialism for socialized roads and for the interstate highway system where the U.S. government used military-socialism as its tardy excuse for following the socialist Hitler and his Autobahn. Snyder's response would be the stale socialist whine "BuT wHo wiLL bUIld muh rOAdz?!?!"

Snyder never blames all the socialist monopolies created and imposed by socialists: socialism's history of electricity monopolies, phone monopolies, road monopolies, utility monopolies. His silence indicates that he thinks socialist monopolies are grand and all fault lies elsewhere.

Change alarmists are being conned. Some capitalists want government to discriminate in their favor and against their competitors -other capitalists. That is what ALL socialism does. Socialism singles out favored industries to be promoted and supported by government against challengers. They make some capitalists rich (at the expense of others) selling books, buildings, software, hardware, medical equipment and more. That includes government schools, welfare programs, mandatory health insurance, and all government action. Programs to "combat climate change" are no different.

Capitalists thrive when socialists throw money at "alternative energy" and "clean technology" and "power conservation products." Some businesses and their politicians only push green politics so they can move high-pollution production overseas for pennies. Socialists are dupes. Socialism is big business.

Similar to socialists, Snyder repeats the vague myth of the "business cycle." He has no comment on the "socialism cycle." Which one impoverishes, enslaves, robs, tortures, and kills more people: his undefined "business cycle" or the well-documented "socialism cycle"? The kleptomaniacs Stalin, Mao, and Hitler provide all the top examples of "Extraordinary Popular Delusions and the Madness of Crowds" even though they were born too late to appear in the older 1841 book with that title by author Charles Mackay (SMH do take top spots in the updated 2017 version of Mackay's book).

Nothing compares to the speculative bubble (or economic bubble) of socialism. No one died during the "Tulip Mania" myth. The socialism cycle holds all the worst world records for mass slaughter. What is Snyder's prescription for the "socialism cycle"?

Anarcho-Capitalism isn't utopian; believing that a tiny percentage of the population can make the best decisions for each individual is utopian.

Socialists are big winners of Darwin Awards: the recognition given to those "who improve our gene pool by removing themselves from it in a spectacularly stupid manner."[134] Darwin Awards commemorate those who perish through some "astonishing misapplications of judgment." The Union of Soviet Socialist Republics was one of the early winners of the epsilon-minus "Honor" in 1917. The Soviets, Germany, and China distinguished themselves with their masochistic drunk history and epic fails. *Slow clap*

Stalin, Mao, and Hitler were also the World's Dumbest Criminals. Socialism shat on the world. Their victims shant be forgotten.

Stalin, Mao, and the Kim scum were trapped on their devolving Galapagos. Socialists prefer being depicted as homicidal evil geniuses rather than overpromoted student council morons. Socialism demonstrates that stupidity is expensive and deadly.[135] Cognitive dissonance is one hell of a drug!

Darwin Awards go hand-in-hand (as if they were conjoined S-letters for "socialism" in the swastika) with

---

[134] For more on socialism's nihilistic "Death Wish" see The Socialist Phenomenon by Igor Shafarevich. It explains how totalitarian collectivism (socialism) has been found in large societies (e.g. Mayans, Incas, Ur, ancient Egyptians) throughout world history.

Pol Pot and his favored Khmer Rouge (KR) comrades were envious of the achievements of the 12th-century Hindu dynasty that constructed the temple area of Angkor Wat and built complex irrigation methods. The KR believed that their work was similar and more important. Angkor Wat remains Cambodia's top sightseeing location; the next most popular attractions are morbid: Tuol Sleng (a KR genocide museum) and the Killing Fields at Choeung Ek, where so many KR serfs were tortured and killed by retarded socialist sadists.

[135] When you are dead, you don't know that you're dead. All the pain is felt by others. The same thing happens when you are stupid.

the Big Whopper Liars Contest. Stalin, Mao, and Hitler were repeat recipients year after year for a long time. Socialists never let the truth get in the way of a shocking story.

Socialism is a big part in the field of agnotology (the study of the spread of ignorance). Agnotology is the study of willful acts to spread confusion and deceit, usually to steal more money (taxation) or to increase the size of government (socialism).

Socialism spread to Germany, Russia and elsewhere with help from the American socialists Francis and Edward Bellamy. Edward's obituary included this: "It is stated that Emperor William purchased 1,000 copies of 'Looking Backward,' which he distributed among the students and working classes of Germany." (obituary dateline Springfield, Mass., May 22, 1898, "The Author of 'Looking Backward' has Passed Away").

Socialism spread from Francis Bellamy at the World's Fair from May 1893 to October 30, 1893, in Chicago. At that fair, the German firm Krupp had a pavilion of artillery (which cost approximately one million dollars).

In January 1892, in preparation for the World's Columbian Fair, the Youth's Companion magazine assigned Francis Bellamy to be manager for the National Public School Celebration of Columbus Day on October 11, 1892.

Columbus Day commemorates the explorer Christopher Columbus in a country named after Amerigo Vespucci, who exposed Columbus' mistaken belief that Columbus had visited Asia or India. In 1492, Native Americans discovered Columbus lost at sea. The country had been previously "discovered" by Leif Erikson and plenty of others, including the aborigines (the 1925 film "The Vanishing American" shows Native Americans being taught the Nazi salute and Bellamy's humiliating chant in a government school).

The Columbus Day holiday inspired Bellamy to write his "Address for Columbus Day" entitled "The Meaning of the Four Centuries," which was part of the program that included the pledge for the Youth's Companion Magazine. Bellamy was hired by James B. Upham's uncle-by-marriage, Daniel S. Ford, to work for the popular magazine where Upham already worked. Upham and Bellamy collaborated to write the pledge.

Upham and Ford were aware of Francis Bellamy's Christian Socialist dogma before Bellamy was hired. Bellamy was a vice president of the Christian Society of Socialists. Bellamy was involved in so much radicalism and subversion that he was forced out of the ministry of his Boston church for his socialist sermons, including topics like "Jesus the Socialist."

The Pledge of Allegiance was a small part of a much larger program (authored and/or supervised by Bellamy) in the Youth's Companion magazine. The larger program included a reference to Rome. The program also included hymns, prayers, and various references to the Bible and God (including the phrase "under God") and more to tie socialism to the cross and Christianity. It was socialism as a religion.

Prayers, hymns, and references to God have never ended in government (socialist) schools, because they are now the Pledge of Allegiance. The pledge compels Americans to worship God and government at the same time.

It is hard to believe that some people object to the pledge only on the grounds of the two-word deification (added in 1954). Some argue falsely that Bellamy would have objected to the phrase and imply that Bellamy was an atheist. People who object only to the two-word deification "under God" are strange and fail to see the forest because they are staring at a single sick tree.

Do not deify government: Defy government.

Bellamy's dogma was the same argument used later by German Christians under Hitler's socialism and under Germany's hooked cross (see Gerhard Hahn, Christuskreuz und Hakenkreuz, Schriftenreihe der "Deutschen Christen" Hannovers, Nr. 1 (1934)). In the German churches, the Christian Cross was next to the Hooked Cross. In American churches, the Christian Cross was (and is) next to the U.S. flag, whose pledge was the origin of the Nazi salute, and whose perfunctory drone continues today.

Another ominous parallel between the German socialist Adolf Hitler and the American socialist Francis Bellamy is that they were both doing what socialists do: using government to make money. Bellamy promoted government schools (socialist schools) in order to sell flags; Hitler was using government to sell his un-sellable book. China's Mao was similar with his "little red book."[136]

The eerie part is that Bellamy's scheme has not stopped. It seems impossible to know how much money the government spends to put U.S. flags (made in China) in government (socialist) schools for the creepy ritual that spawned the Nazi salute and Nazi behavior.

---

[136] Mao pretended to hate property rights (other than his own), so his book was also known by the title "Steal This Book." Instead, the book (and other Mao swag) was outrageously expensive for Chinese serfs. Play stupid games, win stupid prizes. Outside China it was known by the title "Mao's Little-Read Book."

An even bigger number is the outrageous amount of stolen money the government takes to monopolize education. That is another ominous parallel between German socialism and American socialism.

Bellamy's plan to spread his dogma globally was boosted when Bellamy became chairman of a committee to form a World Congress of Youth at the Columbia Exposition in Chicago in 1893. The World's Youth Congress Auxiliary (or World Congress Auxiliary) asked The Youth's Companion magazine (where Francis Bellamy worked) to organize the scheme. A. F. Nightingale was president of the Youth's World Congress. More details are provided in a newspaper article, "Youths at the World's Fair," from the Daily Gleaner on August 22, 1892 ("The Gleaner" continues to publish in Jamaica and states that it was established in 1834). The article explains that the congress would be composed of youths of all nations of the World (and many countries are listed including Germany, Russia, Italy, France and "countries of the Orient"). The youths will "stand before the generation to follow us as witnesses of the humanizing power of the World's Exposition of 1893, and be inspired by its influence to higher and more useful careers, making the fulfillment of its great promises their noblest claim to history." The "humanizing power" that Bellamy brought to the World's Exposition of 1893 (and the fulfillment of Bellamy's "noblest" claim to history) was the Nazi salute and servile chanting to flags daily in military formation in government schools (socialist schools).

The "Brotherhood of man" cliché that is used in the newspaper article was a popular cliché with the international Theosophical Society, which promoted the dogma of Francis Bellamy and Edward Bellamy. The

Theosophical Society also utilized the swastika to promote its socialist dogma.

Bellamy's international aspiration for his World Youth Congress is one of the reasons why Bellamy's original pledge did not reference the "flag of the United States of America." Bellamy wrote his pledge so that it could be adopted by other countries. He wanted to spread military socialism worldwide.

In 1901, Bellamy traveled to Rome, Italy, and met with King Victor Emmanuel III, the man who would appoint as Prime Minister of Italy the long-time socialist leader Mussolini.

Bellamy's scheme to use school children and government schools (socialist schools) to impose totalitarian socialism became a disturbing socialist tactic. Socialists demonstrate the old platitude "Those who can't do, teach." It should be added that "Those who can't teach, teach socialism."

Socialists are gold diggers. Violent gold diggers. The worst form of greed and selfishness is not capitalism, it is socialism (and people who condemn socialism as "selfish" completely misunderstand exactly why socialism is bad).

Did those "coming leaders of mankind" from Bellamy's World Youth Congress include greedy freeloaders who became supporters of the archsocialists Stalin, Mao, Hitler, and Mussolini?

11. KARL MARX & ADOLF HITLER

This chapter contains a list of words and excerpts that shed light on the police state touted by the socialist Hitler in Mein Kampf. Much can be learned from how often some words were used, and about other words that were not used at all.

Startling similarities exist between Hitler and those other notorious German socialists Karl Marx and Friedrich Engels. The following is a review of the books of all three authors simultaneously:

"The angry German ranting of an obscure, small-party socialist, his work was virtually ignored when it was originally published. It is full of anger, hatred, bigotry, and self-aggrandizing. It is the political equivalent of a mean girl's burn book. The work is saddled with tortured prose, meandering narrative, and child-like economics.[137] The author details the means by which his party can gain power. Most people who read it dismissed it as nonsense, not

---

[137] "If socialists understood economics, they wouldn't be socialists" -Friedrich von Hayek.

None of the books pass the Bechdel test.

believing that anyone could -or would- carry out its radical, terrorist programs. Had the author been taken seriously when he was first published, perhaps the 20th century would have been very different. It is foolish to think that the mass slaughter could not happen again, especially if World War II and its horrors are forgotten. If you want to learn about why the world's worst carnage happened, you can't avoid reading the words of the man who was most responsible for it happening. The author, therefore, must be read as a reminder that evil can all too easily grow."

"On The Jewish Question" by Marx was written in 1843, and first published in Paris in 1844 as "Zur Judenfrage" in Marx's own Deutsch–Französische Jahrbücher. In it Marx draws on the stereotype of the Jew as a financially savvy "huckster" and imagines a special connection between Judaism as a religion and "bourgeois" economics. After equating "practical Judaism" with "huckstering and money," Marx argues that "the Christians have become Jews" and that it is mankind (both Christians and Jews) that needs to emancipate itself from Judaism.

Bernard Lewis has described Marx's screed as "one of the classics of antisemitic propaganda." According to Hyam Maccoby, Marx argued that Judaism is a pseudo-religion whose god is money. Some scholars say that Marx considered Jews to be the embodiment of capitalism (anti-socialism) and therefore evil.

The following excerpts from "On The Jewish Question," are often cited as evidence of Marx's antisemitism:

Let us consider the actual, worldly Jew – not the Sabbath Jew, as Bauer does, but the everyday Jew.

Let us not look for the secret of the Jew in his religion, but let us look for the secret of his religion in the real Jew.

What is the secular basis of Judaism? Practical need, self-interest. What is the worldly religion of the Jew? Huckstering. What is his worldly God? Money.

The Jew has emancipated himself in a Jewish manner, not only because he has acquired financial power, but also because, through him and also apart from him, money has become a world power and the practical Jewish spirit has become the practical spirit of the Christian nations. The Jews have emancipated themselves insofar as the Christians have become Jews.

In the final analysis, the emancipation of the Jews is the emancipation of mankind from Judaism...

The same Marxist conspiracy theory was used by German National Socialists to justify killing Anne Frank. It led to another conspiracy theory that proved to be true: the alliance of white supremacist socialism in Germany with Soviet socialism to launch WWII (perhaps the biggest conspiracy theory of that century that turned out to be true).

Marx's white supremacist socialism in "On the Jewish Question" (and in Marx's other works) is a reminder of Henry Ford's "The International Jew." It is likely that Marx influenced Ford.

Marx also influenced Hitler. Hitler wrote: "Everything men strive after as a higher goal, be it religion, **socialism**, democracy, is to the Jew only means to an end, the way to satisfy his lust for gold and domination." (Gemlich letter 1919. Emphasis added). Adolf Hitler's letter to Adolf Gemlich addressed the "Jewish question" 76 years after Marx did so in "On The Jewish Question." The Gemlich letter might be the earliest example of the influence of Marx's anti-Semitism upon Hitler.

Dr. Walter Williams, an economist and author, pointed out that in a letter from Marx to Engels, in reference to his socialist political competitor Ferdinand Lassalle, Marx wrote:

"It is now completely clear to me that he, as is proved by his cranial formation and his hair, descends from the Negroes who had joined Moses' exodus from Egypt, assuming that his mother or grandmother on the paternal side had not interbred with a nigger. Now this union of Judaism and Germanism with a basic Negro substance must produce a peculiar product. The obtrusiveness of the fellow is also nigger-like."

Play that funky music, Marx boy! For Marx, red was the new black. Engels shared Marx's racial philosophy, according to Dr. Williams: In 1887, Paul Lafargue, who was Marx's son-in-law, was a candidate for a council seat in a Paris district that contained a zoo. Engels claimed that Lafargue had "one-eighth or one-twelfth nigger blood." In a letter to Lafargue's wife, Engels wrote:

"Being in his quality as a nigger, a degree nearer to the rest of the animal kingdom than the rest of us, he is undoubtedly the most appropriate representative of that district."

Marx and Engels made reference to the socialist Wholecaust and to the smaller Holocaust (which was a part of the larger destruction). Whereas his forebears carried whiteness like an ancestral talisman, Marx cracked the glowing amulet open, releasing its eldritch energies.

"The classes and the races too weak to master the new conditions of life must give way." – Karl Marx, "Forced emigration" (March 4, 1853).

Marx put the "ass" in "class." His self-righteous diatribe promoted the concept of Eugenics. The theory postulated a crisis of the gene pool. Marx and other bloodthirsty socialists wanted to know: Would the "best" human beings prevail over the inferior ones - the foreigners, immigrants, Jews, degenerates, the unfit, and the "feeble minded"?

Advocating socialism is much worse than advocating racism, according to many. Marx does both and shows how the two are in fact one. Racism is merely a form of collectivism, and Marx was all about collectivism. Marx's myopia viewed individuals as merely members of groups (e.g. classes, races) with stereotypical behaviors.

Marx fomented hatred of individuals/individuality, and he touted the socialist ideal of bigotry, prejudice, persecution of minorities, racism and nationalism, shadeism, colorism, extremism, class-power groups, identity politics, intolerance, anti-Semitism, collective guilt, political correctness, entitlement, objectification of everyone, genetic inferiority, race hustlers, tribalism, herd mentality, class nationalists and red nationalists, hate culture, inequality, terrorism, master races, ethnic classifications and ethnic rivalry, race-baiting and class-baiting, wars and civil wars, cultural upheaval, class economics, castes, violent revolution, self-righteousness, master plans, social ranking, groupthink, red privilege, class supremacy, and race supremacist movements (of every type), socialist supremacy, and the supreme socialist man. It led to the intersectional identity politics of non-binary transocialist redfluid panauthoritarians. Someone should do a master's thesis deconstructing socialist rhetoric.

As Barack Obama explained "No one is born hating another person because of the color of his skin or his background or his religion ... ," because one learns those things from evil people such as the socialists Marx, Lenin, Stalin, Mao, Hitler, Pol Pot, the Kim gang, et cetera. That noble message is magnified by a U.S. leader who killed lots of people, including innocent brown men, women, and children in foreign lands who were drone bombed.

There is no country in Europe which does not have in some corner or other one or several ruined fragments of peoples (Völkerruinen), the remnant of a former population that was suppressed and held in bondage by the nation which later became the main vehicle of historical development. These relics of a nation mercilessly trampled under foot in the course of history, as Hegel says, these racial trash always become fanatical standard-bearers of counter-

revolution and remain so until their complete extirpation or loss of their national character, just as their whole existence in general is itself a protest against a great historical revolution. -"The Magyar Struggle" by Engels in Marx's Neue Rheinische Zeitung (13 January 1849). The phrase "racial trash" (Völkerabfälle) is sometimes translated as "residual fragments of peoples" by critics who want to pretend there are no similarities between the German socialists Marx, Hitler, and Engels.

"The Austrian Germans and Magyars will be set free and wreak a bloody revenge on the Slav barbarians. The general war which will then break out will smash this Slav Sonderbund and wipe out all these petty hidebound nations, down to their very names. The next world war will result in the disappearance from the face of the earth not only of reactionary classes and dynasties, but also of entire reactionary peoples. And that, too, is a step forward." - "The Magyar [Hungarian] Struggle." Containing an apparent reference to WWI as a socialist war. The Slav Sonderbund (separate band) are lower than Marx's lumpenproletariat? Marx was all about bigoted name-calling, labeling, racism; and derogatory terms for all the "classes" (lower, middle, upper, and more) that he concocted. Marx promoted identity politics among socialists. As in, they want everyone to have the same identity. Theirs. They want to turn humanity into unanimity.

Among all the large and small nations of Austria, only three standard-bearers of progress took an active part in history, and still retain their vitality —

the Germans, the Poles and the Magyars.... All the other large and small nationalities and peoples are destined to perish before long in the revolutionary holocaust. -"The Magyar Struggle" by Engels in Marx's Neue Rheinische Zeitung. The word "holocaust" (Weltsturm) is sometimes translated as "world storm" by people who want to pretend there are no similarities between the German socialists Marx, Hitler, and Engels. They encourage you to hate people you don't know from countries you've never been to just because you were born somewhere else. (Nationalism).

Some translators try to distance Marx and Engels from Hitler. Those interpreters never mention how their preferred (non-"holocaust") translations also correlate with higher death tolls under Stalin and Mao (who were inspired by Marx and Engels too). They never discuss the hate mongers Stalin, Mao, and Hitler together PERIOD. They refuse to ever discuss the larger atrocities of Stalin and Mao in regard to Marx's and Engels' "world storm" term (that some translators prefer over "holocaust").

Modern socialists defend Marx and Engels by pointing out that neither used the exact term "holocaust." It highlights another commonality among the German socialists Marx, Hitler, and Engels: the term "holocaust" was not used by Hitler either. Modern socialists never mention that fact.

"Holocaust" in the sense of "the mass murder of Jews by German socialists in the Socialist War that started in 1939 with Soviet socialists" was a term introduced by historians during the 1950s, probably as an equivalent to Hebrew shoah 'catastrophe' (used in the same sense).

It leads back to another link between socialism and

weird stale religious beliefs: "He is to wash the inner parts and the legs in water, and the priest is to burn all of it on the altar. It is a burnt offering, an offering made by fire, an aroma pleasing to the Lord." (Leviticus 1:9)

The German racist socialists Marx, Hitler, and Engels had so much in common in addition to their socialist hate speech. The racist socialists Hitler, Marx, Engels, Stalin, and Mao had much in common too. Many socialists are Holocaust deniers in this regard. They deny both the socialist Holocaust and the larger Wholecaust of which the Holocaust was a part.[138]

Even if the term "holocaust" is removed from the Marx/Engels quotes, the remainder contains the otherwise racist goals of Marx and Engels. The racist prophecies persist despite any alternative translation of "holocaust." According to the two socialist seers there are nations, peoples, races, ruined folks, fragments (or whatever label any apologist wants to use) that are going to be extirpated, be wiped out, or perish. In whatever way it is interpreted, it is what the socialists Stalin, Hitler, and Mao tried by murdering millions.[139] When

---

[138] Another German philosopher, Friedrich Nietzsche, seems to have foreseen genocide from the socialists Marx, Engels, Hitler, Stalin, Mao, and others. In 1885, he wrote of disapprovingly of socialism: "The earth is big enough and man is still unexhausted enough for a practical lesson of this sort and demonstratio ad absurdum - even if it were accomplished only by a vast expenditure of lives - to seem worth while to me." (The Complete Works of Friedrich Nietzsche, Vol XIV: The Will to Power, § 125, p. 102-103).

That is what happens when you think your violence isn't as violent as others' violence. It's easy for people to dismiss evil when they have invested in the ideology so much, it's part of their being.

[139] Who is buried in Marx's tomb? No one. The tomb is empty because his resurrection occurred (Zombie Marx) and he

socialists can't beat your ideas, they'll beat you…to death.

Based on Marx's derogatory comments on "The Jewish Question" it seems Marx thought the Jewish people needed to be wiped out in Marx's holocaust (or whatever any apologist wants to call it).

Marx was raised a privileged white male in a bourgeois family and that, according to Marx, means that all of Marx's opinions are balderdash. Marx lived a bourgie life.

Marx taught everything he knew to Stalin, Mao, Hitler, Pol Pot, the Kim thugs, Castro, etc., and they were still stupid as hell. A Marxist teaching economics is like a faith healer teaching nursing.

You know what socialism is? …Words. Written by academics, preached by demagogues, swallowed by true believers. Nothing beyond words.

Despite his deadly socialist dogma, Marx wanted to be a profit-making capitalist. He dreamed of being a rich author and profiteering from the sale of books. His capitalistic dreams were similar to Edward Bellamy's dream (and similar to Francis Bellamy's scam to profiteer from socialism through flag sales) and to the German socialist Hitler with his notorious book. Marx failed. He died as impoverished as he had lived. But Marx showed the way to riches for Stalin, Mao, Hitler and others. Their product was Socialism - and they became wealthy selling it. They used Marx' business model.

While Marx wrote about workers in factories, calling

---

retreated back to his home planet, having almost accomplished his mission of annihilating the people of Earth. He inspired episode 22 of the Twilight Zone, "The Monsters Are Due on Maple Street."

them slaves, the money he lived on he received from Friedrich Engels. It came from the Engels family's interest in a factory. So, the "slaves" were supporting the Marx family, while Marx sat and wrote speeches. Marx was similar to other socialists such as Stalin, Mao, Hitler, Pol Pot, the Kim thugs, etc.

Hitler's Mein Kampf contains many of the words listed below. Some of the words listed below are followed by comments, and their frequency of use in Mein Kampf may or may not be noted. The information is also impacted by which translation of Mein Kampf is searched. This review is preliminary:

Anarchy: 1 time? It was used in a manner indicating Hitler's disapproval of anarchy. See the original German language edition and the Murphy edition in the English language.

Armlet: 5 times? Hitler explained that his notorious red armbands (and his "Hypnotic magic") were learned from other socialists, including Marxists: "In Berlin, after the War, I was present at a mass-demonstration of Marxists in front of the Royal Palace and in the Lustgarten. A sea of red flags, red armlets and red flowers was in itself sufficient to give that huge assembly of about 120,000 persons an outward appearance of strength. I was now able to feel and understand how easily the man in the street succumbs to the hypnotic magic of such a grandiose piece of theatrical presentation." German socialists were playing catch-up to outlandish publicity stunts that Soviet socialists orchestrated for more than a decade before Hitler's rise to power. Sergei Eisenstein created Battleship Potemkin for Soviet socialism in 1925, about ten years before Leni Riefenstahl's work for German socialism. They would both be outdone by socialist pomp and circumstance in China under Mao.

They were all preceded by pledging allegiance to flags in the USA as another example of such hypnosis (1892).

Aryan: used 58 times? Hitler's concept of the "super socialist man." God's chosen people or race, as compared to others who make similar assertions? Was it a race or a religion or both? Sort of a synonym for goy or gentile? Yet, it was related to the term "Iranian" (what "color" are "Iranians"?). See more on the use of the term "Aryan" near the end of this chapter.[140]

Atheist: 2 times.

---

[140] German socialism's version of the "New Soviet Man" (also parroted by Mao) or "superman." Once again, Soviet socialism started it, and German socialism aped it. Homo Sovieticus (a taxonomic-sounding term, as if socialism would evolve a new super primate species) could be fabricated from "socialist psychology" and eugenics. Soviet socialism relied upon fraudulent Lysenkoism (beginning in 1928, from Trofim Lysenko), a form of Lamarckism, which suited Stalin's stupidity about genetics. Did socialism's stupidity unintentionally demonstrate the urgent need for eugenics? In the USSR, there was only the Age of Endarkenment, and no Age of Enlightenment. The lies were taught for "free" in socialism's outrageously overpriced schools that were paid for involuntarily (nothing is so expensive as when it is free and provided by government). Lysenkoism influenced Soviet agricultural socialism which in turn contributed to crop failures, mass starvation, cannibalism, et cetera. Stalin turned Russians into food kind-of-sewers. Socialism rejects reason in all sciences, not just economics. The archetype Homo Sovieticus became satirized as dispirited sheeple in socialism's police state. They were the true "beat generation" -and beaten down daily.

Blood: ?

Bourgeois: used 191 times?

Bolshevic, Bolshevization, Bolshevism, or Bolshevized, etc. Used 27 times? ("To-day Germany is the next battlefield for Russian Bolshevism"). Hitler often used "Bolshevik" to avoid mentioning the actual name of the majority party in the Union of Soviet Socialist Republics: the Russian Social Democratic Workers' Party (RSDRP). It resembles National Socialist German Workers' Party (NSDAP). Hitler did not want to highlight the resemblance in their declared dogmas, similar to how the misnomer "Nazi" is used by modern socialists as a false flag to cover up their kindred spirit. "Bolshevik" is usually translated as "majority."

The Russian Tsar abdicated 2 March 1917. The provisional government lasted ~eight months, until the Bolsheviks took over in the coupe d'état of Red October 1917. Swastikas appeared on ruble paper currency printed in 1917 and 1918 and used thereafter.

Chinaman: ?

Christ, Jesus, Christianity: multiple times.

Christian-Socialist: 15 times? (and Christian-Socialist Party).

Communist: "For the National Socialist Movement has set itself to the task of converting those communists."

Comrade, Comrades: (Kamerad) 29 times in Ford

translation. It is military socialism with etymology from 1585-95 and Middle French "camarade" and Spanish "camarada" to reference a group of soldiers billeted together in a room (equivalent to cámar). Socialists worldwide call each other "comrade" UN-ironically, e.g.: "If you will not be a comrade too, it means a broken skull for you."

Cross: only once as a reference to the method of execution or amulet of Christianity. This suggests that Hitler is avoiding comparison of the Christian cross to the Hakenkreuz (as a religious idea) and instead promoting the Hakenkreuz as his political idea ("S" letter shapes for "socialism").

Eisner: ? (and Kurt Eisner)

Fascism or Fascist: appears three times? It appears each time as a reference to Italy, and not as a self-description by Hitler. The first quote seems to be a positive reference to the France, Russia, and Italy: "The appearance of a new and great idea was the secret of success in the French Revolution. The Russian Revolution owes its triumph to an idea. And it was only the idea that enabled Fascism triumphantly to subject a whole nation to a process of complete renovation."

The second quote: "The fight which Fascist Italy waged against Jewry's three principal weapons, the profound reasons for which may not have been consciously understood (though I do not believe this myself) furnishes the best proof that the poison fangs of that Power which transcends all State boundaries are being drawn, even though in an indirect way. The prohibition of Freemasonry and secret societies, the suppression of the supernational Press and the definite abolition of Marxism, together with the steadily increasing consolidation of the Fascist concept of the State - all this will enable the Italian Government, in the course of some years, to advance more and more the interests of the Italian people without paying any attention to the hissing of the Jewish world-hydra. (page 486).

Ford: 1. Henry Ford is the only US personality mentioned by name in Mein Kampf. The socialist Hitler envied Ford's success as well as his anti-Semitism. The socialist Stalin envied Ford's success too, and voiced no dispute of Ford's anti-Semitism. Thank goodness socialists in the USA did not make Ford (nor anyone) the official socialist monopoly-government car manufacturer for the USA; and thank goodness socialists in the USA did not impose by law the bunk in Ford's book. Socialists in Germany DID want to have an official socialist monopoly car manufacturer (Volkswagen); and they DID impose by law the bunk in Hitler's book. Socialists in the USSR DID want to have an official socialist monopoly car manufacturer; and they DID impose by law the bunk in Marx's book.

Stalin was nutzier than Hitler and contracted with Ford to oversee construction of a "socialist" automobile plant in Gorky (Ukraine) beginning in 1929. Ford was paid millions. Stalin praised Ford and the American engineers when the "Ford" plant was completed in 1932 (Stalin's praise exceeded that in Nazism's Mein Kampf).[141]

---

[141] Ford was schmoozed by two of the world's worst socialists. They murdered millions and their dogma (socialism) preached the eradication of ALL capitalists. Ford is lucky he wasn't killed by either one of them.

The plant was called "NAZ" (Nizhegorodsky Avtomobilny Zavod) and the first cars were the NAZ-A, and the NAZ-AA (I am not making this up). NAZ-A production commenced in 1932 and lasted until 1936. Most, if not all, of Ford's Soviet cars and trucks went straight to military use under the Soviet military-socialism complex.

It was all downhill from there. Stalin could not make cars even after "stealing" Ford's capitalist expertise. By 1938, Stalin ramped up the killing of American socialists who had been lured by Stalin into the USSR. The "American village" that had been built around the "Ford" plant soon contained no Americans.

In 1939 Stalin and Soviet socialists formed new allegiances -with Hitler and German socialists. Stalin and Hitler were aided by whatever remained of Ford's Soviet automobiles as Stalin and Hitler launched their socialist war together (WWII). Ford pioneered the assembly line for cars; socialists pioneered the assembly line for mass murder.

Hitler's Volkswagen ("people's car") didn't happen until later when it was a capitalist enterprise because, under Hitler, German socialists became preoccupied with killing people and stealing their stuff. Socialists redirected everything to military purposes (military socialism). The VW factory had produced only a handful of cars by the time German socialists joined Soviet socialists to pillage in the socialist crusades.

The capitalist Ford created the *real* "people's car," not American socialists, German socialists, nor Soviet socialists. Oh, and Ford had been doing it since 1908.

As socialists, Hitler and Stalin completely misunderstood everything about Ford's success.[142]

Socialists believe that everything produced by free people in the markets (food, clothing, shelter, medicine, cars, etc) can be taken over as a government monopoly and done cheaper and better. That is why socialism is totalitarian. Millions then suffer and perish.

Socialists did NOT bring humanity the "weekend" or the "8-hour work day." Greedy capitalists (including Ford) did. Greedy capitalists also brought cheap cars, unlike any that Stalin, Mao, or Hitler could finagle.

God: ?

Heil: 4 times? (Hitler mentions hearing "HEIL HOHENZOLLERN" shouted in Vienna). The notorious stiff-armed gesture that had been used in the USA's socialist pledge, and adopted later by German socialists, is not specifically mentioned in Mein Kampf.

Holocaust: does not appear in Mein Kampf.

Kapital: In a German-language edition, the phrase "das kapital" appears in Hitler's book four times; and

---

[142] It is a reminder of the confusion regarding Ford in "Brave New World" (1932) by Aldous Huxley. It is as if Huxley was satirizing Stalin's socialist monopoly-government car scheme (1929) that completely misunderstood Ford's success under capitalism.

Ford's capitalist karma ran over Hitler's socialist dogma. Soviet socialism (under Lenin and Stalin) and Chinese socialism (under Mao) also had car histories that are simultaneously horrifying and laughable. The problems persisted: There were only five million cars in the USSR in 1976 (and that was probably a wild exaggeration); Americans owned nearly 100 million.

Socialists should only travel by trebuchet.

"kapital" appears ~30 times as a word or part of a word. The term "capitalist" appears ~5 times?

Lebensraum: ? "living room/space." While Soviet socialists had announced their goal of taking over the world in their "revolution" for the "New Soviet Man," Hitler's limited version of the plan in Mein Kampf was to head East. In 1939, Soviet socialism and German socialism worked together toward their shared goals.

Left: 5? In the sense of "left" wing.

Marx: The phrase "Karl Marx" appears 3 times? To wit: "And international Marxism is nothing but the application - effected by the Jew, Karl Marx - of a general conception of life to a definite profession of political faith; but in reality that general concept had existed long before the time of Karl Marx. If it had not already existed as a widely diffused infection the amazing political progress of the Marxist teaching would never have been possible. In reality what distinguished Karl Marx from the millions who were affected in the same way was that, in a world already in a state of gradual decomposition, he used his keen powers of prognosis to detect the essential poisons, so as to extract them and concentrate them, with the art of a necromancer, in a solution which would bring about the rapid destruction of the independent nations on the globe. But all this was done in the service of his race."

Marxism, Marxist, etc: ~236 times? Hitler was influenced by Marx and Marxists (Stalin and Lenin), as were so many people (including Stalin, Lenin, Trotsky, Mao, Pol Pot) who were like Hitler in that they also killed millions of Marxists, Communists, Socialists, etc. Socialism provides millions of temptations for schadenfreude that anti-socialists must try to resist.

Mohammedan (sometimes translated as "Islam"): only once? (at 293 Religious Conditions). The only credible comment by Hitler on Muslims (and a minor passing mention whose relevance seems greater now) might be: "The extent to which the general turmoil has spread is shown by a study of the religious conditions before the war. Here, too, a uniform and effective conviction of the world had long since been lost in large parts of the nation. At the same time, the officially resolving followers of the churches play a smaller role than the indifferent ones. While the two denominations [Christianity?] in Asia and Africa sustain missions to bring new supporters of their doctrine - an activity which has shown very modest successes against the advance of especially the Mohammedan faith - they lose in Europe millions and millions of inward followers, Who either oppose the religious life or even change to their own ways. The consequences are not particularly favorable in the moral sense."

Movement 596?

The Movement 193?

Nazi, Nazis, Nazism: does not appear.

Nigger: 3 times?

Pan-German: 44 times? (and "Pan-German Party" or "Pan-German Movement").

Racial 136?

Racialist, race-based: ?

Red: ?

Reich: over 190 times? (but no mention of the phrase "Third Reich").

Right: 1 time in the sense of "right" wing?

Roman: ?

Serb, Serbs, Serbian: 5?

Sieg: ?

Siegfried: ?

Slav: 4?; Slavs: 8?; Slavic: 16?;

slave: 4?; slaves: 10?; slavery: 8?; enslave: 2? Hitler does not remark about the etymological relationship (in German and English) of the terms for "Slav" and "slave" and "Caucasus" and "Caucasian" (The word "slave" originated from Caucasians and other Slavs who were enslaved). The term "Slav" denotes locations where many perished under Soviet socialism and German socialism: Ukraine and the Caucasus (the last word being "Slavic" and the source of the word "Caucasian," so that the word "slave" derived from Caucasians and other Slavs who were enslaved). German socialism aspired to re-enslave the Slavs, and Soviet socialism did re-enslave the Slavs where German socialism had failed.

Storm Detachment: 25?

Swastika: does not appear in the original German language (where "Hakenkreuz" was used), but is always used in translations, and without any explanation of the choice of "swastika" over "hooked cross." The term "Hakenkreuz" translates almost literally as "hook cross" (or "hooked cross") and avoids the confusion caused by translation to "swastika."

Third Reich: Never appears in Mein Kampf.

Vienna: 80 times?

Weltanschauung: used 84 times? Sometimes translated as "race-based society"?

There are popular misconceptions about Hitler's use of the term "Aryan." This section of this chapter examines the use of the term "Aryan" in Mein Kampf. The following analyzes the 1939 Murphy version of Mein Kampf.
....
The following example indicates Hitler is using the term "Aryan" to refer to more than one set of people.
(p 228) "Aryan tribes, often almost ridiculously small in number, subjugated foreign peoples and, stimulated by the conditions of life which their new country offered them (fertility, the nature of the climate, etc.), and profiting also by the abundance of manual labour furnished them by the inferior race, they developed intellectual and organizing faculties which had hitherto been dormant in these conquering tribes."
....

(page 226)? "Within a few decades the whole of Eastern Asia, for instance, appropriated a culture and called such a culture its own, whereas the basis of that culture was the Greek mind and Teutonic skill as we know it. Only the external form - at least to a certain degree - shows the traits of an Asiatic inspiration. It is not true, as some believe, that Japan adds European technique to a culture of her own. The truth rather is that European science and technics are just decked out with the peculiar characteristics of Japanese civilization. The foundations of actual life in Japan to-day are not those of the native Japanese culture, although this characterizes the external features of the country, which features strike the eye of European observers on account of their fundamental difference from us; but the real foundations of contemporary Japanese life are the enormous scientific and technical achievements of Europe and America, that is to say, of Aryan peoples. Only by adopting these achievements as the foundations of their own progress can the various nations of the Orient take a place in contemporary world progress. The scientific and technical achievements of Europe and America provide the basis on which the struggle for daily livelihood is carried on in the Orient. They provide the necessary arms and instruments for this struggle, and only the outer forms of these instruments have become gradually adapted to Japanese ways of life.

If, from to-day onwards, the Aryan influence on Japan would cease - and if we suppose that Europe and America would collapse - then the present progress of Japan in science and technique might still last for a short duration; but within a few decades the inspiration would dry up, and native Japanese character would triumph, while the present civilization would become fossilized and fall back into the sleep from which it was aroused about seventy years ago by the impact of Aryan culture."

....

(p 231) "The Aryan neglected to maintain his own racial stock unmixed and therewith lost the right to live in the paradise which he himself had created. He became submerged in the racial mixture and gradually lost his cultural creativeness, until he finally grew, not only mentally but also physically, more like the aborigines whom he had subjected rather than his own ancestors. For some time he could continue to live on the capital of that culture which still remained; but a condition of fossilization soon set in and he sank into oblivion. That is how cultures and empires decline and yield their places to new formations."

....

(p 232) "The readiness to sacrifice one's personal work and, if necessary, even one's life for others shows its most highly developed form in the Aryan race. The greatness of the Aryan is not based on his intellectual powers, but rather on his willingness to devote all his faculties to the service of the community. Here the instinct for self-preservation has reached its noblest form; for the Aryan willingly subordinates his own ego to the common weal and when necessity calls he will even sacrifice his own life for the community."

....

(p 234) "The Jew offers the most striking contrast to the Aryan."

....

(p 237) "We ought to remember that during the first period of American colonization numerous Aryans earned their daily livelihood as trappers and hunters, etc., frequently wandering about in large groups with their women and children, their mode of existence very much resembling that of ordinary nomads. The moment, however, that they grew more numerous and were able to accumulate larger resources, they cleared the land and drove out the aborigines, at the same time establishing settlements which rapidly increased all over the country."

....

(p 239) "In the Aryan mind no religion can ever be imagined unless it embodies the conviction that life in some form or other will continue after death."

....

(p 241) "A development began which has always been the same or similar wherever and whenever Jews came into contact with Aryan peoples."

....

(p 241) here the term "Aryan" appears to be used simply as a synonym for "non-Jew" (goy, gentile?).

"[The Jew's] commercial cunning, acquired through thousands of years of negotiation as an intermediary, made him superior in this field to the Aryans, who were still quite ingenuous and indeed clumsy and whose honesty was unlimited; so that after a short while commerce seemed destined to become a Jewish monopoly."

....

(p 276) "Those who effectively combat this mortal enemy of our people, who is at the same time the enemy of all Aryan peoples and all culture, can only expect to arouse opposition on the part of this race and become the object of its slanderous attacks. "

....

(p 332) "One thing is certain: our world is facing a great revolution. The only question is whether the outcome will be propitious for the Aryan portion of mankind or whether the everlasting Jew will profit by it.

By educating the young generation along the right lines, the People's State will have to see to it that a generation of mankind is formed which will be adequate to this supreme combat that will decide the destinies of the world.

That nation will conquer which will be the first to take this road."

....

(p 346) "The constructive principle of Aryan humanity is thus displaced by the destructive principle of the Jews, They become the 'ferment of decomposition' among nations and races and, in a broad sense, the wreckers of human civilization."

....

(p 351) "Any party that is led by him can fight for no other interests than his, and his interests certainly have nothing in common with those of the Aryan nations."

....

(p 429) "Catholics and Protestants are fighting with one another to their hearts' content, while the enemy of Aryan humanity and all Christendom is laughing up his sleeve."

....

(p 429) "This pestilential adulteration of the blood, of which hundreds of thousands of our people take no account, is being systematically practised by the Jew to-day. Systematically these negroid parasites in our national body corrupt our innocent fair-haired girls and thus destroy something which can no longer be replaced in this world."

....

(p 429) "For the future of the world, however, it does

not matter which of the two triumphs over the other, the Catholic or the Protestant. But it does matter whether Aryan humanity survives or perishes. And yet the two Christian denominations are not contending against the destroyer of Aryan humanity but are trying to destroy one another."

....

(p 489) "In place of preaching hatred against Aryans from whom we may be separated on almost every other ground but with whom the bond of kindred blood and the main features of a common civilization unite us, we must devote ourselves to arousing general indignation against the maleficent enemy of humanity and the real author of all our sufferings."

....

(p 495) "They would remain as the fertilizing manure of civilization, until the last residue of Nordic-Aryan blood would become corrupted or drained out."

....

(p 309) "A benefit which results from the fact that there was no all-round assimilation is to be seen in that even now we have large groups of German Nordic people within our national organization, and that their blood has not been mixed with the blood of other races. We must look upon this as our most valuable treasure for the sake of the future."

12. SIGNS & SIGNATURES OF SOCIALISM

Hitler changed the Hakenkreuz, and Hitler changed his own signature in a similar way. Rarely seen autographs from Hitler show that he evolved his signature "Adolf Hitler" into "S Hitler." It was a declaration of his socialism every time he signed his name: as if he was signing "Socialist Hitler."[143]

Most people have never seen Hitler's signature. That is because the media never display Hitler's signature and do not want readers to know what it reveals.

Hitler's handwriting has been "analyzed" by "experts" who declare that his evil nature should have been obvious from his penmanship. LOL. They all refer to Hitler as a "Nazi" and/or a "Fascist" and are ignorant of what he called himself and, of course, they all completely overlook the "S" symbolism in his signature.

Ernst "Putzi" Hanfstaengl (an intimate of Hitler's and his foreign press chief), also signed his name with a similar "swastika" flourish. Hanfstaengl, educated in the U.S., might have encouraged Hitler to adopt the

---

[143] Some capitalists use a contrasting style in which "S" letters are signed and spelled as dollar signs ($), as in "$teve $mith."

American Nazi salute, as well as the "swastika" style signature.

German military medals were cast with raised lettering that displays Hitler's "S" style signature.

There are signatures from other Hitler underlings that appear to use a "swastika" style flourish. Sometimes the letter "S" in someone's name is written as the vertical half of a swastika or as one of the "SS" Schutzstaffel symbols. Sometimes it appears as a small "S" lightning bolt substituted for the dot over the letter "i." Leni Riefenstahl's signature during that specific period sometimes displays a stylized "s" letter.

Joseph Stalin's signature sometimes had similar stylized flourishes (especially during that time when he and Hitler were pals and launched WWII together). The name that Stalin signed in Russian was: Иосиф Сталин, but he would only write the first letter of his first name (along with his last name): И Сталин. The initial letter was sometimes scrawled so that the "И" resembles "S" in a swastika style with a lightning bolt flourish. The "Ст" part of his last name was sometimes rendered to resemble the hammer and sickle symbol (the "С" as the sickle and the "т" as the crossed hammer/handle).

In 1920, Hitler decided that the National Socialist German Workers' Party needed its own insignia. The new flag had to be "a symbol of our own struggle" as well as "highly effective as a poster." (Mein Kampf, Chapter 7 of the 2nd volume, sometimes pg. 495).

In Mein Kampf, Hitler described how the Reichsbanner went from Schwarz-Rot-Gold to Schwarz-Rot-Weiß: (p 384) "We National Socialists regarded our flag as being the embodiment of our party programme. The red expressed the social thought underlying the movement. White the national thought. And the swastika signified the mission allotted to us - the struggle for the victory of Aryan mankind and at the same time the triumph of the ideal of creative work..." Another version states: "In red we see the social idea of the movement, in white the nationalistic idea, in the hook-cross the mission of the struggle for the victory of the Aryan man, and, by the same token, the victory of the idea of creative work..." (pg. 496-497).

A dust jacket for Mein Kampf from 1926–27 shows the "old style" swastika, flat on its side as if drawn in a square (not turned 45 degrees as if drawn in a diamond). So, Mein Kampf might have been written before Hitler began turning the swastika and using it for "S" letter shapes. That might explain why Mein Kampf has little to say about the topic.

In German, the quoted reference from Mein Kampf was: "im Hakenkreuz die Mission des Kampfes fÜr den Sieg des arischen Menschen und zugleich mit ihm auch den Sieg des Gedankens der schaffenden Arbeit..."

In his own words, Hitler used the word "sieg" twice and can be interpreted as stating that the hooked cross is a "sieg" sign. Also known as "sig runes," the "lightning-bolt" signs are letters of an ancient Germanic alphabet. An interwebz image search for "double sig rune," "sig rune," "sieg rune," "sigel rune," or "sowilo" provides more examples. The "sieg" rune corresponds with the letter "S" and was used for "S" in other representations.

Hitler's quote has overlapping use of the word "sieg." The word "sieg" means "victory." His swastika sigil represented two "S" letters for "socialism" or "socialism and sieg" (socialism and victory) and is related to "Sieg Heil!" (Hail to Victory) in the sense of "Hail to the Victory of Socialism!" (Hail to the Victory of the National Socialist German Workers' Party).[144] Germany became another example of why socialism is a big "Sieg Fail!"

Hitler's flag quote in Mein Kampf refers to the red color and the "social idea of the movement" (socialism) for which Hitler claimed the National Socialist German Workers' Party was struggling for victory.

The struggle for victory began in 1919 when Hitler joined the German Workers' Party, a socialist group. The group sought a new name that would attract socialists in other anti-capitalist hate groups. Other German socialist groups used terms like "National" and "Socialist" in their titles, and the German Workers' Party adopted "National Socialist German Workers' Party."

Hitler gave the Hakenkreuz the same meaning as the group's new name. For Hitler, the joined "S" letters represented socialists joining together as the National Socialist German Workers' Party. The intertwined letter "S" shapes represent "Socialists" unified, or "Socialist Solidarity" and the victory of the National Socialist German Workers' Party bringing socialists together in one large group.

Hitler also wrote: "Two years later, when our squad of hall guards had long since grown into storm detachments, it seemed necessary to give this defensive organization of a young Weltanschauung a particular symbol of victory, namely a Standard." In German it

---

[144] Americans have "hailed" their flag since ~1812, as attested in the National Anthem (the Star Spangled Banner): "What so proudly we hailed at the twilight's last gleaming..." (Let's not mention what gesture they used after 1892). They continue to hail the flag, though the current gesture is the hand-over-the-heart, as dictated by flag laws written to hide America's scary past, present, and future. Cf. "Hail, Hail, the Gangs all Here!" When the band plays "Hail to the chief," they point the cannon at you.

was: "Zwei Jahre spÄter, als aus der Ordnertruppe schon lÄngst eine viel tausend Mann umfassende Sturmabteilung geworden war, schien es nÖtig, dieser Wehrorganisation der jungen Weltanschauung noch ein besonderes Symbol des Sieges zu geben: die Standarte." Hitler again used the phrase "Symbol des Sieges." In the only remarks on the emblem by Hitler, the Sturmabteilung was specifically referenced.

The Sturmabteilung had well-known Nazi banners that included Hitler's Hakenkreuz-swastika in the old style (horizontal / square), the new style (slanted / diamond), and another banner also utilizing another stylized "S" logo, for the "SA" (Sturm Abteilung).

Hitler mentions "Siegfried" in Mein Kampf. Siegfried is a name for a male in the German language, composed of the Germanic elements sig "victory" and frithu "protection, peace." The name is medieval, and survived into modern times and, after 1876, it enjoyed renewed popularity due to Richard Wagner's "Siegfried," the third of the four operas that constitute Der Ring des Nibelungen (The Ring of the Nibelung), inspired by the story of Sigurd in Norse mythology.

The term "Nazi" was (and is) a term of derision used by people against the National Socialists German Workers' Party. Party members did not use the term "Nazi" to refer to themselves. Party members used the terms "socialist" or "national socialist" or the full name of the party.

In the notorious 1934 film "Triumph of the Will" by Leni Riefenstahl, and in the 1925 book "Mein Kampf" by Adolf Hitler, the word "socialist" is used throughout and the words "Nazi" and "Fascist" are never used -not a single time- in reference to the National Socialist German Workers' Party. In the film, the German socialists refer to each other as "Kamerads" (comrades).

Stylized "S" letters were used in other emblems under German National Socialists including Hitler's "SS" Division which used two similarly stylized "S" letters side-by-side for "Schutzstaffel," as compared with the overlapping "S" shapes of the Hakenkreuz / swastika. The person who created the "SS" and "SA" emblems (Walter Heck in 1933?) understood the alphabetical "S" letter representation of Hitler's swastika.

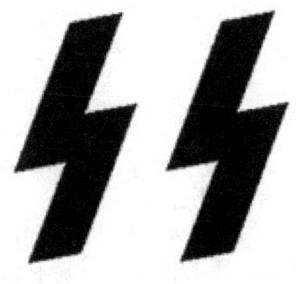

Many people (including "scholars") have written about Hitler's Schutzstaffel (the "SS Division") and its stylized "SS" logo. Some authors have noted that the "SS" insignia uses runes that correspond to the letter "S" as alphabetical representation of the word "Schutzstaffel." All of those authors failed to compare the "SS" emblem to the swastika, and failed to make Dr. Curry's demonstration of the alphabetical function of the swastika for "socialism" under Hitler.

Swastika errors were committed by Carl Gustav Jung in his book "Man and His Symbols" (1964). Jung failed to identify the symbol as a cross (the book identifies Hitler in a photograph next to "Nazi swastikas") and failed to discuss Hitler's symbol in the book's lengthier section about crosses as symbols (thus indicating glaring ignorance about the symbol on the part of Jung and his co-authors).

Alphabetic lettering in a stylized form is shown in other Nazi-Sozi paraphernalia, in Nazi posters, in German medals, flags, banners, and including but not limited to the logos of the "NSV" (National Socialist Volkswohlfahrt), and the "T-O" logo of the Todt Organization; and the Technische Nothilfe (abbreviated as TN, TeNo, TENO; literally: Technical Emergency Help).

Swastika-style symbolism is visible today and every day on the streets as the VW logo. The logo is two identical "V" letters crossed to form the letters "V" and "W" (or a "V" and a "W" letter joined) in a similar "hooked cross" alphabetical style for "Volkswagen." The VW was Hitler's socialist "People's Car" scam that he never produced for "the people" (because he was busy killing them in war).

Franz Xaver Reimspiess, Nikolai Borg, and others have claimed credit for the VW logo. Borg, a young commercial artist, impressed others when he won the competition for the creation of a logo for the "Deutsche Jugendherbergswerk." Borg said that he was invited to draw the Volkswagen car logo in a request from high-up: Dr. Ing. Fritz Todt, with the "Organization Todt" the general inspector for roads and a militarily organized building troop used in the entire theater of war (boasting its own alphabetical emblem in the conjoined letters "O" and "T" for its logo). Borg stated that he made nine drafts with different connections of the crossed "V" letters, to represent the letters "V" and "W" before his final version emerged. Borg has exhibited photographs in which Borg's VW emblem design was placed on top of the swastika image that inspired it, and was created simply by replacing the two crossed "S" letters of the swastika with the two crossed "V" letters (that also form the letters V and W).

Before the VW emblem was created, the logo for Volkswagen was a swastika encircled by a cogwheel. It was the trademark for the organization that controlled Volkswagen, the socialist trade union organization Deutsche Arbeitsfront (DAF or German Labor Front). The swastika of the Deutsche Arbeitsfront emblem was the origin of the Volkswagen logo, both philosophically and stylistically.

A doubter asks "When did any German socialist ever say that the swastika represented overlapping 'S' letters for 'socialism'?" She should be answered with "When did any German socialist ever say that the Volkswagen logo represented overlapping 'V' letters (or a 'V' and 'W') for 'Volkswagen'?" Your mileage may vary.

Similar stylized representation is visible in the meshed "M" letters in the emblem of the Maybach automobile (from Maybach-Motorenbau); and the "S" shaped logo used with the Trabant Sachsenring car from Automobilwerke Zwickau (which also used a revealing "A-Z" logo). Audi's emblem evolved from four car companies that showed similar alphabetical functions in some early emblems.

The "S" symbolism was adopted by the British Union of Fascists and National Socialists (BUFANS) in 1935 when they changed their name from "British Union of Fascists" (the leader Oswald Mosley, former Minister in the pre-WWI Labour Government, added "National Socialists" as Hitler had with his party's name). The BUFANS' symbol was a single "S" shape symbol, mimicking the double "S" symbol of German socialists. Sometimes, the "S" symbol was above the fasces symbol (on their military-style black headwear).

The BUFANS updated its flag with the stylized "S" letter shape for socialism, and discarded their older flag which had a fasces (from 1932 to 1935) on a red background. BUFANS also wore armbands with its "S" symbol to further parrot German socialist armbands. BUFANS also culturally appropriated the American socialist salute to its flag (the socialist Bellamy had desired that his pledge ritual spread globally, and he had designed it for that purpose).

All commentators (including those who post on Wakipedia) pretend that they have no idea why BUFANS' changed symbol corresponded with its changed name; or the same commentators pretend that the changes were of no meaning or significance. They bluff that the BUFANS symbol is merely a "lightning bolt" with no "S" symbolism for "socialism."[145]

The "S" symbolism for "socialism" was adopted by the People's Action Party (PAP) in Singapore. The PAP smeared its way onto the political scene in 1954 when it was formed by English-educated middle-class men who had returned to Singapore from Britain. The PAP became a member of the Socialist International. The PAP logo has a double connotation for "Singapore Socialists." The S-letter is red and thereby consistent

---

[145] For a long time Wakipedia liars also refused to tell readers that the BUF changed its name to BUFANS. In the past, web searches for "British Union of Fascists and National Socialists" showed Dr. Curry's work at the top and indicated that no Wikipedia article existed. Wikipedia gave the mis-impression that the BUFANS never existed, or that its name-change never occurred. It was common comic revisionist history air-brushed at Wakipedia. Later, Wikipedia writers began to use Dr. Curry's work without attribution in apparent attempts to bolster their own credibility.

with the socialist symbolism of the color under German socialism, Soviet socialism, and Chinese socialism. There is evidence that the PAP also adopted the stiff-arm salute from American socialism. The PAP eventually played copycat to the USA again in adopting a hand-over-the-heart gesture. PAP members continue to wear uniforms at their Party meetings, dressing all in the same color and clothing. All commentators (including Wakipedia) pretend that they have no knowledge of the PAP symbol's derivation and no knowledge of the "S" shape's meaning.

The "S" symbolism for "socialism" was adopted by the Brazilian Integralist Action (Ação Integralista Brasileira or AIB) in a unique manner: with an uppercase sigma (Σ) in its center, instead of a swastika. The meaning of the AIB symbol has been overlooked because the Greek letter sigma resembles the English and German letter "E." However, the Greek letter sigma corresponds to the English and German letter "S." There were two main versions of the Greek letter sigma in ancient history. One version of the Greek letter sigma was the AIB's "E" shaped symbol, and the other was the "S" shaped symbol that is also described as a lightning bolt rune-shape. in Germany under the NSGWP (and still today worldwide), the "S" shapes used in the swastika, the SS division and other uses were known as "siegs" or the "sieg rune," and the name is derived from the Greek word "sigma." "Sieg" is also a word in German and was used under the NSGWP as part of its robotic chanting of "Sieg Heil" to its swastika flag, and to its leader with the stiff-arm salute The AIB also culturally appropirated the stiff-arm salute from German socialism and American socialism. All commentators (including Wakipedia liars) pretend that they have no knowledge of the AIB symbol's derivation.

Anyone who doubts that Hitler used the swastika to represent "S" letter shapes for "Socialism" is someone who believes Hitler was blind and that Hitler remained blind throughout the decades that Hitler used the symbol for his National Socialist Party.

Eventually, Dr. Curry's decoding of the swastika will become so well-known and so obvious that no one will believe that Dr. Curry "made the discovery that Hitler used the swastika to represent 'S' letter shapes for 'socialism' " because no one will believe that there ever was a time when people could not see that Dr. Curry's assertion was self-evident. People will not believe that there ever was a time when the world did not see the glaring truth. People of the future will not believe that people of today were so blind and ignorant. It will be a paradigm shift.[146]

A 1935 Youth's booklet from the National Socialist German Workers' Party shows that youngsters were taught about the "S" shapes of German socialist symbols. The entire 35-page book was uncovered by Dr. Curry and it is the only example known to exist. Although the book is in its original German language, the illustrations supplement the text's explanation that common emblems under the National Socialist German Workers' Party often used the "S" shape, including the side-by-side use in the "SS" Division (for "Schutzstaffel") and the overlapping use in the Swastika.

This is a translation of excerpted text in the 1935

---

[146] The same path of doubt, dissemination, and eventual widespread acceptance and paradigm shift will occur regarding Dr. Curry's discovery that the USA's flag pledge was the origin of the Nazi salute and Nazi behavior.

Nazi youth's book:

"Today, we are proud of our Germanic heritage; we wish German custom to again be in the lead over everything foreign, and to demonstrate this, the Hitler Youth has taken the old victory sign, the Siegrune, for their flags and armbands.

From the Siegrune "S" one can easily create an "S" "S" form [illustrations showed a stylized rune "S" next to an English-style alphabetic "S" letter]. And the Leader's Schutz-Staffel, which we abbreviate "SS", carries the double-rune "SS" [an illustration showed the classic stylized rune "SS"] as their badge. This victory and salvation rune may also be found in a stretched version, which looks like this [an illustration showed a longer version oriented horizontally]. Many bear a small line in the middle, [an illustration showed the previous version oriented horizontally and a short notch added in the middle] and is then known as Wolfsangel.

"I know something, I know something," Harmut suddenly explained, taking the pencil from his father's hand. "If you superimpose two Wolfsangels, you get a hooked-cross. This is also two Siegrunes." [an illustration showed a Hakenkreuz (swastika)]

"You have made a nice and meaningful discovery, my son," father happily noted, "because the....." [End of quote from that page of the 1935 Nazi youth book].

Each summer thousands of Hitler Youth marched from their hometowns down German roads to meet en masse at Nuremberg to join in the yearly rally and congress of the Nazi-socialists. Socialism is extremely effective at channeling the energy of ignorant young people in all countries.

The notorious film "Triumph of the Will" by Leni Riefenstahl from 1935 was propaganda for the sixth annual rally of Hitler Youth. The word "socialism" is used in a positive manner throughout the film by the speakers to extol their dogma. The words "Nazi" and "fascist" are never used in the film.

"Triumph of the Will" shows the National Socialist German Workers' Party parading its industrial army of military socialism. In keeping with their socialist dogma, Hitler is praised as the "epitome of altruism" and the speakers refer to each other as "comrades" who will cause a "revolution of the people and workers" to end "class struggle" and create "egalitarianism."

The following words were emphasized as shown (with capitalization) in the book "Look to Germany" by Stanley McClatchie:

"NATIONAL SOCIALISM? What does it mean? The true significance of this name given to the German movement is usually overlooked, and the hasty reader at the breakfast table is prone to see - "National...ism".

THE GERMAN FLAG? What does it look like? The majority of foreigners know that it contains a swastika and believe that this signifies only - "National...ism".

THE FLAG BEARERS? Who are they? The world regards their disciplined ranks, the brown uniforms and reflects - "National...ism".

It is time, however, to wake up!
S O C I A L I S M is the principle word in the title of the Movement. The basic colour in its banner is
R E D and those who wear the brown uniforms are

COMRADES!"

13. USA TRAVELS TO ITALY

Benito Amilcare Andrea Mussolini was named after five different socialists: Mexican President Benito Juárez; Italians Andrea Costa and Amilcare Cipriani; and Mussolini's two parents. He was born into socialism, raised to be a socialist, and became a well-known and long-time socialist leader. Mussolini acquired his title "il duce" -leader- when he was known only as a socialist.

As a socialist leader, he began to mimic American socialists in their use of the stiff-armed salute, martial chanting to flags, the glorification of ancient Rome (or false myths about Rome), and the use of the fasces as an emblem of government and socialism.

In ancient Rome, the fasces was a bundle of sticks fastened together. It signified "union," or people (or states, or nations) banded into a group.

"Fasces" [**fas**-eez] (and its cognates, such as "fascism") are often confused with the word "feces" [**fee**-seez], even though the latter is obviously less disgusting. One is waste matter discharged from the intestines through the anus; and the other is shit. One is a natural daily function for all humans and necessary for health and life; and the other one is dangerous crap.

Manure is useful in many ways, unlike socialism. Guano fertilizes fields to grow food. Socialism destroys food.

The word "fascist" is related to the word "fagot" (or faggot (British)) as a bundle of wood (see the work of the etymologist Dr. Curry) and via the similar early pronunciation of the words "fasces" and "faggot" (the original Latin term "fasces" was pronounced with a hard letter "C" sound or /k/, not the modern soft letter "C" sound or /s/).[147]   It resembles the pronunciation differences between "feces" and "fecal."

The etymology extends to Greece and Aesop (believed to have lived in ancient Greece between 620 and 560 BCE). Fabulous research compares a translation from the Greek writing of one of Aesop's Fables known as "The Old Man and his Sons" or "The Bundle of Sticks." In the fable, an old man on the point of death summoned his quarreling sons around him to give them some parting advice. He ordered his servants to bring in a faggot of sticks, and said to his eldest son: "Break it." The son strained and strained, but with all his efforts was unable to break the Bundle. The other sons also tried, but none of them was successful. "Untie the faggots," said the father, "and each of you take a stick." When they had done so, he called out to them: "Now, break," and each stick was easily broken. "You see my meaning," said their father. And the meaning was supposed to be: Union gives strength.

Mussolini's message was: Individually we are

---

[147] A similar comparison would be the pronunciation of the words "Pisces" and "Piscatorial."

Hard and soft "C" sounds are illustrated in these related words: Caesar, Kaiser, Tsar, and Czar. Following ancient Caesars, Mussolini became a great seizer.

effeminate like a single twig, but in bundles we are mighty faggots.[148] Etymologically speaking, socialists think of themselves as fags.

In another bizarre parallel to "Christian Socialism," the phrase "fire and faggot" described punishment of a heretic by burning in blazes stoked with faggots of wood. Heretics who recanted were forced to display the symbol of a faggot on their shirt sleeve for public humiliation.

Homosexuality was illegal under the old crusades, and under the modern era's early "Christian socialism," and under the modern socialist crusades of the archsocialists Stalin, Mao, Hitler, Mussolini, Che Guevara, Castro, Pol Pot, in North Korea, et cetera.

The derogatory term for a "male homosexual," 1914, is probably from the earlier use for an old heretical woman,[149] and a reference to the "flaming faggots"

---

[148] In the demented documentary "Aim High In Creation" (2013) a North Korean official refers to the fasces symbol as a symbol of their socialism (at ~32:00 minutes in).

[149] "Heretics" under modern socialist Crusades might include Charlotte Corday or Fanya Kaplan. Kaplan undoubtedly hastened the end of Lenin's career and his life by shooting him three times at close range. She proved that the only way to stop a bad guy with a gun is a good girl with a gun. It is a fascinating comparison to what Lenin did to Czar Nicholas and the Czar's family. Sic semper tyrannis!

Kaplan shot Lenin because he had banned other political parties (including Kaplan's Socialist Revolutionaries). She perceived Lenin as "a traitor to the revolution." A capitalist sold Kaplan the gun with which she shot Lenin. It was very Kaplanesque.

After the shooting of Lenin and Moisei Uritsky (also on August 30, 1918) the Bolsheviks worsened with their "Red Terror."

German socialism followed Soviet socialism's template

(homosexuals were also burned at the stake).

The word "fasces" is also related to these words: fascine, fascia, fascinate, fasciatus fish, plantar fasciitis, and many others.

In his book "A History of Fascism, 1914-1945," Stanley G. Payne described the term "fasci" as common among socialists in Italy: "Forming a fascio—the term means band, union, or league—had been standard practice among various sectors of Italian radicalism since the 1870s. Fasci (the plural form) had been organized by trade unions, middle-class radicals, or reformist peasants, the most famous being the Fasci Siciliani, the broad federation of peasants and others in Sicily during 1895–96 that had brought much of the island out in revolt against the existing political and economic structure. Thus, the nomenclature adopted by the new Fascio Rivoluzionario [of Mussolini] was standard practice..."

On December 11, 1914, Mussolini started a political group: Fasci d'azione Rivoluzionaria (Union of Revolutionary Action). It combined two other movements: (1) Fasci d'azione Rivoluzionaria Internazionalista and (2) Fasci Autonomi d'azione Rivoluzionaria (a previous group he started).

Fascism meant "unionism" to the socialist Mussolini. Mussolini's socialist "unionism" mimicked "soviets" (councils) under Russian socialism (the Union of Soviet Socialist Republics). It was Mussolini's version of socialist syndicalism. Both the Italian and Soviet systems were similar to the organization that arose later under German socialism (the National

---

again on July 14, 1933 (after the Reichstag fire), when Hitler declared his Socialist Party to be the only political party in Germany and outlawed other parties.

Socialist German Workers Party).

"Fasci" referred to Mussolini's socialist union for socialist revolution. It is similar to the word "faction" in that Mussolini's group was another of many socialist-inspired unions.

The term "fascio" was the Italian word for workers' groups, peasant organizations, labor unions and the other socialist groups (anti-capitalist hate groups) where Mussolini had developed a large following.

Mussolini's Fascism was Focialism, or Fauxialism, because it was socialism updated with a new name.[150] The long-time socialist leader sometimes used the F-word to trick people into continuing to support socialism.

The Fasci d'azione Rivoluzionaria asserted that it supported socialism, using the famous quote by French socialist Louis Auguste Blanqui, "He who has iron has bread" on the title page of its socialist newspaper, Il Popolo d'Italia.

Mussolini was founder and editor of the newspaper, and he announced under its title that it was the "Socialist Daily" (Quotidiano Socialista). The newspaper began on November 15, 1914.

After some indecision, Mussolini supported World War I by appealing to the need for socialists to overthrow the Hohenzollern and Habsburg monarchies

---

[150] In "The Road to Serfdom" (German: Der Weg zur Knechtschaft) the Austrian economist Friedrich von Hayek challenged the lie among socialists that fascism was a capitalist reaction against socialism. He argued that fascism, National Socialism and socialism had common roots in central economic planning and empowering the state over the individual. Since its publication in 1944, The Road to Serfdom has been an influential exposition of market libertarianism.

in Germany and Austria-Hungary. Mussolini claimed that they had consistently repressed socialism. Mussolini argued that hundreds of thousands of Italians were under Habsburg rule (also spelled "Hapsburg"). He asserted that the defeat of Hohenzollern and Habsburg monarchies would help the working class.

Mussolini explained that the war would bring Tsarist Russia to social revolution. He gleefully supported the deposition of the tsar and he supported the socialist revolution that formed the Union of Soviet Socialist Republics (USSR) in 1917.

Mussolini and Lenin worked together and praised each other's socialist work. Later, Mussolini joined in a pact with German socialism (22 May 1939). Mussolini remained in his Axis pact with the socialist Hitler at the very time that the socialist Stalin joined in a pact with German socialism, mere months later (23 August 1939 - a date that has lived in infamy).[151] Italian socialism, Soviet socialism, and German socialism worked together at the same time. Soviet socialism was on the path to formally join the socialist Axis, and by its behavior had already done so.

In 1919, Mussolini created a new socialist sub-group called "Fasci di combattimento" (also known as the "Fascio nazionale di combattimento"). It referred to his socialist band of combat. It was another use of the word

---

[151] Stalin's fake name means "steel" and so Soviet socialism's pact with German socialism was "The Pact of Steel," or a joining with "The Pact of Steel" (German: Stahlpakt) that German socialism had forged months earlier with Italian socialism. In German, "steel" is "Stehlen." Upon Stalin joining, Mussolini is said to have declared: "Bolshevism is dead. In its place is a kind of Slavonic fascism." The source of this alleged quote is not clear. It is worth noting that the first sentence is not "Socialism is dead."

that is similar to "faction" to designate socialist-inspired unions. Socialism is always faction against faction.

Mussolini's group consisted merely of socialist associates of the socialist Mussolini. In his cleverly titled "My Autobiography," Mussolini stated: "My first article in the Popolo d'Italia turned a large part of public opinion toward the intervention of Italy in the war [WWI], side by side with France and England. Standing by me and helping my work as newspaper man were the Fascisti. They were composed of revolutionary spirits who believed in intervention. They were youths—the students of the universities, the socialist syndicalists…"

The first meeting of the Italian "battle Fascists" took place after Mussolini advertised in his socialist paper. Mussolini stated autobiographically: "I prepared the atmosphere of that memorable meeting by editorials and summonses published in the Popolo d'Italia."

When Mussolini had to turn over the operation of his newspaper, he chose one of his socialist family members: his brother Arnaldo.

Socialism continued to grow in Germany with the German Workers' Party (Deutsche Arbeiterpartei, DAP) and Hitler's membership therein. On February 24, 1920, Hitler decided to change the name of his group (the DAP). On that date, Mussolini continued to be known as a socialist leader in Italy (although he used the term "fasci" for some of his socialist union sub-groups), and Lenin continued to be known as a socialist leader in the Union of Soviet Socialist Republics.

The DAP changed its name to the Nationalsozialistische Deutsche Arbeiterpartei (National Socialist German Workers Party). Hitler did not adopt Mussolini's use of the term "fasci" in any form. Hitler did not name his Party the National Fascist German

Workers Party. Hitler's socialists never self-identified as "Fascists," nor as "Nazis."

On 9 November 1921, Mussolini transformed the Fasci Italiani di Combattimento into the National Fascist Party. The new party name occurred after Hitler had added the word phrase "National Socialist" (not National Fascist") to the name of Hitler's party. Hitler did not re-rename his party, but remained with "National Socialist." There is no evidence that Hitler ever thought about removing "socialist" from the name of his party. Hitler's autobiographical "Mein Kampf" was published on July 18, 1925 and used the term "socialist" as self-identification throughout.

In 1928, Mussolini published "My Autobiography." In it he continued to boast of his work imposing socialism, including: "I think that Italy is advanced beyond all the European nations; in fact, it has ratified the laws for the eight-hour day, for obligatory insurance, for regulation of the work of women and children, for assistance and benefit, for after-work diversion and adult education, and finally for obligatory insurance against tuberculosis."

Mussolini continued to describe Fascism as his version of Socialism: "All this shows how, in every detail in the field of labor, I stand by the Italian working classes. All that it was possible to do without working an injury to the principle of solidity in our economy I have set out to do, from the minimum wage to the continuity of employment, from insurance against accidents to indemnity against illness, from old age pensions to the proper regulation of military service. There is little which social welfare research has adjudged practical to national economy or wise for social happiness which has not already been advanced by me. I want to give to every man and woman so generous an opportunity that work will be not a painful necessity but a joy of life. But even such a complex programme cannot be said to equal the creation of the corporative system. Nor can the latter equal something even larger. Beyond the corporative system, beyond the state's labors, is Fascism, harmonizer and dominator of Italian life, standing ever as its inspiration." (p. 278, My Autobiography).

While his autobiography was published in 1928 and glorified Mussolini's socialist policies therein, Mussolini demonstrated his economic ignorance and also recounted his trite socialist work from years earlier: "In 1923, some months after the march on Rome, I insisted on the ratification of the law for an eight-hour day." [Socialists everywhere applaud brainlessly].[152]

Mussolini summarized his socialism with this classic yawn-inducer: "Over all conflicts of human and legitimate interests, there is the authority of the government; the government alone is in the right position to see things from the point of view of the general welfare. This government is not at the disposition of this man or that man; it is over everybody, because it takes to itself not only the juridical conscience of the nation in the present, but also all that the nation represents for the future. The government has shown that it values at the highest the productive strength of the

---

[152] Mussolini did not reference any Italian version of America's Henry Ford (and others) who, in 1914, years earlier, had instituted eight-hour shifts and higher wages. Capitalism creates shorter work hours and higher wages. Socialism does the opposite. Under socialism, workers waste uncompensated hours in lines waiting for bread, toilet paper, etc.

nation." (My Autobiography, p. 279).

Toward those sleepy socialist tropes Mussolini's autobiography urges the muzzle and leash of every police state: government schools and universities (socialist schools and universities).

Here are some interesting words to search for in Mussolini's autobiography: Corporative state, masons, socialist-masons, popolo (Popolo d' Italia), fasciti, fascismo, capital, bolshevism, Lenin, Russian famine, soviet, sovietist, and internationalism.

Mussolini was aware of mass starvation under Lenin (e.g. the Soviet famine 1921-1922) and did not want to duplicate or exceed it (in comparison, the socialists Stalin and Mao exceeded Lenin's famine gleefully). Mussolini said: "Only some time afterward did the news of the dreadful Russian famine, as well as the information furnished by our mission which had gone to Russia to study Bolshevism, open the eyes of the crowd to the falsity of the Russian paradise-mirage. Enthusiasm ebbed away little by little. Finally, Lenin remained only as a kind of banner and catchword for our political dabblers." Mussolini adopted the conceit of Lenin, Stalin, Hitler, Mao, the Kim scum, and all socialists: Things will swing when I am king!

Lenin's socialist famine also caused Lenin to re-think his own socialist mess, and he decreed the "New Economic Policy" (NEP on March 15, 1921). It was another way in which Lenin influenced Mussolini's socialism with so-called "new" scams.

Lenin described his own humiliating defeat by economics (and his continued effort to glorify his own thievery as "socialism"), while Lenin followed Mussolini's socialist path in their struggle to cling to power and keep up their pretense:

At a meeting of Communist factory groups at Moscow, Lenin said: As regards actual economic relations we observe here in Russia five different economic systems. The first is the patriarchal system, where the peasant works only for himself. The second is small trade, where he brings his own products to the market. The third is the capitalist, where a small amount of private capital is formed, the fourth is state capitalism, and the fifth socialism. If one observes the economic life of Russia one sees all five systems existing alongside of each other. The reason for that is that our great industry is not yet re-established, and that the socialised factories receive only a tenth of what they require. The general decay of the country, the shortage of fuel and raw material, the unsatisfactory transport situation, have brought it about that small industry exists alongside of socialism. Under such circumstances state capitalism amounts to the unification of the small industries. It is natural that uncontrolled trade means the growth of capitalism, but we do not fear this capitalism. We do not fear it because we achieve an immediate increase in production, and that is what we need. In this way a state capitalism will form itself which we do not fear, because we shall determine the boundaries in which it will grow. This capitalism will be under the control of the state. When the state holds all factories, all undertakings, and all railways in its hands capitalism gives no anxiety. The Soviet power must look all things quietly in the eyes and call everything by its proper name. A capitalism which develops under control while the proletariat has the power in its hands in no

way contradicts the idea of Communism. ("Ladder of Communism" Maoriland Worker, Vol. 12, Issue 247; 28 SEPTEMBER 1921).

Benito Mussolini did NOT say: "Fascism should more appropriately be called Corporatism because it is a merger of State and corporate power." That fake quote was commonly attributed[153] to Mussolini until the attribution was debunked by the veteran historian Dr. Rex Curry.

Some people point to Giovanni Gentile (in "La Dottrina del Fascismo") as the person who created the quote that was attributed falsely to Mussolini. "La Dottrina del Fascismo" was written by Giovanni Gentile, and published under Mussolini's name in the Encyclopedia Italiana. However, the only reference to "corporatism" within Gentile's article is in section VIII, and NOT in the words of the quote.

There is no original source in Italian that refers to the quotation. Instead, there is one source in Italian, that translates an American source.

Mussolini never uttered the quote that is attributed to him, and anyone who understands what Mussolini DID say would know that the quote does not describe Mussolini's beliefs.

Mussolini's use of the term "corporatism" did not mean a business corporation and is related etymologically only because both words use the Latin root word for body: "corpus." Christian socialism and

---

[153] Dr. Curry debunked the columnist Molly Ivins, who used the fake quote around 24 November 2002. Ivins showed that she did not understand Mussolini. The fake quote spread rapidly in the US after Ivins' column. The fake quote has probably been repeated on Wakipedia (Wikipedia).

Christian corporatism rely on similar interpretations of the Bible, including the New Testament in I Corinthians 12:12-31 where Paul of Tarsus compares individuals to different parts of one human body, functioning together. Those are the same ideas that influenced Francis Bellamy, the American Christian Socialist, in his descriptions of Jesus as a "socialist." Mussolini's use of the term was influenced by the Catholic church's use of the Latin term "corpus" within the religion and by a Catholic study of corporatism under Pope Leo XIII from 1881.

On July 2, 1926, Mussolini imposed the Ministry of Corporations and soon thereafter the National Council of Corporations. The pompous Italian socialists also created the Istituto per la Ricostruzione Industriale (IRI). They were ominous parallels to Lenin's Soviet socialism at that time, and what would happen later under Hitler's German socialism, and Roosevelt's American socialism.

In 1927, Mussolini touted his "Charter of Labor." In his autobiography Mussolini explained the socialist charter thusly: "It is composed of thirty paragraphs, each of which contains a fundamental truth. From the paramount necessity for production arises the need of an equitable sharing of products, the need of the judgment of tribunals in case of discord, and, finally, the need of protective legislation." (page 280).

The 30 paragraphs are written in socialist babble with various socialist scams including mandated "paid vacations" (written with the classic socialist lie to imply that it is "free" or paid for by someone else and that mandatory "paid vacations" have no downward effect on wages or employment); and numerous other mandated fringe benefits for workers (written with the classic socialist lie to imply that such benefits hadn't previously existed until socialists thought them up and imposed them by law upon everyone; and that such mandatory benefits are "free" or paid for by someone else and that the benefits have no downward effect on wages or employment).

It is a wonder why Mussolini never wrote: "Business owners are greedy, but if you raise minimum wages, increase mandated benefits, and boost taxes, then businesses will magically stop being greedy and won't raise prices to compensate, nor take any evasive action to shift costs." Mussolini assumed correctly that all of his socialist supporters were dimbulbs.

Mussolini's Ministry of Corporations organized the Italian economy into 22 "sectoral corporations" (see the Address to the National Corporative Council on November 14, 1933, and the Senate Speech on the Bill Establishing the Corporations on January 13, 1934). The 22 sectoral corporations were the method via which the socialist Mussolini organized his Unionism (Fascism), and his beloved worker's unions, and the economy. It was not until February 5, 1934, that the 22 "corporations" were defined:

1. Social Care & Credit
2. Internal Communications
3. Sea & Air
4. Entertainment
5. Hostelries
6. Professions & Arts
7. Building Construction
8. Water, Gas & Electricity
9. Mining Industries
10. Glass & Ceramics
11. Grains

12. Vegetable, Flower & Fruit Cultivation
13. Wine and Oil Cultivation
14. Livestock & Fish
15. Wood
16. Textiles
17. Clothing
18. Metalworking
19. Machinery
20. Chemicals
21. Liquid Combustibles & Fossil Fuels
22. Paper & Publishing

They were not capitalist "corporations" as is claimed by many deceitful socialists in the USA. Socialists deliberately lie about what the socialist Mussolini was saying. Socialists misuse Mussolini's term. Mussolini's "corporations" distorted free markets, businesses, industry, capitalism, and bona fide corporations.

Mussolini didn't mean the power of big corporations. He meant the power of a large number of individuals working collectively as a bureaucracy or union. That is what he meant by "corporativismo."

Article 6 of the Charter of Labor explains what a "corporation" is under Mussolini's socialism: "Legally organized trade organizations assure legal equality between employers and workers, maintain the discipline of production and labor, and promote its perfection. A corporation constitutes the organization of one field of production and represents its interests as a whole. Since the interests of production are national interests, the corporations are recognized by law as state organizations by virtue of this representation."

In his autobiography, Mussolini waxes socialist: "In this institution are concentrated all the branches of national production. Work in all its complex manifestations and in all its breadth, whether of manual or of intellectual nature, requires equally protection and nourishment." (page 281).

Mussolini's term is closer to the concept of a municipal corporation, which is a form of socialism: a government entity that imposes a socialist monopoly on the provision of goods and services.

A Socialist declares that she wants to end "corporations" until she is asked, "You want to end municipal corporations?" After she researches the meaning of "municipal corporation" the socialist admits that she supports the worst form of corporations (municipal corporations, and the BBC, the CPB -the Corporation for Public Broadcasting, etc). Socialists continue to share so much with the socialist Mussolini.[154]

Mussolini said, "Some still ask of us: what do you want? We answer with three words that summon up our entire program. Here they are...Italy, Republic, Socialization . . . Socialization is no other than the implantation of Italian Socialism..."[155]

Mussolini said, "For this I have been and am a socialist. The accusation of inconsistency has no foundation. My conduct has always been straight in the sense of looking at the substance of things and not to the form. I adapted socialisticamente to reality. As the evolution of society belied many of the prophecies of

---

[154] Compare that to the socialist Pol Pot who daftly believed that cities were bad capitalism, so he forced people to move to the country. Millions died. Billions of lives were ruined.

[155] Speech to a group of Milanese Fascist veterans on October 14, 1944, Op. Cit., Spampanato pp. 682-683, and Revolutionary Fascism, Erik Norling, Lisbon, Finis Mundi Press (2011) p. 43.

Marx, the true socialism folded from possible to probable. The only feasible socialism socialisticamente is corporatism, confluence, balance and justice interests compared to the collective interest."[156]

Mussolini pointed out that Marx's predictions did not occur. Marx's fantasy about the future was similar to that of Edward Bellamy: utterly wrong and the cause of poverty, suffering, and death.

How many times do the words "Fascism" and "Fascist" appear in Marx's books "Das Kapital" and "The Communist Manifesto"? Marx never used the words in print or speech because Marx died before the words were coined. Marx did not foretell any Fascist revolution, even though many people claim that such revolutions have occurred in Italy, Germany, and elsewhere. If so, then that means that Marx was incorrect about what kind of revolutions would happen.

Marx and Mussolini had much in common. They both camouflaged their failed socialist dogma with new labels: Communism and Fascism. The main philosophical difference between Communism, Fascism, and Socialism is the spelling.

Mussolini (and all modern socialists) were inspired by the socialism used in ancient Rome by Gaius Julius Caesar to maintain support: He made people dependent upon him by pretending to give everyone "free" stuff.

Mussolini was inspired also by the socialist Gabriele D'Annunzio. A web search for "Gabriele d'Annunzio was also a socialist" (or in Italian "Gabriele d'Annunzio fu anche socialista") reveals his socialist history (Don't bother with Wikipedia; it will never tell readers that

---

[156] As quoted in "Soliloquy for 'freedom' Trimellone island," from Ivanoe Fossani's interview of Mussolini, March 20, 1945, from Opera omnia, vol. 32, one of Mussolini's last interviews.

Gabriele d'Annunzio was a socialist. The anonymous bulletin board posters on Wikipedia do not want anyone to know. The rest of the web reveals what wakipedia hides). Few know that the poet was deputy of the Socialist Party, and even a candidate in 1900.

Mussolini used the term "Duce" as a socialist, as well as socialism's stiff-armed salute. He acquired "Duce" from D'Annnunzio's use of the title. D'Annunzio set up the short-lived Italian Regency of Carnaro in Fiume with himself as Duce.

D'Annunzio's socialist scams were evident in Fiume when he coauthored a constitution. The constitution established a socialist state with nine sectors of collectivization to represent the so-called different sectors of the economy (workers, employers, professionals), and a tenth (D'Annunzio's invention) to represent the "superior" human beings (heroes, poets, prophets, supermen). It established a Technical Council of Labour. The Carta also declared that music was the fundamental principle of the state.

The American socialist Edward Bellamy (1850-1898) was the source of Mussolini's and D'Annunzio's dogma from the grave, via Bellamy's international bestseller "Looking Backward" (1888) and other Bellamy preachings. Dr. Curry unmasked Edward Bellamy's "military socialism" as the blueprint for Mussolini's and D'Annunzio's departments and dictatorship. Bellamy touted "10 great departments" in his "industrial army." D'Annunzio's followed Bellamy's ten departments quantity, and il Douche' (Mussolini) more than doubled it.

Bellamy's book offers these excerpts of socialism's kindergarten economics: "Now the entire field of productive and constructive industry is divided into ten great departments, each representing a group of allied industries, each particular industry being in turn represented by a subordinate bureau, which has a complete record of the plant and force under its control, of the present product, and means of increasing it. The estimates of the distributive department, after adoption by the administration, are sent as mandates to the ten great departments, which allot them to the subordinate bureaus representing the particular industries, and these set the men at work. Each bureau is responsible for the task given it, and this responsibility is enforced by departmental oversight and that of the administration; nor does the distributive department accept the product without its own inspection; while even if in the hands of the consumer an article turns out unfit, the system enables the fault to be traced back to the original workman. The production of the commodities for actual public consumption does not, of course, require by any means all the national force of workers. After the necessary contingents have been detailed for the various industries, the amount of labor left for other employment is expended in creating fixed capital, such as buildings, machinery, engineering works, and so forth."

Bellamy touts his "military socialism" here: "The general of his guild holds a splendid position, and one which amply satisfies the ambition of most men, but above his rank, which may be compared--to follow the military analogies familiar to you--to that of a general of division or major-general, is that of the chiefs of the ten great departments, or groups of allied trades. The chiefs of these ten grand divisions of the industrial army may be compared to your commanders of army corps, or lieutenant-generals, each having from a dozen to a score of generals of separate guilds reporting to him. Above these ten great officers, who form his council, is the general-in-chief, who is the President of the United States."

Bellamy's fairy tales are similar to those told by the socialists Mussolini, Stalin, Mao, Hitler and many others. The militant socialists Stalin, Mao, and Hitler were similar to the socialist Mussolini and their underlings: They all suffered from socialism's military-industrial complex. It was the authoritarian ideology touted by the Bellamys from 1888: Military Socialism and National Socialism.

Here is another excerpt from Edward Bellamy:

"The President, I suppose, is selected from among the ten heads of the great departments," I suggested.

"Precisely, but the heads of departments are not eligible to the presidency till they have been a certain number of years out of office. It is rarely that a man passes through all the grades to the headship of a department much before he is forty, and at the end of a five years' term he is usually forty-five. If more, he still serves through his term, and if less, he is nevertheless discharged from the industrial army at its termination."

Each one of Bellamy's and Mussolini's socialist bureaucracies has one or more extant twins among the thousands of huge faceless socialist monopolies in the United States including: the Department of Commerce (1903, 1913); Department of Labor (1903, 1913); Department of the Interior (1849); Social Security Administration; Federal Communications Commission; Department of Health and Human Services; United States Postal Service; Department of Agriculture (USDA 1862);[157] Bureau of Land Management;

---

[157] In "The Grapes of Wrath," author John Steinbeck ignored

Department of Transportation; Federal Trade Commission; Federal Aviation Administration; Department of Education; Army Corps of Engineers; Army, Navy, Air Force, Marines. Many predated and influenced Mussolini's socialism. Many predated and influenced Franklin Delano Roosevelt (FDR), or were concocted by him. Many continue to cripple the USA.

FDR completed the hydroelectric dam started by the socialist President Herbert Hoover. Both presidents were following Stalin's Dnieper Hydroelectric dam engineered by Colonel Hugh Lincoln Cooper (from the US), who was awarded the Order of the Red Star (the first time that such a prestigious medal had been given to a foreigner).[158] The Dnieper dam's construction began in 1927 (it opened October 1932); The Hoover dam's construction began in 1931 (it opened in 1936).

FDR created the Farm Security Administration (FSA) in 1935 as part of his New Socialist Deal. It socialized land owned by poor farmers and engaged in relocation of them to group farms. Critics strongly opposed the FSA because it was socialist agriculture similar to that which caused long-term shortages, squalor, and starvation under the socialists Stalin and Lenin.

German socialists expanded on the American socialist example with their first ghetto in 1939, while

---

the Department of Agriculture's role (in the dust bowl, in food shortages, et cetera), to the detriment of millions of readers then and now.

[158] Which was more prestigious (or which medal is prettier): the Order of the Red Cross medal awarded to Col. Cooper under Soviet socialism (1932); or the Grand Cross of the German Eagle medal awarded to Henry Ford by German socialism six years later (1938)?

Hitler was conspiring with Soviet socialists to divide up Europe and relocate people. War is just one more big government program under the military-socialism complex. Later, Chinese socialists used "labor camps" to imprison and murder for Mao, expanding on earlier examples under many other intolerant socialists including Stalin, Hitler, and FDR.

FDR imposed the Civilian Conservation Corps (from 1933 to 1942; and segregated in a racist manner), and similar camp scams were used to intern Japanese (1942 to 1946).[159] Thus, FDR's camps over-lapped in time the camps of Stalin. Some of FDR's camps preceded Hitler; some overlapped, or followed. FDR's message via the work camps was that work makes you free, even when the government gives you a socialist make-work job. Under German socialism the same Marxist concept was "arbeit macht frei." Who was learning from whom? It was mutual?

FDR's FSA is notorious for its photography program, 1935–44, that includes a photograph of Brownies (junior Girl Scouts) saluting the flag with the Nazi gesture within a relocation farm compound (dated February 1942, in Tulare County, California, by photographer Russell Lee).

In 1946 the FSA was replaced by the Farmers Home Administration. It continued as part of Lyndon Johnson's

---

[159] Did Americans fight the "Nazis" so that those Americans could be called "Nazis" for having the same views as they had when they fought the "Nazis"? Did Americans fight the "Nazis" so that their children and grandchildren could be called "Nazis" for having similar views to their grandparents who fought the "Nazis"? If the Americans who fought German socialism expressed their beliefs today, they would be called "Nazis." This is an awkward moment to bring up the pledge gesture in the USA around that time.

socialist programs in the 1960s, with an expanded budget, of course.

Mussolini's doppelganger in the USA was Roosevelt (FDR). The twin-brothers suckled like wolves on the public teat, competed to be degenerate statists, raced to create new bureaucracies, and spread the roaming mythology of socialism. Both were influenced by the Bellamy cousins.

FDR grew up doing the stiff-armed socialist salute (during the Pledge of Allegiance and also outside of the pledge) long before the socialist leader Mussolini learned it. FDR was merely one in a long line of presidents and other famous Americans who helped teach the notorious gesture (and the deadly dogma behind it) to Italy and the world.

From 1892, Italian children (and all foreign children) in the USA had been brainwashed to accept government (socialist) schools along with Nazi salutes and Nazi behavior therein.

An Americanization rally was held on April 27, 1917 at City Hall in New York City. A photograph shows children dressed in costumes of different countries (including Italy) with flags of the different countries as a woman stands with an American Flag on the steps of City Hall (Bain Collection). The children are rendering the first part of the gesture in the early Pledge of Allegiance.

Another breath-taking photograph of the same Americanization rally shows a sea of thousands of students rendering the Nazi salute to the U.S. flag (entitled "1917 American School children saluting the Flag Stars and stripes Washington High School New York").

The conditioning of foreign students in the U.S.

continued for decades. Another example of the training is shown in a photograph of French preschool age children performing the initial gesture of the old pledge salute at L'Ecole maternelle francaise in New York, New York (dated June 6, 1944, D-day, and photographed by Howard Hollem, Edward Meyer or MacLaugharie). The children are being taught to make the gesture toward the French flag -not the U.S. flag- in the New York school. That behavior was entirely consistent with Bellamy's plan from 1892 to spread his socialism and his pledge worldwide. It was consistent with Bellamy's desire to "Americanize" foreigners in the U.S. (under Bellamy's reasoning, a student was "Americanized" when he/she embraced Bellamy's socialism, including socialist schools and daily worship of government therein).

As Mussolini began his fascitization of socialism, he also culturally appropriated the American stiff-armed salute and the accompanying automatic group-speak already prevalent under U.S. socialism. Mussolini did more than dictate America's stiff-armed gesture in Italy: He imposed the gesture along with knee-jerk chanting to the flag in government schools (socialist schools) as had been the practice in the USA since 1892. On January 31, 1923, the Ministry of Education imposed a sycophantic incantation to the flag in Italian schools and the creepy scene was immortalized by the photographer Stefano Stagnoli in his photograph "The Promise to the Fatherland."

Mussolini learned the American stiff-armed salute early in his socialist career, and he learned of it from the socialist Gabrielle D'Annunzio, who probably learned it from old early movies (from the USA) that utilized the widespread gesture in the United States' Pledge of

Allegiance to the Flag (the practice had been occurring for about three decades in the USA -from 1892).

Mussolini died on 28 April 1945, but his long-time work promoting socialism lived on in Italy and worldwide. Before Mussolini's death, German socialists created the Italian Social Republic (not the Italian Fascist Republic) in northern Italy and installed Mussolini as prime minister (23 September 1943). It lasted 19 months.

Mussolini was executed by firing squad and then he was hung upside down for display outside of a gas station in Milan. Two days later, Hitler committed suicide (April 30, 1945), to escape Mussolini's fate. Hitler had left prior instructions for his remains to be doused in petrol, and set ablaze. Whatever was left of his burnt remains -at best unrecognizable, ghoulish, and fragile- they were not hung upside down at any gas station.

14. USA'S AUGUST LANDMESSER

August Landmesser[160] is best known for his appearance in a photograph wherein he refused to perform the stiff-armed salute under German socialism during the launch of a naval training vessel (the Horst Wessel) on 13 June 1936.

No article about Landmesser points out that the same gesture (and persecution of anyone who refused the gesture) was happening in the United States[161] at the same time that it was happening in Germany to Landmesser and others; that the pledge to the U.S. flag was the origin of the gesture that Landmesser defied. Only in the comments section do people reference the academic work of Dr. Curry showing that the U.S. was the origin of the Nazi salute and Nazi behavior from the American socialist Francis Bellamy.

No article about Landmesser points out that the same behavior continues in the USA, where only the gesture has changed. Every day in government schools (socialist

---

[160] There appears to be compelling evidence that the person is Gustav Wegert, and not August Landmesser.

[161] It is no wonder that individuals outside the U.S. sometimes refer to citizens of the United States as "Statists" or "Statesians."

schools) children sycophantically intone en masse on command. The gesture changed to hide the pledge's unseemly past. Children are kept ignorant of the history of the quotidian ritual that they are led to perform.

No article about Landmesser explains that a growing wave of students refuse to be bullied into the brainwashing and are learning the truth about the pledge's shocking past. No one celebrates their bravery. They are ordinary heroes in extraordinary times. Such students attract abuse from people who praise August Landmesser and who have nothing to say about the fact that Americans were persecuted (at the same time that Landmesser was persecuted in Germany) for refusing to perform the nazi salute in the Pledge of Allegiance (POA) in the USA.

No article about Landmesser includes photos of Americans circa 1936 that are very similar to the Landmesser photo. Has anyone in the media printed such a photo, or do any of them even have that knowledge?

There are court cases involving prison for Americans who refused to do the Nazi salute for the USA's pledge or who otherwise showed "disrespect" to the U.S. flag. Americans were beaten, imprisoned, even lynched.

The government and government schools deserve blame for that photo of Landmesser. Francis Bellamy deserves blame for Landmesser's predicament.

The photo of Landmesser is powerful and would be more powerful if Americans were not so ignorant of the history of USA's Pledge of Allegiance as the origin of the Nazi salute and Nazi behavior.

15. YESTERYEAR'S INDOCTRINATION

Francis Julius Bellamy died on August 28, 1931, in Tampa, Florida. Tampa was also the city where Bellamy's Pledge of Allegiance died. A plaque memorializes him and his pledge at the house where he resided on 2926 Wallcraft Avenue.

Although he died in Tampa, Bellamy's remains were moved to Rome, New York, the origin of the "ancient Roman salute" myth that developed from his pledge.

He lived long enough to see the government schools (socialist schools) that he wanted to impose on everyone. He lived long enough to see those schools impose segregation by law and teach racism as official policy and force children to perform the Nazi salute and slavish chanting daily for 12 years of their lives, upon threat of violence or punishment. He lived through a time when people were beaten, arrested, jailed, imprisoned, and even lynched for defying his pledge.

No evidence has been found that any of the above bothered him, nor that he considered any of the above to be inconsistent with his dogma of "Christian socialism" and "Military socialism."

His work continues to haunt the world. The American Nazi salute continues to be used in many places, including Mexico, China (including Taiwan), and Russia, North Korea,[162] along with persecution of dissenters.[163]

It is funny that some Americans complain if the USA's iconography of ignorance is recited in the Spanish language, instead of the English language. They are correct that the Pledge of Allegiance (POA) should not be chanted in Spanish. It should only be chanted in German, Russian, or Chinese.

Or better yet, just say "Nein!" to the pledge. Don't Jewish that all Germans had said that? Nein out of ten people support Hitler's socialism today.

Another subtitle for this book could be "To see or not see Nazi reality." The real "not sees" are people who do not see the socialist imagery of the swastika and the PoS who chant the USA's POA. This book was written to educate modern "not-sees."

The cult of socialism was the same as the occult

---

[162] North Korean children use a modified version that begins with (1) an altered Nazi salute thrust outward and then (2) retracted back toward the head so that the hand stops in an almost vertical orientation near the forehead, in an odd military salute (see the film documentary "Under The Sun"). Photographs often only show the vertical part (the final part) of the gesture.

[163] India's supreme court ordered cinemas across the country to display the flag and play the national anthem before films and the court also directed that moviegoers should "stand up in respect" while the anthem is played (November 30, 2016). The military salute (British) is often used to salute the flag in India (The military salute to the flag was a practice that began in the US and was the origin of the Nazi salute). A movie-goer was dragged to cops for not standing up during the anthem (Times of India, Feb 3, 2017). Should theaters in the US play the National Anthem and lead the pledge before all movies?

nightmares whispered about Nazism. The swastika was a sign of "socialist" identity. The chosen people of the National Socialist German Workers' Party were a bizarre para-military fraternity that wanted to evolve and impose a new world order [#nwo], creating a utopian future, resembling the Military Socialism and Christian Socialism of American socialists (including Francis Bellamy and Edward Bellamy).

People who adopted the "Double S" and its dogma of socialism preached the sacrifice of everyone. They called it a brave new world, but it was a grave new world.

The misanthropes, necrophiliacs, and cannibals caused millions of deaths. Socialism is misanthropy incarnate.

Some critics argue about the exact number of millions of people murdered in the socialist Wholecaust (of which the Holocaust was a part) under the Reich of Stalin, Mao, Hitler, and other socialists. After all, Who's counting? Socialists weren't counting. Millions of people murdered in various socialist countries adds up. But the socialists retort: it only adds up if someone adds it up. The socialists are a reminder of a retort from the ethicist Dr. Rex Curry: "A million murdered here, a million murdered there, pretty soon you are talking a lot of people." Here are estimates: ~50 million under the Union of Soviet Socialist Republics?; ~40 million under the Peoples' Republic of China?; ~20 million under the National Socialist German Workers' Party?[164] In

---

[164] Socialists disputed those death estimates so adamantly that if anyone publicly disseminated those figures in those countries then he would be killed too.

As socialists say, it is less horrifying if you focus instead on all the millions of people that they DIDN'T kill.

addition to the body piles, billions of lives were ruined.

Those deadly eras are known as the modern socialist inquisitions, the modern socialist Dark Ages (and their inhumanity and death tolls exceeded that of the previous Dark Ages and of all prior inquisitions). The Age of Endarkenment resulted in the worst death toll in human history and was so large that all Holocaust Museums could quadruple in size and scope by adding Wholecaust Museums to document the entire socialist slaughter.[165]

Socialists fancied themselves as the "illuminati," but they were the "deluminati." Today, on world maps, they are the countries where the least light shines at night. Their psychopathology set and holds the worst records for extinguishing the life-lights of so many.

The socialist psychopathy of the Bellamy cousins continues in the USA today. Many Bellamy policies caused the oppressive domestic government. The pledge continues along with laws mandating that teachers lead the clownish intonation every day for twelve years in the life of each child.

Some people say that freedom is promoted by children who are tread upon to submissively drone daily to the national flag in government's schools. They also say that you can eat yourself thin, and drink yourself sober.

The anti-libertarian government continues to own and operate schools, including the same schools that imposed segregation by law and taught racism as official government policy. The USA's practice of imposing segregation by law (in government schools) and teaching racism as official policy even outlasted the

---

[165] The House of Terror is a museum located at Andrássy út 60 in Budapest, Hungary. It contains exhibits related to both German socialism and Soviet socialism. www.terrorhaza.hu

National Socialist German Workers Party into the 1960's and beyond.

After segregation in government schools ended, the Bellamy legacy caused more police-state racism of forced busing that destroyed communities and neighborhoods and deepened hostilities. Those schools still exist. Also extant are the same governmental bodies and their busing systems.

Segregation and discrimination continues under socialism. It occurs geographically, via zoning, districting, funding, maintenance, and more. Racism occurs via refusal of bilingual education (e.g. Spanish, Hebrew, et cetera) or by providing only one hour of a language.

When a student enrolls, Government schools demand social security numbers (socialist slave numbers or "SS numbers") that were given to students as newborn infants to track and control them for life, stealing the whole way. The Ponzi scheme is one of many ways that socialism has taught parents how to rob their own children, including unborn grandchildren.

SS numbers were imposed in 1935, and many of the USA's slaves gleefully tattooed their numbers into their skin. That was years before tattooed numbers were used at Auschwitz under German socialism. SS number 535-07-5248 is tattooed on Thomas Cave in a 1939 photograph by Dorothea Lange. That was before similar tattooing occurred in concentration camps in Auschwitz, Poland. Cave's tattoo is near his right bicep. Did some Americans tattoo the SS number on their left forearms (where Auschwitz tattoos were usually placed)?

Were there any instances of Americans burning their SS cards in protest against the US police state?

Lange also photographed children performing the

pledge of allegiance (with the hand-over-the-heart) shortly before they were relocated to an internment camp in 1942, after the racist socialist President Franklin Delano Roosevelt (FDR) followed the modus operandi of the socialists Hitler and Stalin. FDR ordered the relocation of 120,000 Japanese-Americans. It was another one of FDR's many socialist pogroms or programs (seven years earlier, in 1935, FDR began the popular modern police state program whereby Americans are numbered so that they can be tracked and taxed from cradle to grave). FDR remains one of the most popular presidents in the US, and he might be as popular as the robber barons Stalin, Mao, and Hitler were as leaders in their socialist hellholes. FDR might be as popular in the US today as the mass murderer Mao is in China. All seriousness aside, FDR can't be that adored can he?

Lange's hand-over-the-heart photograph should be compared with another photograph that shows Japanese-Americans performing the stiff-armed salute to the flag inside one of FDR's internment camps. Another photograph (credited to Library of Congress/Corbis/VCG via Getty Images) shows the gesture performed by "Japanese American Students at Graduation" in Santa Anita, California in June 1942 (# 640459801). Shortly after their graduation ceremony they were sent to a relocation camp.

Is George Takei in any of those photographs?[166] The

---

[166] Takei tweeted: "History shall record that you [Donald Trump] are not only the stupidest, most incompetent president ever, but also the cruelest and pettiest." Other tweets reminded Takei that FDR literally put Takei in a camp. Set phasers to not-that-stunned. There are not many people like Takei who can boast that they vote for and support a

notorious gesture was probably performed by actor George Takei (Sulu in the television series Star Trek) when he resided in a relocation camp from 5 to 8 years of age.

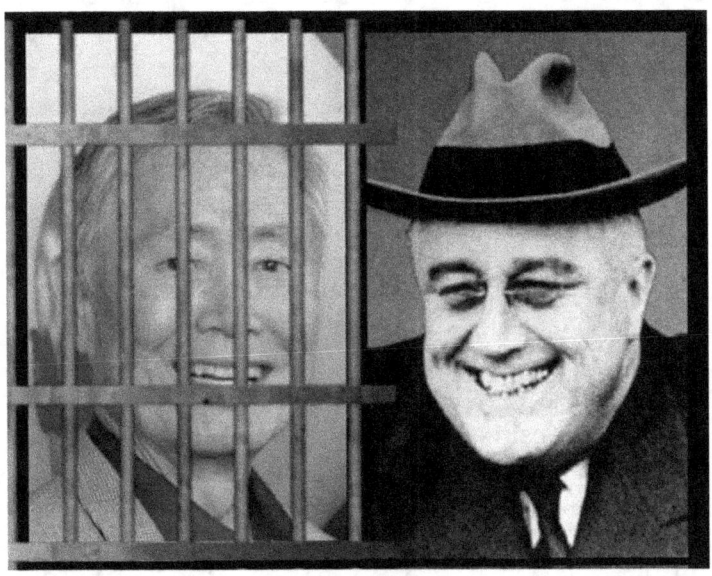

Takei's camp experience inspired his Broadway musical "Allegiance." Even so, Takei is not known to have ever commented on the early gesture for the Pledge of Allegiance (inside his camp or out).[167] The gesture

political party that put them, personally, in an internment camp. Stockholm syndrome? Socialism is a psychological issue akin to Stockholm Syndrome. The POA is part of the syndrome. Why don't Japanese-Americans claim the "lingering effect" of the relocation camps impedes their ability to succeed? How about tearing down statues of FDR, and renaming bridges and schools?

[167] It is not known if Takei or his parents received their Social Security numbers while in the camp. It is not known if any campers were so proud of the number that they had it

would have made the musical more surprising for audiences ("Allegiance" closed in five months).

The hand-over-the-heart continues today in G-schools (government schools) where each classroom contains a flag, and where small children are conditioned with a soldierly chant at the daily ring of a bell, as if Pavlov's dogs.

The school ritual led to flags in churches and temples. Flags in religious establishments also evolved from the "Christian Socialism" and "Military Socialism" of Francis Bellamy and Edward Bellamy.

Inside mosques, there are not flags of ISIS, Al-Qaeda, or of terrorist organizations. In government schools, most Muslim students feel it is improper to pledge allegiance to the flag (or to anything or anyone other than God).

In non-Muslim churches and temples you will find the flag of the USA (and memorials to the government traveling around the world killing people).

Bellamy's pledge is different from the Bay`ah (Pledge of Allegiance) in Islam, where a Muslim pledges obedience to the ruler of a region.[168] The

---

tattooed to their forearm or other body part.

[168] Non-religious people quip that when the veil is lifted then this truth is revealed: The religion of Islam is stupid because it is based on Judaism and Christianity.

Some historians praise Islam for promoting science long ago. Muslims needed science to calculate the many mandatory times for screaming calls to organized robotic chanting (prayer) each day; and the direction of Mecca to pray toward; and the prohibition of the depiction of the human form (including @8{> sideways Mohammed emoticons) meant that they had to produce intricate geometric patterns to decorate their buildings. See? And you thought religious stupidity produced no scientific benefits.

Muslim pledge is only recited once, whereas Bellamy's Bay`ah is recited by little children synchronically and every day for 12 years as prescribed by state laws. Muslims pray daily facing mecca. Americans pledge daily facing the flag (and they should face DC).

After the Pulse nightclub was attacked in Orlando, Florida in June of 2015, the government released transcripts of a 911 phone call with the culprit's "pledge of allegiance" that was censored so heavily that it was not clear whether or not the culprit pledged allegiance to the U.S. flag.

The pledge continues as enforced infantilism for simpletons. It is an anachronistic Nazi artifact that was written more than a century ago for kindergartners. Bellamy's juvenilia (and juvenalia) is intoned by almost every man-child today. [Googoo gah gah]. The flag ritual makes non-participants feel like the only adult in a room full of children. Intelligent grown-ups imagine that they are in second grade again. It is the daily blue pill.

Always try to see things as they are, not as others want them to be. Better to be silent and thought a fool than to robotically chant the pledge and remove all doubt.

How did so many people over the decades write about the USA's Pledge of Allegiance and the swastika and fail to make the discoveries that were made by Dr. Curry? What caused the forgotten history? How could those writers (some of whom viewed historic photographs of the early pledge's Nazi salute), have failed (or refused?) to even ask the questions: (1) Was the Pledge of Allegiance the origin of the Nazi salute and Nazi behavior? (2) Did it impact Germany and other countries at all?

The societal amnesia is the fault of government's schools (socialist schools) that will never ask these questions about the daily pledge ritual and its relationship to socialism in Germany and worldwide. The government's schools have conditioned researchers and writers not to ask or answer the questions that have been answered here.

The word "Nazi" is used to hide the true origin of "Nazi": it means "national socialist." The word "Nazi" evolved from the first two syllables of the German word "national" in the term "national socialist." Hitler did not call himself a "Nazi"; he called himself a "national socialist." Bellamy did not call himself a "Nazi"; he called himself a "national socialist." The word "Nazi" continues to be used to conceal connections between German socialism and American socialism. Francis Bellamy was a Nazi; he was an American Nazi.

Those are some of the reasons why government schools are unconstitutional: they violate the First Amendment right to freedom of speech and freedom of the press. The government schools (socialist schools) tell everyone what to think and say and write.

If government made cars, G-schools would have you believe there would be no cars without government.

Innovators and creative geniuses cannot be molded in government schools (socialist schools). They are precisely the individuals who defy what the government has taught them.

"The Greatest Mistake in American History: Letting Government Educate Our Children" was written by Harry Browne. Some other countries (including Germany) ban home-schooling. In other words, Germany continues to do what the socialist Hitler did. When the state tells you that you can't pull your children out of school, it is immediately time to pull them out of school.

The flag pledge is a fundamental part of the USA's police state. It is a daily Milgram experiment, a witch hunt, and it demonstrates the banality of evil (and the evil of banality). Litigation continues to occur concerning the persecution of people who refuse.

Government schools have been losing students, respect and money faster than you can recite the Pledge of Allegiance (if you still cared to do so).

Many people who read this book have already rejected the salute and the POA's daily juvenile drill.

After reading this book, they also stop standing up.

Of those who still stand up, many of them stand up only to leave the room wherever the hypnotic veneration is slavishly directed.

Many of them stop returning to any room or meeting if the childish vow is repeated in the future.

Many of them abandon attendance and membership in groups that persist in the bizarre brain-washing.

Many of them create better groups where free people do not engage in the outlandish ritual of worshipping government.

Fight antidisestablishmentarianism. Please help stop the Pledge of Allegiance (POA) and the socialism that it promotes and perpetuates. Remove the pledge from the flag, remove flags from schools, and remove schools from government.

Support the "Stop the Pledge of Allegiance Foundation." Take the pledge not to pledge. Don't fellate the state.

16. BACKGROUND FOR THIS BOOK

The author Jonah Goldberg in the book "Liberal Fascism: The Secret History of the American Left, From Mussolini to the Politics of Meaning" cites Dr. Curry. The following is an excerpt:

Religion was the glue that held this American national socialism together. Bellamy believed that his brand of socialist nationalism was the true application of Jesus' teachings. His cousin Francis Bellamy, the author of the Pledge of Allegiance, was similarly devoted. A founding member of the first Nationalist Club of Boston and co-founder of the Society of Christian Socialists, Francis wrote a Sermon, "Jesus, the Socialist," that electrified parishes across the country. In an expression of his "military socialism," the Pledge of Allegiance was accompanied by a [stiff-arm] salute to the flag in American public schools. Indeed, some contend that the Nazis got the idea for their salute from America. (page 216).

...The story of the Pledge of Allegiance and its National Socialist roots is a fascinating one. Dr. Rex Curry, a passionate libertarian, has made the issue

his white whale. (page 440, n. 25).

Goldberg cites Dr. Curry's breakthrough regarding the pledge, but he does not mention Dr. Curry's other accomplishments, such as the swastika as an alphabetic brand for "socialist."

Is Goldberg unaware that German socialists did not call their emblem a "swastika"? (He never explains their emblem's name and its alphabetic representation, even though it would bolster his arguments about "Liberal Fascism"). His ignorance explains why he failed to make Professor Curry's discovery about the swastika.

Goldberg is hopelessly trapped in the ludicrous left-wing/right-wing political classification that is taught in government schools (socialist schools).

The term "Third Reich" appears throughout "Liberal Fascism," even though Goldberg does not explain it, and provides no citation to Hitler ever using the catchphrase. Dr. Curry made the discovery that writers provide no credible reference to show Hitler ever used the idiom, and that there are no references to show Hitler employed it as a common byword. Goldberg and other writers provide no example or explanation, even though their books repeat the term as if it were one of Hitler's favorite phrases in his many speeches of which there are film and audio recordings.

Does "Liberal Fascism" fail to clarify for readers that "Nazis" did not call themselves "Nazis" nor "Fascists"? The book uses the term "Fascism" in its title which appears on its cover above a smiley-face cartoon adorned with a Hitler moustache.

The book "From a 'Race of Masters' to a 'Master Race': 1948 to 1848" by the author A. E. Samaan (2013) states:

Dr. Rex Curry, the professor and attorney from Florida, has debated and largely proven the unavoidable evidence that Hitler's National Socialism was significantly influenced by Bellamy's 'nationalistic' form of 'socialism.' Curry is famous for making the claim that Hitler adopted the 'stiff-arm salute' from Francis and Edward Bellamy. (page 589).

Thus, Dr. Curry's claims that much of the fanfare and propaganda we now attribute to the Hitler Youth and the Nuremberg rallies actually originated with American customs, are definitely sound. (Samaan at page 590).

Professor Curry ... has been researching the link between Hitler's National Socialism and Edward Bellamy's 'socialistic' form of 'nationalism.' (Samaan at page 594).

The Sonoran News in Arizona explained the following in an article by Linda Bentley:

....Dr. Rex Curry, a libertarian lawyer who has done vast research on the Pledge's socialist roots, provides pro bono services nationwide to educate students and teachers about 'the right to reject robotic ritualism.' The history of the Pledge simply proves Upham and Ford were able to capitalize on the promotion of Bellamy's socialist agenda, and it's not over yet.

From the Daily Herald, in Provo, Utah, with Randy Wright, the Executive Editor:

Dear Dr. Curry -- Thanks for your help on short notice last night. The subject of the Pledge of Allegiance came up in connection with a rally at a local college in support of the phrase 'under God.' Your material made a terrific sidebar. Little known facts from the past.

From "God Save the South: A Treasure Chest of Forbidden Information," By John Thomas Nall:

The Pledge of Allegiance (1892) was the origin of the raised arm salute adopted later by the National Socialist German Workers Party (Nazis). The Pledge was written by Francis Bellamy, cousin to Edward Bellamy (the author), and both were self-proclaimed national socialists in the United States. The original Pledge began with a military salute that was then extended out toward the flag. In practice, the second gesture was performed palm down. The gesture was not an ancient Roman salute. All of these are discoveries of the symbologist Dr. Rex Curry (author of "Pledge of Allegiance Secrets"). (page 208).

In "Cosmic Evolution: The Accelerated Human," the author James B Lawrence wrote:

...new discoveries show that American soldiers used the swastika as their symbol early in World War I, and up to 1941, against Germany. The symbol was used by Americans in the French Escadrille

Lafayette, by the 45th Infantry Division, and on Boeing P-12 planes. The discoveries are in the growing body of work by the historian Dr. Rex Curry (author of 'Swastika Secrets'). He has previously shown how socialists in the USA originated the modern swastika as overlapping 'S' letters for 'Socialists' joining together in a utopian 'Socialist Society.' During the time when American soldiers adopted the swastika, the symbol was associated in the USA with the growing popularity of 'military socialism,' a dogma touted by Edward Bellamy, the American author of the international bestseller 'Looking Backward,' (1887) known as the bible of National Socialism. The symbol was also famous in the USA as alphabetical symbolism for socialism in the Theosophical Society (TS), from 1875. In 1888, the Theosophical Society teamed up with Bellamy's Nationalist movement for military socialism. The 'Bellamy swastika' spread. By 1915, the symbol was also widely popular as an ornamental 'Good Luck' symbol, as in a 1915 postcard showing the American flag posed favorably with a swastika. (Introduction page ix and in works cited).

Pastor Alvin H Franzmeier: "...the Sig-Rune became an 'S" and two together became the swastika and represented socialists joining together to form the National Socialist German Workers' party. In 1935 the swastika flag became official for Germany. The swastika symbol was not called that, but rather a HakenKreuz or hooked cross. This was Hitler's attempt to unite the church with the state, especially since German culture was strongly influenced by Christianity. You can find more on these topics on

Rex Curry's website and its various pages. He has some interesting things to say about the use of the swastika also in America up to the start of WW II, as well as the open hand salute. The symbol was used by various socialist groups, not only in the USA, but also in the USSR."

Matt Crypto: "Before Dr. Curry's work, I had never viewed photographs nor film footage showing the early Nazi salute of the Pledge of Allegiance. At that time, I did not even know that the Nazis were the 'National Socialist German Workers Party' and that they did not refer to themselves as 'Nazis.' I once doubted the greatness of His Excellency Professor Doctor Sir Rex Curry, but he sure put me in my place. Never flag in the fight for freedom!"

From Wikipedia: "The American socialist Francis Bellamy's Pledge of Allegiance to the U.S. flag was the origin of the Nazi salute and Nazi behavior (e.g. robotic chanting to flags) under Hitler's German socialism. German socialists used the Nazi flag's symbol to represent crossed 'S' letters for their socialism (see work of the historian Dr. Rex Curry)."

Jimmy Wales, Wikipedia's founder, has also mentioned the influence of Dr. Curry's scholarship on Wikipedia. The discoveries have been publicized and verified by many readers and writers on Wikipedia.

It is unfortunate that Wikipedia is an anonymous bulletin board that changes by the millisecond. That is because anyone can participate and "anyone" includes Neo-Nazis on Wikipedia who delete historic documentary film footage and other factual material showing Professor Curry's erudition (regarding the U.S.

as the origin of the notorious stiff-armed gesture via the military salute in the early Pledge of Allegiance; and the swastika as an alphabetical mark for socialism). Wikipedia is notorious for displaying lies despite the efforts of many other noted historians and writers (including Timothy Messer-Kruse, John Seigenthaler, Philip Roth) to correct the glaring falsehoods.

From the Tampa Bay Times Newspaper (TBT): **"Hi Dr. Curry, Thanks for your help today on our column exposing the early salute of the Pledge Of Allegiance."** (with columnist Robyn Blumner).

Despite the thank you note, TBT covers up the National Socialist German Workers Party and the origin of its dogma, symbols, and rituals. Perhaps that is because the TBT building is adorned with swastikas and a huge U.S. flag put on a pole out front every day.

Walter Duranty won a Pulitzer Prize covering up for socialists at the New York Times (NYT). TBT follows Duranty's prize-winning strategy of fake news and alternative facts. The NYT started in 1851, and the TBT started ~1898, and ever since then TBT emulated the NYT's crapaganda.

TBT is upset about recent talk of a Pulitzer Prize (that will NOT go to TBT) for *exposing* socialism and the Pledge of Allegiance as the origin of Nazi salutes and Nazi behavior.

After the writer Daniel "LaRouche" Ruth was fired by the former Tampa Tribune (another bay area newspaper), TBT hired him. TBT did so despite his history of Nazi-style name-calling. After LaRouche's loss in a public debate challenge the local response against the crackpot was so great that LaRouche said he was labeled a "Dork, anti-free market statist, $#%!&,

Dummkopf, liberal, daffy, dolt, stupid, dunce and, oh by the way, socialist." Ruth's nickname could be "Duranty" (instead of "LaRouche").

Not long after the "socialist" crack, Ruth's former employer/newspaper the Tribune said to the kook: "Uh, Daniel Ruth? Start packing your bags!"

On another occasion, Ruth admitted publicly that locals have labeled him "bigot, prejudiced, hateful and ignorant." Good Grief, even Lyndon LaRouche was not that crazy!

Ruth supports bleating the socialist Pledge of Allegiance to the Flag and said so with his Nazi-style name-calling. He publicly harassed a small group that didn't want to chant. It is revealing to note that the TBT hoists the flag every morning in front of its swastika-decked crib; flag hag LaRuth is NOT out front to bleat his sacred flaggotry. Bleating only takes 12 seconds a day for life, so why not, LaRouche? Government's cock will not suck itself; That's what the media is for. While pestering others, LaRuth forgot to ask all TBT personnel join him (and government school students) each morning outside to mumble at TBT's flags. If hypocrite LaRuth begins bleating his quotidian propaganda, then he can use the earlier gesture that he prefers (he was schooled about it from educational outreach programs about Dr. Curry's discoveries).

TBT's USA flag pole sits beside another pole for Florida's state flag, designed to pay homage to the confederate flag. Ruth could write a pledge for the state banner (and have it imposed by law in schools, with TBT's support). He could promote it by chanting daily immediately after his USA flag ritual. What gesture would Ruth select for his state flag pledge?

Ruth is another example of how TBT has always

been duped by the World's Dumbest Criminals and the world's dumbest dogma (socialism) from Stalin, Mao, Hitler and their fellow travelers.

On the domestic level, TBT reinforced its masthead, "America's Dumbest Newspaper," when it was duped by America's Dumbest Criminals. Thereafter, America's Dumbest Newspaper duped its readers (both of them): America's Dumbest Readers.

Both Tampa Bay area newspapers were always notorious for their "2 girls, 1 cup" journalism. Self-loathing news. They have been consistent enemies of the people and their goal has been to expand always the existing socialist police state. Readers are kept ignorant with fake news and false flag propaganda. That is why the Dead Writers Club put the Tribune out of business in 2016.

The Tribune declined for years and its death seemed near and dear to observers. Yet, it never whined to the government for a bailout, nor for "historic preservation" as the city's long-time newspaper, or to be outright socialized (similar to the fake news outlets at NPR, PBS, CPB, BBC). Instead the Trib went under while having its money stolen for competitors (NPR, PBS, CPB). The Tribune's silence seemed inconsistent in light of its decades embracing socialism all around it, and begging for more socialism for everything else, including the pettiest things: a socialized football stadium and other socialized sports trash. Heil socialism!

The failing TBT is not doing well either (it bought what remained of the crippled Tampa Tribune). It continues to print sometimes a small section of newspaper that it labels "Tampa Tribune" in an effort to keep the Tribune's past alive.

The Tribune's past includes this racist quote: "We are

not fully informed as to Mencken's color and race, but his remarks about Negro superiority in the South lead us to believe that he must be a Negro by inclination if not by birth. He is, as a matter of fact, far inferior to the average Southern Negro" (From "Menckeniana -A Schimpflexikon" 1928). The book contains selections from editorials, reviews and general hate mail printed about H. L. Mencken when he was in his mid-40s (during a time when socialist schools imposed segregation by law and taught racism as official policy more than they continue to do so today).

That past complements the TBT's past. In 1935, TBT published a "Negro news page," and in 1948 the page became a daily part of the paper (at that time known as the Saint Petersburg Times). The paper would also use the term "darkies" and headlines such as "Police Quell Negro Riots."

During that time, photos of the Pledge of Allegiance would have included the early American Nazi salute.

It is a wonder why anti-racist protestors have not vandalized the swastika building or physically torn it down.

TBT displays its swastikas across the street from a Holocaust museum. I am not making this up.

In the past, TBT had an employee cafeteria on the property, but it is now a Hofbräuhaus. I am not making this up. It's German-themed, the attendants dress in German attire, and people sing German songs.

Holocaust museum tourists can cross the street to the Tampa Bay Times and see its swastikas, salute its flags, and then sing German songs at the Hofbräuhaus.

Dr. Curry is cited in the book "By Faith Isaac" from the author Elsa Henderson (November 1, 2013).

"He was one of the first people to publicly burn his social security card…" – State Library and Archives of Florida, Deborah Thomas Collection; Florida Flambeau Newspaper, Florida State University. (the Archives of Florida resemble archives in other states in that the hundreds of thousands of searchable old photographs contain no historic examples of the early Pledge of Allegiance gesture by any public officials, politicians, school students, or anyone ever anywhere. Are the photographs removed from archives and destroyed?)

Newdow v. Rio Linda Union Sch. Dist., 597 F.3d 1007 (9th Cir. 2010), a case litigating the constitutionality of the phrase "under God" in the pledge, mentions Dr. Curry. In the case's related litigation, the United States Supreme Court was schooled about Dr. Curry's achievement showing that the pledge as the origin of the Nazi salute and Nazi behavior (Dr. Curry pointed out that some justices might have a conflict of interest or bias in favor of the pledge because some of the justices were old enough at that time to have actually performed the Nazi salute while chanting the pledge)

Professor Curry's scholarly work was adopted and cited in "Loose Cannons: 101 Myths, Mishaps and Misadventurers of Military History" (October 20, 2009) by Graeme Donald although Donald inserted at least one error: Donald did not comprehend that Bellamy's original pledge did NOT describe the hand-over-the-heart gesture nor the classic stiff-armed Nazi gesture (Donald repeats the error in his book "On This Day In

History"). As a consequence, Donald did not understand (and was unable to explain) how the original pledge's use of the military salute (as its initial gesture) CAUSED the Nazi salute as the pledge's second gesture, during actual performances of the pledge.

Amazon.com (and other websites) adopted as its policy the recommendations advocated by Dr. Curry. Amazon's web site deletes and discourages use of the common 4-letter shorthand n-word ("Nazi")[169] for "National Socialist German Workers' Party" within Amazon's reviews, product information, tags and other uses. By fighting the shorthand term, Amazon encourages customers to learn and to use the actual accurate name of the group: National Socialist German Workers' Party.

For a long time, Dr. Curry has exposed widespread ignorance in the media and in the general public about what the 4-letter abbreviation abbreviates. That etymological ignorance has grown through overuse of the hackneyed shorthand term in print and in government schools (socialist schools). The shorthand term should be avoided, unless it is used in conjunction with the full actual name of the Party. Amazon is helping the doctor reverse the ignorant habit within the media and the public.

eBay (and other websites) agree with Dr. Curry's discoveries that the Pledge of Allegiance was the origin of the Nazi salute and Nazi behavior. eBay will remove from sale old historic photographs of the early American

---

[169] It is also important to stamp out the public's widespread derogatory use of the offensive G-word. (Ginger)

Pledge of Allegiance (with the Nazi salute) on the grounds that such photographs are in fact "Nazi artifacts" that violate Ebay's terms.

A comic meme (graphic image) displayed a still shot from the movie "Downfall" in a scene where Hitler is frantically screaming into a phone handset. The meme's punchline is shown in Hitler's dialogue balloon: "There's no crying in Nazism!"

Dr. Rex Curry was the only person on the planet who viewed the meme and posted "The meme is funny; and the humor is heightened even more by the fact that Hitler did not use the word 'Nazism.'"

Because of government schools (socialist schools) no one else on the internet recognized the meme's error. The most ignorant respondents reacted with anger at the idea that Hitler did not use the word "Nazism." They had no idea what words Hitler used to describe his dogma.

17. FIGHT THE PAST & PRESENT

Two embarrassing "Pledge of Allegiance" cases from the U.S. Supreme Court are: Minersville School District v. Gobitis, 310 U.S. 586 (1940); and West Virginia Board of Education v. Barnette, 319 U.S. 624 (1943). Gobitis originated in 1935 and held that children could be persecuted for refusing the servile incantation and the one-armed salute of USA's flag pledge. Gobitis was not overturned until the case of Barnette (1943). It was one of the fastest self-reversals by the U.S. Supreme Court.

Barnette is often cited as holding that "you do not have to say the pledge." The holding was more than that. The holding in 1943 was also that you don't have to perform the American Nazi salute (or whatever other bizarre gesture your socialist school dictates).

People similar to the Gobitis kids were being persecuted in Germany and the USA at the same time. The National Socialist German Workers' Party had been in existence since 1920, and had electoral breakthroughs in 1930, and dictatorship in 1933. At the time (1940) when the Gobitis decision upheld mandated daily droning of the socialist's pledge in the USA, the German socialists were allies with Soviet socialists in a pact to divide up Europe, invading Poland together, spreading

WWII, and leading to the socialist Wholecaust (of which the Holocaust was a part). "News" outlets in both countries rhapsodized about the two countries joining together in their shared socialist kampf. Finding examples of that old harmonious propaganda is almost as difficult as finding old photographs of America's stiff-arm salute.

G-schools have been a part of every authoritarian regime in the past. They are part of the prison planet, including the police state in Germany (as it was under Hitler's socialism) and in the USA.

Government schools remain a part of the police Reich and they have police officers permanently assigned to the schools today. Government schools are unconstitutional for that reason, and for many other reasons, including the following:

1. Government schools violate the First Amendment right to freedom of speech and freedom of the press. The government schools (socialist schools) tell everyone what to think and say and write. The pledge is part of that statal indoctrination. Schools will not teach children that they can refuse the pledge, but bully them into obedience every day.

2. Government schools violate everyone's right to due process of law and to a fair jury trial. Government schools tell everyone which political parties to vote for, and to submit to taxation (theft),[170] to socialism, to unjust laws, and to render verdicts of "guilty" against people charged under unjust laws.

3. Government schools violate the 4th Amendment

---

[170] Due to school brainwashing, if you say "Taxation Is Theft" it is like saying "Hitler was right." Make the first maxim your motto.

right against unreasonable searches and seizures. They will not teach students to exercise their right to remain silent, and to refuse to answer questions from police and other government employees; to refuse to consent to searches of their persons, possessions, lockers, and cars. Government schools evade the "expectation of privacy" standard that exists outside of schools. Schools are day-prisons for kids.

All students (and all adults) should learn to evade the police state.[171] The way to evade the police state is: evade the police.

Do not talk to the police.

Do not consent to any search of any kind.

Do document encounters with police by video recording them.

Police officers are often video recorded during traffic stops. The videos are often recorded on cell phones by drivers who are stopped by police. Other videos are recorded by dashboard cameras installed on police cars, or by body cameras worn by police officers.

Video recordings of police are often posted to the world wide web on the internet and viewed by millions of civilians. Some videos expose illegal searches, improper arrests, shocking violence, thefts, corruption, and more. The videos make drivers want to avoid becoming victims of the USA's police state.

Any driver who cannot afford to install a video recording system in his/her car should visit a thrift store and buy broken cameras that look like digital recording cameras. The cameras can be positioned using Velcro in

---

[171] Every true American commits at least three felonies a day. The author of this book consistently tops seven. And that is *before* lunch. That's how you fight the police state.

the rear window and on the dashboard above the steering wheel facing toward where police stand outside of the driver's window. The rear window camera serves as a warning sign to discourage some police from even pulling a car over. If a cop does approach the driver's window, the driver can gesture at the cameras and state "I have cameras" (which technically is not a lie, even though the cameras don't function).

Drivers should pro-actively prevent cops from following behind them in traffic. Police have ticket and arrest quotas that have led to the planting of drugs, to corruption, and to deaths.

If you are able to see a cop in your rear-view mirror (no matter how far back the cop is), then you should turn and either take a different route, or circle the block, or pull into a gas station or convenience store.

If you are on the highway and it is possible to take an exit, then do so. If possible, re-enter the highway after the officer has passed.

If there is a cop at an intersection ahead of you in a position where you will pass and he might end up behind you, preemptively turn before you pass the cop's location. Change your route, or circle the block so that the cop will have proceeded elsewhere, or so that he will be ahead of you.

It should go without saying: Don't ever pass a cop. If a cop appears in front of you, then you should remain a long way back, or take a different route. Don't pass.

If you turn and the officer follows you, then you should immediately find a place to stop (e.g. pull into a gas station, convenience store, or fast food location, then exit the car and go inside).

In other words, prevent cops from being in a position to read your tag, and prevent them from being in a position to pull you over.

At night, it is difficult to identify police cars from a distance. Many people minimize night driving in order to avoid having a police car sneak up on them.

Similar prophylactic behavior is wise at home: if there is a knock at the door and the person knocking is a cop (or looks like a bureaucrat or anyone from the government), do not answer the door. Do not speak. Wait for the person to leave.

Just like politics, law enforcement attracts people with sociopathic tendencies who enjoy having power over others. Sometimes they are ex-military who have learned to hate the populaces they patrolled, and they returned home to treat Americans the same bad ways. Veterans are probably the worst people to become police, yet many people think they are ideal candidates (police departments set up recruiting booths in military bases).

"But some police officers are good cops," is a common response. It is impossible to know in advance whether a cop is one of the violent sociopaths or not. You have to assume the worst and avoid potentially dangerous situations.

Some police officers become enraged by anyone who asserts his/her constitutional rights to not answer questions, not waive the 4th Amendment (not consent to searches), and request a lawyer. Such an officer is angered more if a civilian seems nervous/frightened (completely normal responses) or if a civilian suffers from "Police Tourette Syndrome" (PTS -a disease manifested by uncontrollable coprolalia whenever its victim is stopped by a cop).

The information above might save your life and the lives of those who are with you.

MADNESS

18. UN-EARTHING POLICE DOG FRAUD

Drug dogs are used for lies. They are used to fabricate "probable cause" to search cars (and other conveyances, objects, and packages).

Judges write clueless opinions in which they wonder about how accurate drug dogs are, and they overlook this point: Police can lie and say that the dog alerted when the dog did not alert at all. It does not matter how accurate drug dogs are.

The most common excuse for police dogs is modern prohibition: the insane War on Drugs. At this time, we would like to pause and congratulate drugs for winning the war on drugs.

The word "police" is related to the word "policy" because police enforce the policies of deranged politicians on the local, state, and federal level.

The word 'politics' is derived from the word 'poly' meaning 'many', and the word 'ticks' meaning 'blood sucking parasites.' They often engage is parasitoidism.

Blood-sucking parasites on dogs compare favorably to blood-sucking parasites who use dogs for lies in order to steal millions of dollars from law-abiding citizens under the police state and its asset forfeiture laws. Cops are robbers.

Cops lie like dogs. Cops lie like rugs. According to grammar rules, the second sentence is ungrammatical because, for rugs, the word should be "lay," and not "lie." And dogs are not dishonest, but they do want to lie on the floor. Cops tell lies about drug dogs, and they use drug dogs to tell lies about humans. Perhaps this tweaks it: Cops lie like a dog on a rug during a July day in Florida. In other words, they lie a bunch.

Everyone should feel sorry for drug sniffing dogs at airports and police stations. Imagine being a dog and being forced to have a job.

Drug dogs are natural libertarians with no interest in modern prohibition, and they have to be constantly taught and reinforced (brainwashed) to detect drug odors, and to approach peaceful humans and search them so that humans can be arrested, handcuffed, and imprisoned for decades. That is not an easy trick to teach a dog. It is easier to teach humans.

Drug dogs are a reminder of similar police-state tactics and obsessive Gestapo behavior under the National Socialist German Workers Party.

Police officers should not be forced to endanger their own lives (and the lives of innocent dogs) enforcing modern prohibition and initiating violence against peaceful people engaged in non-violent consensual conduct.

The following paragraphs describe how narcotics dogs are used as ruses against humans, to violate constitutional rights against searches and seizures -

* NEVER CONSENT TO A SEARCH. Consenting to a search means that the driver is waiving his rights under the Fourth Amendment of the U.S. Constitution. If consent is given, and the police either find or fabricate a

reason for an arrest, then any motion to suppress based on an illegal search will be opposed by the prosecution with the truthful argument that the victim/defendant "consented" and waived his rights. If a victim/defendant consents and then tells his lawyer "they had no reason to search my car," part of the lawyer's response will include this: "It does not matter because you consented to the search. You waived your rights. That makes it more difficult for me to help you."

*Cops ask to search cars for no reason at all during routine traffic stops. Cops ask to search because they know that most victims are ignorant of the fact that drivers should "just say 'NO!'" (most drivers are know-nothings about constitutional rights). Drivers who do know are often too frightened or meek to say "NO!"

It is unknown how often cops ask for consent to search. It is unknown how often consent is given under duress or ignorance. Drivers who do not complain roadside will not complain later, and will not learn, and will not litigate later.

The police use of "consent searches" has inspired opponents of the practice to educate the public with the slogan "Say No To Searches!" and "Say No To The Police State."

* If drivers say "no," then cops tell drivers that a K-9 unit has been requested by police radio, and a sniffer dog is coming to the scene and a longer ordeal is, therefore, inevitable if the driver will not "consent" to a search of the car. That warning is often a lie to induce consent. There is no police dog on the way.

* Whether or not a dog is in transit, some cops add

additional lies to make drivers think that there will be a long wait and that the driver must stay until a dog arrives. Cops rely on driver ignorance of the fact that evidence will be suppressed if drivers are detained longer than it takes to complete the traffic stop (e.g. write the ticket). Drivers are induced to consent to search to avoid a long wait based on lies. Cops will say things like "You should consent to search because the dog is going to scratch your car up," which is a threat of property damage made to induce consent, and it is also an indication of a badly trained drug dog (if it is true), and a bad handler.

* Learn to say "AM I UNDER ARREST? OR AM I FREE TO GO?" Some cops let drivers think that they are obliged to stay even when the cop has no reason to detain drivers any longer. Cops rationalize that drivers inexplicably loiter roadside with cops, or that drivers enjoy waiting for dog sniffs. Cops take advantage of drivers who are too stupid (or too meek) to ask if they are free to go. Drivers "consent" (in the cop's rationalization) to unwarranted detention by not leaving.

* Cops lie about how long it takes to write tickets or to obtain radio responses, tag inquiries, license inquiries, or other causes for delay that cops dream up. If a dog is truly en route, then some cops complete tickets very slowly, until the dog arrives.

* Even after the dog arrives at the scene of a traffic ticket stop, cops still try to obtain "consent to search" because cops think that they can more easily avoid suppression of evidence motions that expose the cop's falsehoods, reveal the dog's inaccuracy, destroy the

dog's future credibility, and force the dog to be retired, and necessitate a new dog (puppet) to replace it (until that new dog is exposed). With the dog at the scene, cops will repeat statements such as "You should consent to search, because the dog is going to scratch up your car."

*What happens if a dog is discredited in a court proceeding that reveals the dog to have a high error rate? There appears to be little that prevents police from re-naming the dog, moving it to another location, or taking other actions to continue using the dog for its originally intended purpose: as a ruse to fabricate "probable cause" for searches.

*Another reason why police use drug dogs is the same reason why felons use large menacing dogs: as substitutes for guns, in order to threaten and terrorize people. Video recordings of some drug dogs makes it appear as if they have been trained to bark continuously and to leap and lunge. Some "drug dogs" are also trained to be attack dogs. That can be dangerous if the dog becomes confused about its purpose in a particular situation involving a civilian.

* Police ask for consent because they have no "probable cause" to search. When victims persist in refusing to consent to a search, police take advantage of court cases from judges who opine that police can gain "probable cause" if a properly trained and properly handled drug dog gives a bonafide "alert" indicating that the dog smells the presence of illegal contraband in the car. A search is forced against the driver's will.

*Police fabricate "probable cause for a search" by lying and claiming that a canine alerted when the dog did not alert. A search is then forced against the driver's will. Video recordings on the web show these police lies, including videos where the dog handler parks his car behind the victim's car, and walks the dog to the front of the victim's car (where the dog handler deliberately hides from the police car's dashboard camera), and the dog handler loudly proclaims that the dog is alerting, while there is no view of any alert by the dog on the video.

The police show that the dog alert is fake because they immediately go to the car's doors and start searching the passenger area. Sometimes they NEVER search the front of the car where the dog alerted.

If drugs are not found hidden at the front of the car (and drugs usually are not found there) then that fact should be used in a motion to suppress evidence because it shows that the dog did not alert, or that the dog's alert was an error. The same argument should be made whenever drugs are not found near the spot where a drug dog allegedly alerted on the car.

*Police manufacture "probable cause for a search" by cuing a drug dog, to induce it to "alert," if the dog is not alerting on its own. Police lie and claim that the dog properly alerted. A search is forced against the driver's will. Victims need to pay close attention to the dog and its handler, make a video recording (and also use any police dash camera recording) to uncover the truth.

Cuing can be deliberate or subconscious (dogs may imagine that the handler desires the dog to alert). Sometimes it is not clear whether the cue is deliberate or subconscious. For example, if a dog handler repeatedly walks the dog around a car it could be cuing that is deliberate or subconscious. The handler might know from past experience that if he walks the dog around the car enough, the dog will eventually interpret that as a cue and alert. Motions to suppress evidence should argue that a dog should circle a car once (because if drugs dog are as amazingly accurate as cops claim, then one circle is enough). Any additional circling is cuing (because the cop is angry that the dog did not alert on the first walk).

* Many errors by drug dogs cause lawyers to wonder if police carry drugs to plant scents so that drug dogs will alert. Some news items support such speculation in cases where drugs have been planted by police. Drug prohibition is wrong, and its wrongfulness is compounded by government during enforcement of "modern prohibition."

* If a narco dog alerts and nothing is found in the resulting search, then cops will never record that as an error by the dog. If confronted by the apparent error under cross-examination, cops will testify (testi-lie) that the dog detected lingering odors of contraband that were recently present. Cops will testify that dogs never make mistakes, never have and never will, and that apparent errors are, in reality, the dog's skillful detection of residual odors of contraband.

No one can question a dog about whether the cop is lying or mistaken, and it is usually a waste of time to ask a cop the same types of questions.

Police like dogs because the dogs cannot be cross-examined. Defendants are denied their constitutional right to confront witnesses against them.

A motion to suppress should be filed because experts will testify that drug dogs can be trained (and should be trained) to ignore residual odors. Dogs that are not trained to ignore residual odors should be considered incompetent to provide probable cause for a search.

* Motions to suppress in court should argue that the drug dogs cannot provide probable cause because "drugs are everywhere." Drugs are on the ground (in restaurants, bars, streets) and can transfer to shoes when people step on the wrong spot. Drugs are then transferred to cars from shoes. Drugs can be on the ground underneath the spot where a car is stopped by police. Drugs are on roads and in parking lots and can transfer to the tires and underbelly of passing cars (this is an explanation of why a dog would alert on parts of a car where no drugs are found). Drugs are in the air, blown by the wind, to land on passing cars. Drugs can be in the rain that falls on cars and dries, leaving a residue. Drugs can be on the hands and clothing of police from earlier arrests. Drugs are on paper money and then transferred to the hands, pockets, and clothing of innocent people who handle the money later.

* Drug dog fraud is about more than cops stealing drugs. It is also about cops stealing cars, money and other valuables. Under the police state's civil forfeiture laws, police will lie and claim that large sums of money are "drug money." Police will steal the money, even if no drugs were found and no arrest was made. Police will bolster their lies that the money is drug money with additional lies that a dog alerted on the car or on the money (even if no drugs were found). Police use asset forfeiture laws to steal cars, money, real estate, and

other valuables. Under civil forfeiture laws, police can engage in theft without finding drugs, without filing any criminal charges, and without convicting anyone of a crime. Regardless of any criminal charges, the theft of the victim's property becomes a separate nightmare.

19. NARCOTICS DOG TRAINING

"I was Mao's dog. When he said bite, I bit!"
-Jiang Qing (3/19/1914 – 3/14/1991)
the fourth wife of Mao Zedong.

Drug dogs are similar to humans in that dogs must be taught to approach peaceful people and search them, so that humans can be arrested, handcuffed, robbed, kidnapped, and imprisoned for decades under modern prohibition. That is not an easy trick to teach a dog. It is easier to teach humans.

Sniffer dog skills are often overestimated because people anthropomorphize dogs.

A dog's skills should be under-estimated because the most humanlike quality that dogs have is that they are natural libertarians with no interest in the war on drugs.

Drug dogs are trained by playing a game. The dogs are taught using toys. The toys are hidden with drugs to trick the dog into a game of searching for its toy by associating the toy with drug odors.

A drug dog's training is not unique or complicated. Many canine house pets will search for a toy that is hidden under a sofa pillow or a coffee can. The toy can be hidden with a package of cinnamon or some other item with a unique odor. After a few weeks, the cinnamon can be hidden alone, without the toy, and the dog will find the cinnamon via its smell, a smell that the dog was taught to associate with its toy. [toy squeaks, dog barks]

Many errors can happen due to the training method. There is always the danger that a drug dog will alert on anything that resembles or smells like its toy (towels, tennis balls, car carpet, etc.).

Errors occur if a dog smells anything it desires, or wants to attack, or wishes to investigate: if a cat was carried in the car [grrrr]; if another dog has ridden in the car; if there is the odor of food in the car.

A Reuters news report stated that a San Diego arena was evacuated for about two hours, delaying a first-round game in the hugely popular national college basketball championship, after a hot dog cart attracted the attention of a bomb-sniffing dog. [Bark! Bark!]. Thousands of fans arriving for a game between Marquette University and the University of Alabama were kept outside. Authorities cordoned off part of the building. It was meat, and not explosive heat, attracting the dog's attention.

Many drug dogs are so inaccurate that they could be replaced with the "drug coin." Flip the "drug coin" and if it lands on "heads," then that means that there is an alert and that there is probable cause to search. If it lands on "tails," then that means there is no alert, and that there is no probable cause (but a search occurs anyway).

Drugs dogs often bark up the wrong tree. In the U.S. Supreme Court case of *Illinois v. Cabelles*, Justices Souter and Ginsburg dissented, pointing to studies showing that drug dogs frequently return false positives (12.5 to 60% of the time, according to one study).

Sniffer dogs are trained to detect only specific contraband (e.g. cocaine and marijuana). Some dogs are trained to detect only a single drug (e.g. only marijuana). To attack a K-9, determine what drug(s) it was trained to detect. If an arrest was made based on an alert for a substance that the dog was not trained to detect, then that should be part of a motion to suppress arguing that the alert was an error, or that it was a lie. One example would be: if a dog trained to detect only marijuana allegedly alerts and a search reveals only cocaine, then an arrest will occur for the cocaine despite the apparent error by the dog. Police will not volunteer any information about the fact that the dog was only trained to detect marijuana.

If an arrest is made based on a search by a drug dog, then a motion to suppress the evidence should be filed based on the arguments in this book including any evidence of cuing, the behavior of the dog at the scene, inadequate training of the dog, inadequate maintenance of the dog's training, a history of false positives (or a lack of record keeping regarding the dog's false positive rate) and various other problems that might be evident based on the timing and conditions during the detention of the victim and the search.

If a search occurs via the use of a drug dog, and no arrest occurs, then the police should be sued civilly based on the arguments in this book.

Under the current statist quo [sic], if contraband is found then the arrest will probably stand. If nothing is found, the driver leaves shaken, but there are few cases where the driver complains or sues. Bad police are emboldened by the fact that people will not take action after bad searches.

It doesn't matter whether a drug dog is accurate. The

dog is present at the scene as a cover-up so that when the officer is called to testify he will "testalie" in court. Dogs are perfect pets for perjury.

Any case that lacks a videotape of a dog's actions on the scene should result in rejection of testimony that the dog alerted, or that the dog alerted without cueing.

Drug dogs differ from humans in that the natural libertarianism of drug-dogs always resurfaces, and must be suppressed constantly by law enforcement retraining. Without constant reinforcement, the dogs lose interest, and skills they actually have will deteriorate further.

Record-keeping is indispensable for knowing whether dogs are guessing, or seeing cues. A record must be kept of every instance when the dog alerts and whether drugs were found. That is the only way to know the dog's error rate (how often the dog provides false positives) or to discover whether the dog is merely used for official lies. Only with record keeping and independent testing can any judge draw any conclusion from the dog's "game playing" out on the street.

Any criminal case with inadequate record-keeping about a dog should result in suppression of the evidence and dismissal of the charges against the defendant.

Dogs approximate humans in that they go along with the system to avoid disapproval from peers. Humans crave approval from supervising officers, other police, teachers, classmates, friends, et cetera. Drug dogs crave approval from their police handlers. Dogs play the game, and will try to guess and read cues (subconscious cues or deliberate cues), because the dogs are searching for approval, not for drugs.

Dogs mimic humans in that they can be trained (brainwashed) to do hurtful things – such as passing the 18th amendment (the old prohibition) in the case of humans. In the dogged pursuit of modern prohibition, some dogs are slow learners, as are some humans.

The government's war on drugs is a dog chasing its own tail. The war is a jobs program for unskilled laborers who otherwise would be blowing leaves or dropping fries for a living.

Let's liberate drug dogs. Return them to protecting people from violence and theft, which is also the only proper purpose of law enforcement. Dogs should be man's best friend, not man's persecutor.

"...a tattoo is positive identification. No one should ever do anything to help the police..." - George Carlin

20. HISTORY OF DRUG DOGS

Drug dog fraud was encouraged in January 2005, under the U.S. Supreme Court case of *Illinois vs. Caballes* (not one of Dr. Curry's cases), holding that a dog sniff during a traffic stop was not a "search." *Caballes* involved an allegedly "legitimate" traffic stop for speeding (that turned into 12 years in prison for marijuana).

Caballes is interpreted to mean that cops can take dogs fishing. *Caballes* and similar cases turn canines into props for lies. When dogs are used as props for lies, it doesn't matter whether dogs are well-trained.

The *Caballes* case from the U.S. Supreme Court foreshadows more police-state possibilities: Uniformed law enforcement marching through neighborhoods with German shepherds on leashes sniffing anything and everything -every car parked on or near the street, the air emanating from homes, neighbors walking outside.

Imagine the same thing at any place of business or employment, and police marching German shepherds through parking lots, car to car, for no reason other than fishing expeditions. Imagine the same nightmare in any shopping area or a downtown street area, a festival, a bar's parking lot. Uniformed agents on the streets with

German shepherds sniffing and searching purses, pockets, bags, cars, anything. The uniformed harassing the uninformed.

Police-state tactics were witnessed worldwide via videotape from Stratford High School in Goose Creek, South Carolina, where police used dogs in a surprise "raid" for students inside of a school.

No drugs were found in the raid of the Goose Creek school.

In other schools, classes have been interrupted and the children were marched out and lined up to be harassed by a dog.

What next? Cops with growling German Shepherds marching through classrooms at the ring of the bell to sniff herded children as the students bark the Pledge of Allegiance in the police-state camps known as government schools? Require that matriculates micturate each morning for lab analysis? If so, that would give the government another excuse to re-impose the pledge's earlier Nazi salute. That will be another way in which the U.S. police state resembles the National Socialist German Workers Party (Nazis). It would delight Hitler and his beloved Shepherd Blondi.

The police state in the U.S. is nothing new. Francis Bellamy (the pledge's author, and the origin of the Nazi salute and Nazi behavior) wrote the pledge to promote the government's takeover of schools. Bellamy was a self-proclaimed socialist and touted (along with his cousin Edward Bellamy) what he called "military socialism."

The Bellamy cousins wanted government to use socialized schools to achieve their goals. They inspired trite propaganda in which every "problem" spirals into a war: the War on Drugs, the War on Poverty, the War on

Crime, the War on Illiteracy, the War on Terrorism, et cetera. They inspired the use of government force and violence for any and all purposes. Today, the U.S.'s military-socialist complex and its aggressive military socialism is the Bellamy dogma.

The government's schools will not teach children about their Constitutional rights, including their 4th Amendment rights against searches (including the right to refuse to consent to searches, to say "NO!" to searches), and their right to remain silent (to refuse to answer questions when a police officer barks at them).[172]

Massive non-compliance does more for liberty than votes ever will.

Civil disobedience is not the problem. Civil *obedience* is the problem.

The Pledge of Allegiance is obedience training for humans: stand, speak, sit, roll over, attack, play dead....

Guardians of groupthink believe that any American who "loves freedom" must vocalize hypnotically, salute and sing whenever someone barks a command to do so.

---

[172] The government says: "If YoU RnT DoInG AnYtHiNg WrOnG yUo DoNt HaVe aNyThInG tO hIDe." If that is true then shouldn't the government declassify everything?

21. POLICE DOG RESEARCH

In an article entitled "Free the Drug Dogs!" at the History News Network (of George Mason University) the writer Keith Halderman stated, *"... attorney Rex Curry, who was one of the first libertarians I ever met, and who helped transform much of my thinking, developed a case that may be headed to the Supreme Court. [The case], which he won, involves a challenge to the veracity of drug dogs searches. The state of Florida is appealing and the issue is on the high court's docket."*

A professional dog trainer wrote about Dr. Curry: *"... you did our profession a great favor. Maybe we can get rid of the B.S. trainers and the monkey-see-monkey-do method to training, and apply the science behind it."*

DrugSense Weekly journal published an interview asking, *"Given the problems with drug dogs explored in your work, why do you think they are so popular with police departments and municipal government?"*
Dr. Curry's answer was, *"Oh that is easy. You have to remember that there is a strong incentive for law enforcement not to CARE whether the dogs are*

accurate. The dogs can simply be props for lies, in that the dogs are there to overcome refusals to consent to search, and the dog provides law enforcement officers (LEOs) with the ability to say that an alert occurred even if there was no alert. And here is another angle: some LEOs do not want a 'drug dog,' they want a 'car dog,' in that they want a dog that when shown a car will alert, as if to say 'yes that is a car.' For some LEOs the goal is to search whenever the LEO desires, period. The dog is simply a ruse to do so. That is why the dogs are so popular. Do not be confused with the idea that there are 'problems with drug dogs.' For some LEOs those are not problems at all. And again, that is why some LEOs have no interest in maintaining records about their dogs."

Many people write with responses to the ongoing research about drug dogs, including this one: *"I discovered a vacant lot where some dog-cops were meeting and I saw them signal training the dogs to 'GO OFF' on cue with very slight hand motions. Then I saw them walk dogs around a COP car they used (this shows it will work in any situation) and when the cop made this little twitch with one finger extended, the dog would bite at the door handle and tires and stand on its back legs and bark at the windows etc..."*

The Libertarian Lawyer was interviewed about drug dogs in Playboy magazine, and that prompted another drug dog expert to quip: *"Dr. Curry made it into Playboy Magazine without taking his clothes off."*

The police state (and the use of drug dogs) is becoming an international problem, as evidenced by this excerpt of a communication from abroad:

"I wonder if I could please ask for some help? We are a children's civil rights organisation based in the UK. As you are probably aware, there has been a rise in the use of drugs sniffer dogs here. In some schools, dogs are taken in to perform routine searches, and it is now commonplace in London to have dogs posted at the exits to London underground trains.

While we have been concerned about the use of dogs and had objected on various civil liberties grounds, we had naively assumed that dogs were pretty accurate! We've found out the hard way that this isn't true: two of our (non-drug-using) teenaged members have now been stopped by dogs at stations, and then searched. They were both pretty upset by the experience.

We want to find all the research possible about the accuracy of sniffer dogs and intend to bring out a report to publicise what is going on. – quite honestly, we are more likely to stop the practice of going into schools with dogs in this way, rather than by arguing civil liberties (not a major concern of the British public!) [from "Action on Rights for Children"]

The description of the police-state in the U.K. (from the comments above) are similar to the U.S.'s police state. People in Britain and worldwide witnessed police-state tactics in the U.S. via videotape from Stratford High School in Goose Creek, South Carolina, where police used dogs in a surprise "raid" for students inside of a school. Those images are available in any web search.

Similar behavior may be in store for the UK if it has not already happened there.

A lawyer revealed: *"A judge in my local county was*

stopped for speeding and was treated like dirt by the cop. That's one judge who woke up."

Government's attitude toward your liberty is like a dog at a fire hydrant. The difference is that the government will pee on your head and tell you that it is raining.

Don't "Howl Hitler" – instead, stop the U.S.'s police state.

22. LOCK YOUR DOORS

Big banks advise their employees to do the following after the bank is robbed and the robber has left: rush to all doors and lock them immediately. The advice is intended to prevent the robber from returning and taking hostages, or taking lives.

There is more to the explanation that the banks don't tell employees: If there are police outside, they might shoot at the robber and drive him back inside the bank. Police can turn what would have been a short incident, into a protracted killing spree. If the robber runs back inside the bank, then hours might elapse before police decide to "rush" in. During those hours, people who are already injured might bleed to death; other people might be executed or injured by the robber; the newly injured victims might bleed to death waiting for police help.

That is why banks advise employees to lock the door BEFORE calling the police. Locking the door is the very first action to take. Do not alert police until AFTER the doors are locked. Locking the door is more important than notifying police because police might make things worse.

The advice of the banks applies anywhere that a violent attack occurs: bars, restaurants, night clubs, dance venues, stores, or anywhere. After an attack occurs and all criminals have exited, the doors need to be locked until it is clear that all criminals are far away or dead. There are many examples of police causing a violent criminal to re-enter and take hostages and kill more victims, and causing people who were already injured to bleed to death waiting for aid.

Even if a criminal has left, or has committed suicide, the police might not know it, and they will sometimes wait a long time before entering a safe location. Police will order injured people to remain inside, where the injured will bleed to death waiting for police help.

Locking the door is especially important in any government-mandated "gun-free" zone, where hoplophobes have disarmed the victims. Governments often disarm their victims. Victims were disarmed by Stalin, Mao, Hitler, Pol Pot, North Korea et cetera.

Victims are disarmed in Florida at bars and nightclubs. Places that sell alcohol are often forced to be "gun-free zones" under state laws. 49 people were killed and 53 were wounded in a government-mandated gun-free zone in Orlando, Florida in 2016 at the Pulse nightclub. There were armed, off-duty police officers and bouncers at Pulse to enforce the law that disarms patrons.

After disarming customers, police might have compounded the lethal situation. Much of the killing occurred after the criminal re-entered the area of his initial attack, after he fled from police near the front exit route, according to some accounts (at the time this was written, government officials would not divulge the details). The culprit was driven deeper into the building where he took hostages and murdered more people over the course of hours before police attacked. Some victims died while waiting for medical help during the tragedy.

An astonishing part of the Florida disaster is that all the patrons seem to have obeyed the law that made concealed firearms illegal inside. Not a single customer inside the bar had a gun that was used in self-defense. There is a high price to pay for obeying laws that restrict self-defense. Disarmament nuts have bloody hands from the millions of defenseless people murdered (by guns and by all other methods).[173] Socialists force many people to remit that steepest payment, as under the egomaniacs Stalin, Mao, and Hitler.

Some bars are so rough that a bouncer at the front entrance frisks everyone for weapons and will not allow entry to anyone who has a weapon.

Other bars are even rougher. At the roughest bars, if the bouncer frisks you and discovers that you are NOT carrying a gun, then he loans you one. "You can't go into this bar without a gun! Are you crazy?" they ask.

---

[173] Ever notice how socialists babble about any non-government "mass shooting" and never mention that the number of people killed was less than the number killed by guns in "guns-are-banned" Chicago about every month? About. Every. Month.

They also never mention how many people the U.S. government killed last month (e.g. outside of the U.S.). The number is probably in the thousands. Do they have any idea how many people the government kills every year? They won't discuss banning government and socialism.

And then there was Waco, Wounded Knee, Sand Creek, Colfax, etc.

If there were 50 "mass shootings" each day, and 50 people died each time, and it went on for 100 years, that would approximate the number of people killed by socialism in the 20th century. That does not include the number injured by socialism in the 20th century.

If you don't have a gun, then you are not allowed to enter.

Some state legislatures are considering statutes that would require a person to carry a gun into places where laws now ban guns (e.g. dance clubs). They think that civilians need to be nudged to defend themselves. Only stupid people go into dangerous places without a gun. Some people learn the hard way and pay with their lives. The police would not go into such places without a gun. Why should you? Cops are exempt from laws that disarm everyone else.

After a shooting incident, there are often public remarks from the worst active homicidal maniac in the USA (the President). His/Her body piles (including children, women, and other innocent non-combatants) while in office exceed that of any shooter in the nation ever. DC is a breeding hive for the criminally insane.

In the case of Barack Hussein Obama (and many other presidents) the toll of death and misery would include his earlier political career (in Congress) expanding military socialism and the police state. BO preferred to kill brown people. He would wear his Nobel Peace prize while he bombed children and innocent civilians.[174] Obama still holds the record for

---

[174] As a comparison, Chinese socialism joined German socialism (under Hitler) as the pair of socialist countries that had Nobel Peace Prize laureates die in state custody.

I don't personally dislike Obama any more than I personally dislike other people who murder children (and then joke about it). One estimate claims that in Obama's last year in office, the US dropped 26,172 bombs in seven countries. But to be fair, they were humanitarian bombs.

Charles Manson died 11-19-2017. He wasn't convicted of *personally* killing anyone, but he was "responsible" for deaths caused by others. How tiny does his death toll seem

most children killed by a Nobel Peace Prize recipient. Obomber is the first Nobel Peace Prize winner to bomb and kill other Nobel Peace Prize winners (Doctors Without Borders).[175]

The deadliest mass shooting on American soil was the battle of Gettysburg with ~10,000 dead under President Lincoln.

Presidents make arrestable serial killers seem angelic in comparison. Comedy ensues when the Murderer-in-Chief pontificates in press conferences about "why are people so violent?" Presidential butchers are surrounded 24/7 by men with guns (and more) and they want to reduce your ability to defend yourself against anyone (including him).

---

compared to that of presidents and socialists worldwide? Manson tattooed the symbol of German socialism to his forehead.

Obomber is a reminder that "Veterans Day" was originally "Armistice Day" and was intended as a celebration of peace and the end of war. The USA's military-socialism complex grew so large, and its non-stop violent globetrotting too, that "Armistice Day" became an awkward embarrassment, and was renamed to accommodate the government's constant warfare and to discourage people from thinking about peace and small government or no government at all (anarchy).

[175] Were Stalin, Mao, Hitler, Pol Pot, the Kim thugs, etc., ever considered for Nobel prizes? They were socialists too. Perhaps Stalin was in the running for a peace prize due to his "non-aggression pact" with German socialism. If not, are there posthumous awards?

Stalin worked hard to bring so much of the world "together" and to provide "free" food, clothing, shelter, healthcare, etc., in his socialist paradise.

No socialists, we're not giving up our right to self-defense unless you come with armed people and kill us, which of course would further illustrate why we won't give up our right to self-defense.

After the Orlando killings, the President and the Secretary of State had the audacity to call for yet more gun control (for others, not for themselves). They believed that the victims had not been disarmed enough.

In the Orlando case, more people would probably have survived if, at the beginning, the police had been disarmed.

The above is why you should do what the police do: arm yourself. It is a reminder of the book entitled: "Dial 911 and Die." When seconds count, the police are only minutes away. And even if the police are closer than minutes away, they might cause more casualties.

There is no duty to protect. The social contract theory was debunked in the court case Warren vs. District of Columbia.

There's a long list of jobs more dangerous than being a cop. There are few things more dangerous than calling a cop.

23. PAST & FUTURE POLICE STATE

Officer Allen pulled his patrol car onto Central Avenue. As usual, all the traffic ahead of him began turning off of Central Avenue. Within moments, the avenue was empty. Allen drove for about a mile and then turned north (right) onto Main Street. Again, all the cars ahead of him began turning off of Main Street until he was alone.

Officer Allen looked in his rear-view mirror and in the distance he could see some cars cautiously re-entering the street in back of him and keeping a large distance, pacing him from behind, never approaching, never passing.

He remembered back when it wasn't this way. People were different until that day when a meme was posted on the internet under the title FYL (For Your Liberty) "Pro Tip." This is that meme:

Never let a police car advance into a position where the police officer can signal for you to stop. Drivers should pro-actively prevent cops from following them in traffic. This is defensive driving.

If you are able to see a cop in your rear view

mirror (no matter how far back the cop is), then you should turn and either take a different route, or circle the block, or pull into a gas station or convenience store.

If you are on the highway and it is possible to take an exit, then do so. If possible, re-enter the highway after the officer has passed.

If there is a cop at an intersection ahead of you in a position where you will pass and he might end up behind you, preemptively turn before you pass the cop's location. Change your route, or circle the block so that the cop will have proceeded elsewhere, or so that he will be ahead of you.

It should go without saying: Don't ever pass a cop. If a cop appears in front of you, then you should remain a long way back, or take a different route. Don't pass.

If you turn and the officer follows you, then you should immediately find a place to stop (e.g. pull into a gas station, convenience store, or fast food location, then exit the car and go inside).

In other words, prevent cops from being in a position to read your tag, and prevent them from being in a position to pull you over.

The information above might save your life and the lives of those who are with you.

The meme above went viral and seemed to spread for years. Soon, it was altering the way people behaved, changing the way they drove.

But it worsened.

First, it worsened at the strip clubs. The police had

harassed the striptease clubs for decades. One day, a nude dance club put a lock on its entrance and dark tinting on the window next to the door. A doorman inside would hit a button to unlock the door for customers.

But they wouldn't let cops in.

And police outside could not see inside the club, or see if the doorman was there or who he was, or whether anyone was inside or not.

It was the buzz-in system that jewelry stores had used for years. Soon, the jewelry stores wouldn't let cops in either. At least not unless the jewelry store had just been robbed and specifically called for the police. Then they would let the cops in. But jewelry store robberies were rare.

Eventually, bars and other businesses began putting electronic buzzer locks on their doors and stopped letting in anyone who wore a uniform or looked like a bureaucrat.

It was time for lunch. Officer Allen pulled into an alley. He began to change his clothes to civilian attire.

It was the only way he could gain entry to a restaurant for lunch![176]

---

[176] This story is a reminder of "The Weapon Shops of Isher" by A. E. van Vogt which began with the sudden appearance out of thin air of a futuristic gun store. A police office attempted to open the front door but it was locked. A news reporter then tried the door and it opened and he entered with the door shutting behind him. The cop tried the door again, but it was locked. No employee of the government could enter.

24. GUNS & HISTORY

Police states disarm individuals in order to prevent resistance to socialism's violence and theft. Government schools (socialist schools) will not teach students about the 2nd Amendment, nor about firearms.

A recent school shooting was described as the worst massacre in American history. It added to the growing number of deaths attributable to government schools and those people who maintain existing gun laws that disarm the innocent. Even so, the number of deaths caused by the government in that school shooting was greatly exceeded by the government's death toll at Waco, Texas, a much worse massacre in American history. And the all-time worst was more than 100,000 innocent men, women, and children killed in the blink of an eye by the government in 1945.

School violence demonstrates that government's schools are unconstitutional under the Second Amendment right to self-defense against violent predators (whether such predators are in the government or out). Government's schools are victim disarmament zones and create ignorance of the Second Amendment Right to Keep and Bear Arms.

Martin Niemöller was famous for his poem "First

they came..." and for his opposition to German socialism and its police state under Adolf Hitler. Niemöller's legacy also serves to remind everyone to oppose victim disarmament zones.

Niemöller, a German Protestant minister, was persecuted in Germany while it was under the influence of the National Socialist Workers Party of Germany and its socialist swastika. The charges were trumped up and he spent the duration of World War II in Dachau (where there were many other people - including other ministers, monks, nuns, and priests - many of whom did not survive). They had all been disarmed.

The beginning of Niemoller's verse is often misstated as "First they came for the Socialists." Niemoller never said "First they came for the Socialists..." (see the work of Dr. Curry). The ignorant use of the term "socialist" in the verse is common because of widespread ignorance that "Nazis" did not call themselves "Nazis" (they called themselves socialists).

Niemoller was an early supporter of Hitler's socialism, so Niemoller would not have written "First they came for the socialists" (unless his poem was a cynical inside joke about how socialists have set world records killing other socialists as under Stalin and Soviet Socialism; Mao and Chinese socialism; Hitler and German socialism, et cetera. In that sense, the phrase would have been accurate).

Socialists lie about the poem (they use the "socialist" version) in order to hide the fact that Hitler's supporters called themselves "socialists" and did so while speaking and writing at length about their deadly dogma.

Some websites (e.g. Wikipedia) concede the "socialist" phrase's lack of support (on the wakipedia page entitled "First they came for..."), yet those websites fail to explain the illogic of the phrase. It is a glaring omission due to the cowardice of wannabe intellectuals. That failure exists because dedicated liars on wikipedia do not want to explain that Hitler's supporters called themselves "socialists."

Wikipedia begins by finessing the phrase as "First they came for..." in the title and leaving off the term "socialist."[177] Yet, on Wikipedia's page for "Martin Niemoller" the false version ("First they came for the socialists...") tops the page, and the rest of the page is designed to hide the fact that "Nazis" did not call themselves "Nazis," but called themselves "socialists" (this is a common method of deceit throughout Wakipedia). Of course, Wikipedia changes by the millisecond, so by the time anyone reads this and views Wakipedia, its deceits might have been buried. Wakipedia tricks readers because its name rhymes with "Encyclopedia" (and its slogan is: "The Free Encyclopedia") even though it is merely an anonymous bulletin board where anybody can post anything (including lies and the lying liars who tell them). Wakipedia and other websites cover up for socialism.

According to one interviewer, Niemoller (1892–1984) himself conceded that he did not use the term

---

[177] A recent discovery purports to reveal on older first draft of the poem that DID contain the word "socialists." That preliminary version was discarded at the time because it was considered too short. It has never been published before now. Here it is:

First they came for the socialists, and I did not speak out - because I was not a socialist.
Then …they didn't come back for anyone else. Everything was pretty much alright.
[END]

"socialist." No one can cite an original source for Niemoller using the term "socialist" in the popular misrepresentation of the poem.

Niemöller survived Germany's socialism, and it is odd to note that later in his life Niemöller seemed seduced by socialism despite his personal suffering under the socialist Wholecaust (of which the Holocaust was a part): ~50 million killed under Soviet socialism; ~40 million killed under Chinese socialism; and ~20 million killed under German socialism. Billions of lives were wrecked.

Mao killed more Chinese than any foreign government ever did. From Mao to now: Comic relief comes from Mao's mugshot mocked on "filthy" money (the Yuan/Renminbi) used for capitalist trade. On the bill, he is modeling fashion for his socialist "free" clothing program: Mao's matching pajama uniforms for China's inmates. The quizzacious impact would increase by pairing Mao's pic with his pal Stalin's portrait, and then adding Stalin's pal Hitler on the same paper currency. They helped create our prison planet.[178]

Russia's Central Bank had the good taste to phase out ruble bills bearing Lenin's satanic goateed portrait.

The fact that Mao was never murdered will be a badge of shame for China for a long time. Ditto for Soviet socialism in regards to Stalin (an old socialist

---

[178] Which is more philosophically funny to print on money: Mao's face or "In God We Trust" (IGWT)? Both? Add IGWT to Mao's money?

It is the 21st century and some countries continue to print money decorated with mass murderers. In the USA, there is currency bearing the portraits of the racist killers Lincoln and Grant. But Mao's kill rate makes them seem angelic in comparison.

joke known as the Soviet reversal: "In America, you kill leader. In Soviet socialism, leader kills you!"). And Kim Jong-un is living proof that everyone in the penal colony known as North Korea has been disarmed.[179] [gun cocks]

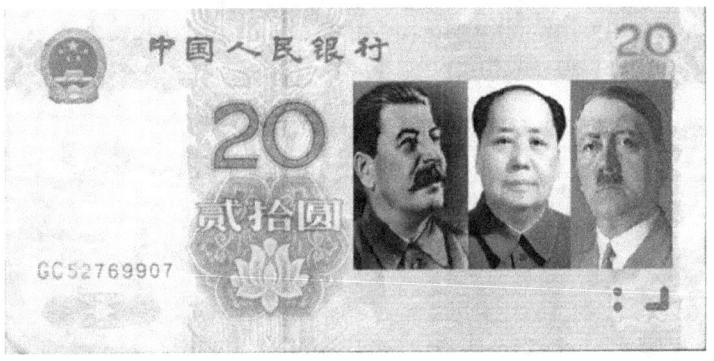

Mao and Stalin believed that only police agencies should have guns. Mao and Stalin demonstrated that socialists are inherently racist/murderous. Today's socialists preach oxymoronic beliefs that (1) police are inherently racist/murderous, and that (2) only police should be armed.

Socialism demonstrates the importance of the individual right to own guns for self-defense (against socialism, etc). Politicians support restricted access to firearms because they do things for which they should be shot. Disarming individuals makes it easier to steal from them. Socialists and their ilk are the reason why "happiness is a warm gun." Guns don't kill; socialists do.

Socialists provide more than a dozen reasons why high capacity clips and magazines are important: (1)

---

[179] No L.A. riot roof Koreans there.

Stalin, (2) Lenin, (3) Mao, (4) Hitler, (5) Pol Pot, (6) Mussolini, (7) Kim Jong-un, (8) Kim Jong-il, (9) Kim Il-sung, (10) Ho Chi Minh, (11) Che Guevara, (12) Fidel Castro. They want "prosperity for all," but will kill anyone if it will bring them an inch closer to their pipe dream. The people who literally kill millions with assembly line shots to the head, want to ensure that you cannot shoot them in the head.

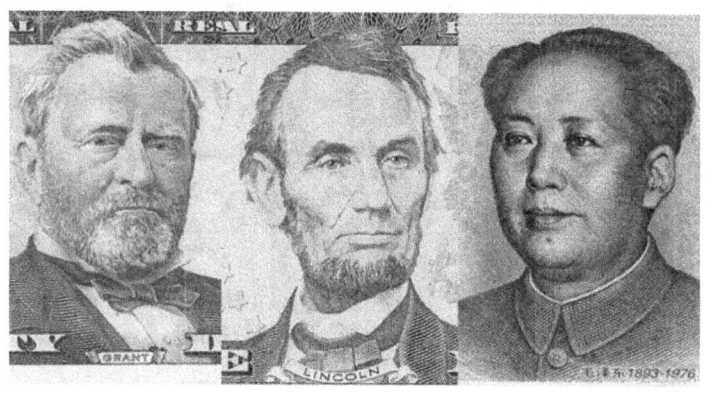

Gun grabbers are logical in the following sense: they want to control the government; they want the entity they control to be the only armed entity; and they're pretty cozy with the idea of snuffing everyone who doesn't agree with them. In fact, they yearn to do so.

ProTip: Every time somebody says you don't need a gun, buy another gun. If the government says you don't need a gun, YOU NEED A GUN!

More government means you need more guns. It inspired the bumper sticker "The more I learn about government, the more I like my guns." Buy a gun with your tax refund.

During Niemoller's suffering under German socialism, similar dogma permeated government schools (socialist schools) in the USA. The U.S. government followed Germany in becoming allies with Stalin and Soviet socialism. Socialist dogma continues to permeate the same schools today, and the Pledge of Allegiance is one example of it.

The pledge to the flag was written by a socialist and it was the origin of the Nazi salute and Nazi behavior.

A better stiff-arm salute is one in which a gun is held in self-defense against violent attackers (whether they are in the government or out). Guns rights stop violent socialism and violent socialists.

The following poem ("First They Came For The Machine Guns") was inspired by Niemöller's poem:

First they came for the machine guns, and I didn't speak up- because I had no machine guns.

Then they came for the "assault weapons," and I didn't speak up- because I had no assault weapons.

Then they came for the rifles, and I didn't speak up- because I had no rifles.

Then they came for the handguns, and I didn't speak up- because I had no handguns.

Finally, they came for my double-barreled shotgun- and I only managed to kill two of them.

(before they mowed me down with their machine guns, assault weapons, rifles, and handguns (while I was trying to reload)).

MADNESS

25. NOT SEE NAZI SOCIALISM

Poetry about the (former) National Socialist German Workers Party:

To say "Nazi"....
to say & not see.
Not see Nazi reality.
not see, not see, Not See
Don't say "Nazi" !
Do not say and Not See
say "National Socialist German Workers' Party."

The preceding poem is about "Not-Sees." Modern "Not-Sees" are the ones who don't want people to see that Hitler and his supporters called themselves "Socialists" and that they did not call themselves "Fascists," nor "Nazis." That is why they will never point out that the swastika was used by German socialists to represent crossed "S" letters for their dogma of socialism. Modern "Not-Sees" are anti-semantic.

Hitler's trademark was a type of cross, a "Hakenkreuz" (hooked cross); he did not call it a "swastika." The misnomer "swastika" was used (and continues to be used) to conceal Nazism's origin in American Christian Socialism, via Francis Bellamy and his cousin Edward Bellamy (author of "Looking

Backward" -the origin of the National Socialist movement).

There are many Not-Sees regarding the links of American socialism to German socialism, Italian socialism, Soviet socialism, Chinese socialism, and global socialism (e.g. links via the Bellamy cousins). There are also Not-Sees about the U.S.'s Pledge of Allegiance as the origin of the Nazi salute and Nazi behavior (see that and other discoveries revealed in the book "Pledge of Allegiance & Swastika Secrets").

Help to unmask Not-Sees. The preceding poem inspired the "Not Say Nazi" movement to stamp out widespread ignorance and to abolish the N-word and the F-word.

Not-Sees also want people to not see that Soviets called themselves "socialists." Not-Sees use the phrase "Stalin's Russia" in order to obscure the actual name of the country: Union of Soviet SOCIALIST Republics. If pressed, Not-Sees insist that the USSR was "communist," and Germany was "fascist," and they were complete opposites. Stalin and Mao and their ilk demonstrated that socialists and communists were considered to be the same thing, and that the word "communist" was an interchangeable synonym for "socialist."

Not-Sees never mention that German socialists and Soviets socialists were allies in a plan to divide up Europe, and invaded Poland together in 1939, launching the Socialist War (World War II), and leading to the socialist Wholecaust (of which the Holocaust was a part). If they mention that time at all, they only mention that the "Nazis invaded Poland," and they hope that the reader is ignorant about the alliance of German socialists and Soviet socialists.

MADNESS

26. TRAINING DOGS & LIZARDS

Earlier chapters in this book explained that a drug dog's training is not unique or complicated. Many canine house pets will search for a toy that is covered with a pillow or a coffee can. The toy can be hidden with an edible treat or some other item with a unique smell. After a few weeks, the snack can be hidden alone, without the toy, and the dog will find the snack via its odor, an odor that the dog was taught to associate with its toy, in a similar manner to how drug dogs are taught to associate the smell of a drug with their toys.

Yard lizards can be trained. The lizards look and behave like tiny Dachshunds. They can be trained to eat out of your hand. With enough training, they will climb up a lawn chair, jump in your lap and stare at you until you give them their favorite treat: mealworms.

Mealworms are available at most pet shops that sell snakes, iguanas, and other reptiles. The worms are sold in small plastic containers and they can be kept in the refrigerator for a month, where the worms stay dormant.

Mealworms make great conversation starters on salads.

Be sure to buy the smallest mealworms, about half an inch maximum length. Yard lizards, formally known as anoles (a-NO-lees), can't eat big mealworms.

Lizards also will eat live crickets; however, crickets jump about and are difficult to use in training.

To begin training, sit on the ground in an area where the lizards sun themselves and watch humans. If the mealworms have been refrigerated, let them warm up to reach maximum wiggliness. Wiggliness excites reptiles.

Start by tossing the worms near the lizards and sit still while the anole watches the worm wiggle and then rushes over to grab it. Then try placing the worms nearer to you, slowly closing the distance. Eventually, hold a wiggling worm in your fingers and lay your hand on the ground. Next, move on up to placing a wiggling worm on your forearm while laying your hand on the ground to serve as a staircase, so that the lizard can crawl up the arm to take the worm.

Some lizards are easier to train (hungrier) than others. In some yards, the animals can be coaxed to take a worm from the hand in one sitting. In other yards, the lizards are skittish and require multiple sessions. Lizards are skittish in areas with cats that prey on them.

The very act of tossing a worm will scare away some lizards. In such yards, a worm can be slowly placed about one yard from a lizard, and within clear view of the reptile. The human should back off to let the creature approach.

Soon, your pets will be happy to see you come outside, and will approach you and other humans. You can call to them and they will come trotting over to you. You are the lizard wizard. If your chicken eats one, it will be digested in her gizzard. Dress the male ones in women's clothing to impersonate Eddie Izzard.

They will chase each other and fight each other to win your worms. They will perform peculiar territorial dances wherein two lizards will circle each other repeatedly with their tails rhythmically curling. They will do other crude things for your viewing pleasure. A carefully placed mirror can also prompt lizards to engage in displays to their own reflections.

So, if your child says he wants a new pet, just buy him a box of mealworms open the back door and say "knock yourself out, kiddo!

27. DOG ECONOMICS 101

Peter was walking with his Doberman "Lobo." They had grown to love these woods over their six years together.

Suddenly a deadly poisonous snake bit Lobo. Peter frantically pulled out his cell phone and was relieved to hear his dog's veterinarian answer. The vet calmed Peter and explained that although the bite is lethal without treatment, there is 100% cure by injection for $2000 if Peter rushes Lobo to the office.

A shocked expression came over Peter's face as he ended the call. The dog was prostrate on the ground whimpering as if asking, "What will happen to me?"

Looking down at his dog, Peter explained, "The vet said you're gonna die."

28. HISTORY OF SOCIALIST PROGRAMS

Have socialists in your city created a "community bicycle program" (CBP)? Some cities turn abandoned bicycles into "community bicycles" available to anyone for temporary use in downtown areas.

Community bicycles are all painted one loud color to help users distinguish them from private bikes. Safety-orange is the color sprayed on by bureaucrats in some towns. Then they call it the "Orange Bicycle Program" (OBP).

In my town, it was a short-lived program. The orange bicycles went unused until they were stolen and, it is hoped, repainted.

Politicians are inspired by programs like "community bicycles," even though they never ride the bikes, nor use government buses, nor government schools.

The same officials will be inspired by these programs:

Community Umbrella Program: Everyone gets caught in the rain without an umbrella. This program attempts to solve that problem. It is unfortunate that "Honor system" umbrellas have been tried with results similar to that of "community bikes," in that the umbrellas are given permanent homes elsewhere. The theft problem might be reduced a tad by painting the umbrellas safety orange.

Community car and RV program: Rain, heat, and other bad weather discourage use of community bikes. Confiscated and abandoned cars and recreational vehicles (RVs) can be painted Day-Glo orange and left with on/off starter switches (to prevent lost or stolen keys). The RV's would also allow folks to catch a nap or even stay overnight if necessary. Instead of a new government rail mass-transit boondoggle, it would be cheaper to leave enough orange cars about for all predicted rail-riders.

Community food, clothing and shelter programs: Food, clothing, and shelter are the three basic necessities and the following programs address them:

Community Refrigerators: community bicycles make riders hot, thirsty and hungry. Old refrigerators can be painted orange, filled with food and beverages, and placed near street corners and bike stands so that riders, pedestrians and anyone else can avail themselves of food and drink, which could be eaten en route to another destination, leaving uneaten portions in another orange refrigerator for others, or for later. This program has the added advantage of allowing people to add their own food and drink to the refrigerators, thus contributing to the program and ensuring its success and longevity.

Community clothing program: Orange jumpsuits can be borrowed from nearby county jails where the orange clothing program is already being enjoyed by many residents (similar to the fashion of Guantanamo Bay detention camp), some of whom have already enjoyed the orange bike program. When the clothing is not being worn, it can be left in orange boxes attached to the top of the orange refrigerators, available to any other clothing-challenged persons.

Community Houses program: For the temporarily displaced. Instead of tearing down crack houses and condemned structures, paint them Day-Glo orange and add them to the other community programs. These free and open houses would work on the honor system, only to be used overnight or so long as it takes the user(s) to find "normal" housing.

Community Sex Toys: Believe it or not, there already are Day-Glo orange dildos (or so I have been told), and that makes this outreach program a no-brainer. Perhaps the playthings can be kept in the boxes on top of the refrigerators (when they are not in use), next to the free orange condoms. This project will cut down on sexually transmitted diseases (STDs), and that will excite community leaders to line up and get behind it. Critics claim that the devices will have to be chained to the sidewalks to keep them from sprouting feet and running off. However, leashing them will limit their range of use.

29. WATER'S SOCIALIST PAST

This motion was actually filed in court against a citation (imposing a monetary fine) alleging lawn-watering on an improper date and time. The citation was dismissed.

MOTION TO DISMISS
WATER CONSERVATION CITATION
FOR IMPROPER LAWN WATERING

The undersigned Defendant moves to dismiss the "Water Conservation Citation" in this case which was recently issued for the alleged watering of a lawn on a day or time not specified by government edict.

This motion to dismiss would be filed with the same arguments if, in addition to socializing water, the local government also socialized food, clothing, shelter, oil, phosphate, phone calls, electricity, lumber, land, milk, natural gas, gypsum, gasoline, football, coal, concrete, chalk, cement, computers, crops, cable TV, toilet paper, or any other goods and services. Those goods and services (food, clothing, shelter, et cetera) will hereafter be abbreviated -
"FCSOPHPHELLMNGGGFCCCCCCCTVTP"

In support of this motion to dismiss, the Defendant states the following:

FCSOPHPHELLMNGGGFCCCCCCCTVTP are a few examples of goods and services, besides water, that government is not supposed to own, sell or monopolize. If Government sold the other items, it would cause the same disastrous results that it has caused in water: shortages, misery, soviet-style rationing and the use of police and courts to restrict everyone's purchases and uses. The more goods and services that government socializes, the more totalitarian society becomes.

Government water is a true monopoly because the government bans competitors by law. In comparison, Bill Gates' computer company is not a monopoly here because there is no law that bans others from selling computers in the same geographical area. It is fortunate that the local government did not take over the computer business, or the same sad results would have occurred as they have with water: shortages, misery, soviet-style rationing of computers, a controlled internet, and the use of police and courts to restrict everyone's purchases and uses.

The government's dihydrogen monoxide monopoly creates the overuse problem and then tries to solve it with more antidisestablishmentarianism via "tiered pricing." Tiered pricing is price gouging under a socialistic system.

Water is too important for the government to be involved. Only under a free market system do higher prices encourage competitors to find and provide more water or other alternatives.

People who support watering rules are chumps who promote waste by propping up the socialized system, helping wasteful individuals evade the true costs of wastefulness, costs which would otherwise be levied in market prices among private firms just like other goods.

The government water monopoly is a violation of every individual's right to "life, liberty and the pursuit of happiness," and a violation of personal freedom and economic freedom.

The purpose of government is to recognize and protect private property rights in all resources, and to protect property rights from violence and theft, so that individuals are free to own and distribute water, food, clothing, shelter, oil, phosphate, phone calls, electricity, lumber, land, milk, natural gas, gypsum, gasoline, football,[180] coal, concrete, chalk, cement, computers, crops, cable TV, toilet paper, and all other goods and services.

It is not the purpose of government to provide water, food, clothing, shelter or other goods and services, and any attempt by the government to do so always involves theft and violence. Government water involves police state tactics of soviet-style rationing in its most petty form. Government water involves theft and violence and is, therefore, illegal.

---

[180] American football (and its many socialized and tax-subsidized stadiums) is a reminder of this global description of statists: no matter how bad "your" team is, you bootlickers always support it anyway. The NFL is sucking the military's dick so hard right now lmao. So glad that DVR enables everyone to skip the demented flags, troops, anthem worship. Western socialists like socialism the way that fat guys in a bar like sports. The psychology of loving a state and a football team seem to go hand in hand.

30. WOODMAN SPARE THAT OLD $10 TREE

Popular songs often misrepresent property rights and economic freedom. Such misrepresentations are sometimes intentional and at other times are a result of sheer ignorance of free market economics. The famous song "Woodman, Spare That Tree" is an example.

The song tells the tale of how a sentimental man prevented the chopping of a familiar tree. The lyrics imply that the tree was saved by emotional pleas and even by an implied threat of violence against the woodman. The libertarian historian Dr. Rex Curry has pointed out that the poetic plea is pure fiction and omits the most important truth: the tree was saved because the woodman was paid $10 to not cut down his own tree on the privately-owned property.

The song originated from a poem written in 1837 by George Pope Morris, a well-known journalist, and poet who founded the New York Mirror in 1823 with Samuel Woodworth. In 1830 Morris wrote that he and a friend were walking in Manhattan when they saw a tenant of a property preparing to cut down a "grand old elm" (the elm became an oak in the song) for firewood. As the story goes, Morris and his companion talked to the woodman and negotiated to pay him $10 to let the tree stand.

Morris' poem misrepresented the event in other ways, in addition to omitting the pecuniary act that actually saved the tree. If any of the parties present remembered the tree from childhood, it was more likely the anonymous woodman. And if any of the parties promoted the progress that removed trees from the landscape of Manhattan, it was Morris, founder of the New York Mirror, as much as the poor tenant.

Morris claimed that the elm tree was still standing as late as 1862.

However, economic myopia might have blinded Morris from seeing if the tenant used the $10 to start a new business, the Manhattan Firewood and Tree Clearing Corporation, which went on to make Manhattan a treeless wonderland, thanks to Morris' seed money. Morris was oblivious to the economic reality that the tenant presumably requested $10 in order to purchase an equal or greater amount of firewood from someone who presumably felled some other tree(s) somewhere else (say on the next block?). In other words, Morris' act may have resulted in the death of one or more older, grander trees elsewhere.

Morris' histrionic misrepresentation has misled many environmentalists who act as if every tree is priceless, as implied in Morris' poem. Yet Morris easily arrived at a price with the tenant and the price was only $10. A better title for Morris' poem would be "Money talks and whining walks."

Edward Bellamy repeated Morris' fiction in the article "Woodman, Spare That Tree!" for the newspaper where Bellamy was an assistant editor (Springfield Daily Union, July 7, 1873: 4, col. 6). Bellamy was the notorious founder (1888) of "National Socialism" and

"Military Socialism" in the United States. He was the cousin and comrade of Francis Bellamy, author of the Pledge of Allegiance (the origin of the Nazi salute and Nazi behavior, as revealed in the book "Pledge of Allegiance + Swastika Secrets").

The poem was set to music by Henry Russell and other musicians. Various examples of the melody can be found by searching the web.

To his credit, Irving Berlin, in comic fashion, restored a more accurate version of the story in the song "Woodman, Woodman, Spare That Tree!" from the Broadway Show "Ziegfield Follies of 1911" (Irving Berlin / Vincent Bryan).

Below are the lyrics to the Russell song. There are two alternate added stanzas authored by Dr. Curry. The first alternate stanza more completely describes the grand finale of free-market environmentalism that saved the tree. The second alternate stanza describes the sad situation of what most people do today with tree ordinances and watering restrictions. At the end is Irving Berlin's treatment of the original story.

Woodman, spare that tree!
Touch not a single bough!
In youth it sheltered me,
And I'll protect it now.
'Twas my forefather's hand
That placed it near his cot:
There, woodman, let it stand,
Thy axe shall harm it not!

That old familiar tree,
Whose glory and renown
Are spread o'er land and sea,

MADNESS

And wouldst thou hew it down?
Woodman, forbear thy stroke!
Cut not its earth-bound ties;
Oh, spare that aged oak,
Now towering to the skies!

When but an idle boy
I sought its grateful shade;
In all their gushing joy
Here too my sisters played.
My mother kissed me here;
My father pressed my hand --
Forgive this foolish tear,
But let that old oak stand!

My heart-strings round thee cling,
Close as thy bark, old friend!
Here shall the wild-bird sing,
And still thy branches bend.
Old tree! the storm still brave!
And, woodman, leave the spot:
While I've a hand to save,
Thy axe shall harm it not.

Here is the addendum that describes what actually happened:

For woodman, see my hand,
ten dollars we agreed;
contracts are always grand
with private property.
both bill and tree are green,
and both are made of wood.
socialism is mean.

MADNESS

capitalism: good!

Here is the more likely modern addendum based on what people (especially those people inspired by Morris' misleading poem) actually do to each other today through tree ordinances, watering restrictions and other government action:

I rush to city hall
and socialists I'll find,
to steal your property
and treat it as mine.
We'll tell you what to do
with trees, water and all;
resistance will bring you
a costly vicious brawl!

The following are Irving Berlin's Lyrics -

[1st verse:]
A great big tree grows near our house
It's been there quite some time
This tree's a slipp'ry elm tree and very hard to climb
But when my wife starts after me, up in that tree I roost
I go up like a healthy squirrel and never need no boost
The other day a woodman came to chop the refuge down
And carve it into kindling wood, to peddle 'round the town
I says to him, "I pray thee cease, desist, refrain and stop
Lay down that razor, man, chop not a single chop"

[Refrain:]
Woodman, woodman, spare that tree
Touch not a single bough

MADNESS

For years it has protected me
And I'll protect it now
Chop down an oak, a birch or pine
But not this slipp'ry elm of mine
It's the only tree that my wife can't climb
So spare that tree

[2nd verse:]
I said to him, "You see that hole
Up near that old treetop
I've got five dollars there, that's yours, if you refrain to chop
No beast but me can climb that tree, 'cause it's too slippery
I can't get up myself, unless my wife is after me
So get my wife and I'll call her a very naughty word
And then you'll see me give an imitation of a bird
You may not know just where to go, when my wife gets around
But when she comes, remember this, if I'm not on the ground."

31. TREE LAWS MAKE TREES HISTORY

Lawyers are often consulted by property owners who want to remove trees without fear of tree preservation laws. Attorneys cannot advise clients to ignore laws (though tree laws often seem easy to ignore). Clients can be told about what a lot of people do: they don't plant any trees that are protected by tree laws. Under tree ordinances, if a tree is small enough to be killed legally, then the tree is killed. Trees are not allowed to grow large enough to enter the web of the law.

Tree laws make treeless property the safest route. That is because tree ordinances can be expanded in the future. Therefore, every existing tree is a potential risk that a property owner will be restricted by government in the future alteration of his property. Removing trees is the only way to be safe when tree laws are a possibility.

Tree laws kill trees, as every libertarian knows. And rightfully so, because tree laws violate private property rights by "socializing" trees.

The following is a popular joke about the endangered species act: if a property owner sees an endangered species on his property he should "shoot, shovel and shut up." The joke is based on the truth that if the government becomes aware of an endangered species on your private property, then you will lose your property rights, and be treated very badly.

Under tree-preservation laws the joke can be altered to warn property owners to "chop, chip and chill."

Tree laws illustrate the fatal conceit of socialism and its unintended consequences.[181] Tree-huggers must have fallen out of a stupid tree and hit every branch on the way down. If public officials were any more stupid, they'd have to be watered weekly. If their antidisestablishmentarianism continues then more "protected" trees will die.

Tree laws prove that socialism is environmentally disastrous. Government built roads through forests, straightened rivers, drained wetlands, cut canals, and subsidized other agricultural uses with taxes and other socialism. The government has already done more environmental damage than private enterprise could ever have afforded to do. Socialism is collective Munchausen Syndrome.

Capitalism saves trees from socialism's destruction. Capitalists farm trees for paper, and other uses. Capitalists created alternative forms of power to replace the burning of wood.

The best environment is a capitalist environment. Mother Nature is a capitalist. [#ancap]

Trees prove that the color of a healthy environment and the color of money are the same. Capitalists are the true greens.

Even so, Government threatens tree owners on private property with tree laws. Tree laws fail to distinguish non-violent private acts from theft and

---

[181] Are there really unintended consequences for socialists when everyone warns them about the consequences (which are well known) and they keep doing it anyway?

violence. With tree laws, the government threatens theft and violence against peaceful people.

The following is poetry about a tree (or poetree) -

I think that I shall never see
a tree-law as beautiful as a tree
and if the tree-laws do not fall
I may not see a tree at all

32. SKIPPY GETS SCHOOLED

Once upon a time, there was a brave little boy named "Skippy" who decided to end bullying at his school. All the teachers at Francis Bellamy Elementary School were supportive when Skippy set a date to launch his anti-bullying campaign. He was going to give all the other children fun rubber wristbands colored red, white, and blue, with the embossed phrase "Say No to Bullies!" Small American flags on little sticks were similarly embossed. The fun freebies were patterned after the red, white, and blue colors of the giant flag painted on their school's exterior, the regular flags in each classroom, and after the large flag waving on the pole in front of their school.

When the big day came, Skippy was at school early in his homeroom class as the teacher began the day with the Pledge of Allegiance. The teacher, Miss Fulford, noticed that Skippy did not stand for the pledge as he always had in the past.

Miss Fulford interrupted the pledge and asked "Skippy, why do you remain seated during the Pledge of Allegiance?"

In his childish voice, Skippy said, "The Pwedge of Aweegiance is part of my campaign against bulwying.

Children think that they have to chant the pwedge. The pwedge is the first bulwying that begins everwy day for wus."

"Do you have some new wacko religious beliefs that have turned you so naughty?" the teacher demanded of Skippy.

"No, Miss Fulford," said Skippy, "I wesearched the histowy. Nazi salutes came from the pwedge!"

"Well, we'll have none of that mister!" the teacher warned, "Even if you won't join everyone else, then you will stand up in respect, and keep your allegiance hole shut!"

There was an awkward pause, as Skippy stared at the teacher, and the teacher glared at Skippy. Red-faced, Miss Fulford realized that Skippy would not move from his seated position. With a vein popping out of her forehead, she pointed at the door and screamed, "TO THE PRINCIPAL'S OFFICE!"

Later that day, all the children rejoiced as they helped the school lynch Skippy. His lifeless body was left to hang from the flag pole, underneath the heroic star-spangled banner that Skippy would dishonor never more. As the sun set on Old Glory, the entire school (or rather, what remained of it) intoned the Pledge of Allegiance, as a murder of crows gormandized until they were satiated. Skippy's little feet and hands had been bound with his own kid-sized rubber bracelets that said: "Say No To Bullies!"

33. TRIANGLE SHIRTWAIST FACTORY FIRE

Ignacia Del Fuego typed during the morning break, finishing her manuscript about the Triangle Shirtwaist Factory fire that killed her great-grandmother and 145 other garment workers on March 25, 1911.

Gazing northeast from her 91st-floor office in Manhattan, "Iggy" could see the area where the inferno occurred near Washington Square in Greenwich Village. Only the top three floors of the ten-story building had been damaged in the fire; the refurbished "Brown Building" was now part of New York University. Two blocks from NYU is the apartment where Iggy resides with her teenage daughter, Tiffany.

The final chapter of Iggy's book explained how the historic Shirtwaist fire, and her great-grandmother Frieda's untimely death, spurred legislation that improved safety for all.

"My book needs a grand finale," Iggy whispered to herself as her brown eyes fixed upon an odd plane on the horizon. It was flying fast and low. The passenger aircraft was racing toward the towering office building next to hers.

Iggy screamed as the plane slammed into floors 94 through 98 of the northern facade next door. She had backed up to the far wall of her office as the fireball exploded 138 feet away from her.

Within moments, Iggy realized that, as in 1911, there was no municipal fire truck with rescue ladders that could reach those people above the conflagration in the adjacent building. The distance was ten times higher than her great-grandmother's garment factory. It was the first time that the thought had ever crossed Iggy's mind during the nine years she had occupied the skyscraper and written her manuscript.

During the fifteen minutes that Iggy stared in horror at the first tower, a second commuter jet slammed into her office tower from floors 78 through 84, only ten floors below Iggy's. The earthquake sent her staggering toward the stairs.

"Go up! Run to the roof!" yelled a feminine voice in the smoke-filled stairwell. Everyone was headed upward, and Iggy joined the rush.

At the top, the roof door was locked. It was another page from Great-Grandma Frieda's requiem.

If the door had been unlocked, it would not have mattered because the government had no plan for helicopter rescues to the tallest buildings in Manhattan.

Everyone had assumed that the government was providing protection. That is why no one in the building had a BASE jump parachute (even though daredevils had parachuted from the towers many times in the past).

Smoke filled Iggy's lungs and she fought to remain upright. Iggy saw the outline of a young lady in the enveloping fumes. Iggy heard the girl sob, "Our government killed us. Its violence did this."

Iggy gasped, "Frieda?" as she struggled to remain conscious, and watched the female walk toward a window that had shattered open.

At least 200 people fell or jumped to their deaths from the burning towers, landing on the streets and rooftops of adjacent buildings. Iggy was one of them.

Hours later, both buildings ceased to exist. The next day, Iggy was part of the soot and dust that coated the Brown Building where it stands today, where Iggy's great-grandmother died, two blocks from the apartment where Iggy's daughter lives. Her ashes were there too.

In the years that followed, thousands more Americans died in growing violence from Iggy's government worldwide, far surpassing the death toll of 1911, as well as surpassing the death toll of 2001. Now, as then, there are no municipal fire trucks that reach that high, no helicopter rescue plans, and no one with BASE jump parachutes in Manhattan's skyscrapers.

Iggy's daughter Tiffany plans to write a book. It will say the opposite of her late mother's lost manuscript.

34. CROSSWORDS

After her mother's death, Tiffany habitually wore a gold crucifix that Iggy had presented on Tiff's seventh birthday. The constant reminder around her neck made her notice crosses in her favorite thrift stores. She collected more jewelry bearing the icon -rings, bracelets, broaches, and more neck chains.

When people complimented her religious trinkets, she beamed. One day, after a freckled kindergartner asked to touch one of her newer crucifixes, she took it off, put it over his head, and said "I want you to keep it. It will enlighten you." After that, she began wearing two necklaces; a nice one paired with an inexpensive one to give away. One to keep and one to share.

Tiffany's curiosity about crosses grew. She studied their history. As her obsession spread, she created crossword puzzles with the iconic shape.

1 DOWN – where dead German socialists live

2 ACROSS – related to the word "Fascist"

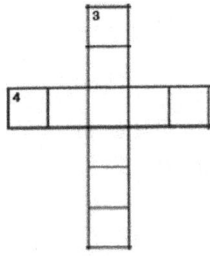

3 DOWN – Stalin's pal in 1940
4 ACROSS – Goring's nickname

Home-made crosses and crucifixes became Tiff's new hobby. Colorful polymer clay from arts and crafts stores hardened when baked, and made each gift one-of-a-kind. Cheap string served as each necklace's chain; but later, Tiff switched from string to wire embedded into the clay. It was easy to implant things in her artwork.

Lin, one of Tiffany's few female friends, texted information to Tiff's cell phone about a new "oddities and antiques" shop in town. En route at 38th Avenue, Tiffany glanced in the rear-view mirror and noticed a cop car a block behind her. She immediately hit the turn signal and detoured right at the next street.

It was a brick street lined with weathered wooden telephone poles strung together with wires at the arms of their crossbeams. She thought they were more likely power lines now instead of phone lines (as capitalism's cell phones had annihilated the government's old hand-picked phone franchise -a socialist monopoly that had crucified so many for so long). Each pole was a cross, and they glided by as hypnotic ghosts while her Volkswagen passed.

Loose gravel slid under her tires in the empty handicapped parking space outside of the Mosley Motel. Tiffany stepped out holding her latest smart phone and clicked some quick pics of the old telephonic poles, the salvation army of marching crosses. One photo showed the sidewalk as a female pedestrian in shorts and purple knee pads sauntered away.

The sound of someone crying came from the inn. Mr. Rogers had not prepared Tiffany for this neighborhood.

35. THE CRUCIFIX

Tiffany gave the naked guy at the seedy roadhouse a crucifix necklace and he stopped crying. Her gift of jewelry was made of bright white clay and cheap but large. Sometimes a kind gesture is enough.

"WheRe'd yOu gEt tHe crUCIfix?" he murmured, his green eyes widening, as he struggled to stand up from the small rain-puddle on the dank hallway's floor.

"Why are you …uh… naked?" Tiffany stuttered, hoping he would forget his question about the crucifix's origin.

"WheRe. dID. YoU. GeT. thE. CrOSs?" he demanded through clenched yellow teeth while he used the wall to remain upright.

Tiffany tensed up as she parried with: "Why were you crying?"

"WHeRE DId YOu GEt THiS SWastIKA?!?!?" he screamed, echoing off all the doors of the 1st floor.

Her right hook across his left chin hit so hard that he collapsed back to the moist concrete.

Tiffany took the crucifix from the naked guy in the motel as he started crying.

36. MORE CROSS WORDS

That wasn't the first time Tiffany had punched a male. Her mother had taught her how to do it. She put her hips, abs, legs, her whole body into her swinging fist. Iggy also taught her what to do immediately after she hit anyone: RUN. Don't stick around to see what happens next. That could be deadly.

The unknown derelict had looked like a thin crappy version of Dr. Bob Zarry, the guy who was dating Tiffany's hot friend Lin. She wondered: *Could the vagrant be his older brother?* The next time she saw Bob, she would pay close attention and search for signs of resemblance.

Tiffany zipped to the Hollander Bistro, a breakfast joint several blocks South. The oddities shop would have to wait until she stopped shaking. She ordered her favorite morning meal: "Bacon and coffee." Bacon helped her write. She munched strips of the heavenly finger food in her left hand while she scribbled on paper napkins with her right.

Tiffany's love for bacon began when she was a young girl and her mother would say "Knowledge is Power ...Francis Bacon." She understood it as "Knowledge is power, France is bacon." For more than a decade she wondered about the meaning of the second part and what was the surreal linkage between the two? It made bacon sound important, cosmopolitan, and mysterious. It made her crave both knowledge and bacon. It made her want to visit France.

Whenever she repeated the quote to someone, "Knowledge is power, France is bacon" they nodded knowingly. Or someone might say, "Knowledge is power" and she would finish the quote "France is bacon," and they wouldn't look at her like she'd said something odd; they would thoughtfully agree. Once, she asked a teacher "What does 'Knowledge is power, France is bacon' mean?" Tiff's instructor spent ten minutes explaining the "knowledge is power" bit, but not a word on "France is bacon." When Tiffany prompted further explanation by asking "France *IS* bacon?" the teacher merely replied "yes." Tiffany didn't have the confidence to press it further. The knowledge eluded her. For years, she just accepted it as something she'd never understand.

Her dream of visiting France came true on a Rheinfahrt she booked from Amsterdam, through Germany, and then briefly near Strasbourg (in the historic region of Alsace), and ending at Basel, Switzerland. In Strasbourg, French bacon was different from the USA's. However, the poitrine fumée, double smoked and double salted, was delicious.

One of her favorite ways to eat bacon was a BLT – a bacon, lettuce, and tomato sandwich. Sometimes Tiffany spread guacamole from avocados next to the bacon on her delicacy. She loved LGBTs.

Turkey bacon was a BOGO at Publix one day, so she bought it. She'd seen the fake food served at a Bar Mitvah in New Jersey the year before. Even her brilliant idea of frying the kosher strips in bonafide bacon grease did not do enough. But it helped.

Tiffany passed through a phase in her life when she practiced the religious ritual of fasting often; but that was back when she thought fasting meant "eating fast." She mistakenly believed the word "fasting" was derived from an Old English spelling of the word "feasting" but with the letter "e" missing. She ate a lot of bacon back then. She enjoyed fasting for years until a Muslim explained what the word "fast" really meant. Bacon influenced her decision to not try true fasting. Ever.

Roses are red
So is bacon
Poetry is hard
……bacon

Bacon's salty yumminess had created so many infidels and apostates. Bacon was the forbidden fruit. Millions had been tempted into reason by people eating tasty pigs. *How much atheism had bacon caused in the world?* Tiffany asked herself.

The nude bum's cross words puzzled Tiff too, as another pink packet of artificial sweetener poured into her refilled mug of coffee. He inspired her to compose another word game -

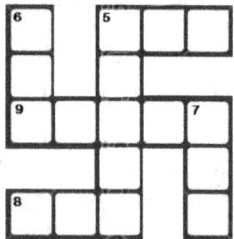

MADNESS

DOWN
5 what Jesus was feeling before he died
6 often precedes "Humbug!"
7 singular nominative pronoun for Tiffany

ACROSS
8 possessive pronoun for Bob's property
9 extra parts on the NSDAP's cross
5 VW was German socialism's _____

A week later, when Tiffany uploaded her new puzzles to a crossword website, she typed up the answer sheet:

1 DOWN - Hades (where dead German socialists live)
2 ACROSS - fag (related to the word "Fascist")
3 DOWN - Hitler (Stalin's pal in 1940)
4 ACROSS - Fatty (Goring's nickname)
5 ACROSS - car (VW was German socialism's ____)
5 DOWN - cross (What Jesus felt before he died)
6 DOWN - Bah (often precedes "Humbug!")
7 DOWN - she (singular nominative pronoun for Tiffany)
8 ACROSS - his (possessive pronoun for Bob's property)
9 ACROSS – hooks (extra parts on the NSDAP's cross)

37. SHE WAS TEMPERAMENTAL

"Not yet," Avocado whispered to Bob; "Not yet. But soon!" she teased him. Bob's love for her was so large he could barely contain himself.

As the days passed, Bob tried not to pester Avocado. He knew that Avocado would warm up. It would just take a little time. One day soon Avocado would be ready, and oh what a glorious day that would be.

On Friday, Bob was in the bathroom, engaged in good personal hygiene, the details of which will not be elaborated here. Suddenly, Bob could hear Avocado scream... "I'M READY!" He could not believe his ears. Again, Avocado's screaming came "HURRY!" Bob quickly dropped what he was doing and pulled up his pants. "EAT ME ... NOW!"

Bob jerked open the bathroom door and, clutching his unbuckled belt, he sprinted down the hall toward the kitchen which was, now ...eerily ...silent.

Bob was too late.

As soon as he ran in, Bob could see that Avocado had changed. She looked sick. She had become quiet.

Avocado whispered sadly, "...too late. Too late. Toooo
late."

It was over.

38. 2 GIRLS 1 CUP

It sure is difficult giving a blowjob while you are crying, Tiffany thought. Yet that is how she had always done it. Guys don't seem to care either. That included Bob.

Perhaps it was because Bob was reclined on his pool's pink lounge chair with his head tilted up at the sunny 2 PM sky and his eyes closed as he murmured "MMMmmmmm." Bob's small dog watched Tiffany hungrily.

Sometimes, to slow her weeping, she would sing to herself in her head over and over again a song that she had been taught long ago in grade school about a patriotic little boy lynched by anti-pledge bullies setting fire to flags in all the classrooms. He gave his own life to defend the nation and save all children:

Me and Skippy
Skippy and Me
God how happy
We will be
Pledging all across our schools
Me and Skippy
Skippy and Me

The ode didn't help Tiffany today. Her tears

continued to drip.

The sky might cry with her. Distant thunder rumbled softly though the sun shined brightly. A pleasant pre-storm breeze cut through the usual scorching summer heat. News on Bob's big-screen TV updated the path of a growing hurricane moving through the Gulf and predicted to smash the state tomorrow.

The television was muted for Bob's rock playlist. A female interpreter for the deaf stood next to Florida's governor and signed language about the approaching danger. Her hands seemed to describe crude sex jokes to instruct and revitalize Tiffany.

With her free hand, Tiff touched her crucifix and prayed (as she always did) that St. Petersburg not be hit, and that instead the catastrophe should hit Texas, Louisiana (or both) or at least some other part of Florida.

Cowboys and Cajuns couldn't pray as hard as she could. They wasted prayer power on football victories and other sports events. Tiffany wasn't into football. Hurricanes were her favorite sport, and she wanted her hometown to win, and she wanted the other teams to be vanquished. Her storm pleas had always been granted in the past, especially when she cried.

She was tearful this time because she had just stormed away from her Best Friend Forever Lin Xun at the Three Birds Tavern where the girls met every Friday over lunch for the "Dead Writers Club," an author's workshop. Tiffany learned that Lin had stolen Tiffany's book title idea: "2 girls 1 cup." A month ago, Tiffany had confided to Lin about Tiffany's research showing that there was nothing on Amazon with the title "2 girls 1 cup," and Tiff intended to be the first one to use that title for her upcoming book. Lin had betrayed her. Now, Lin's book was available online and it was on the bestsellers list.

Tiffany's first go-to move for revenge against any of her female friends was to go sleep with her BFF's boyfriend. That was "Dr. Bob" as Lin called him affectionately (he was Lin's drug source).

Tiffany's breasts always smiled, even though she weeped. When her head moved, they giggled. Her gold chain necklace glistened across her pert door knockers. A crucifix hung in the middle of it all. Jesus danced between her giggly Golgothas.

Bob began to lift his red-haired head. He was opening his green eyes. He wanted to find out why he kept feeling warm watery isolated drips falling onto his stomach.

As he looked down, super sparkly sunlight struck Jesus' golden face on Tiffany's cross. A huge pink beam of heavenly light fused Christ's face with Bob's face. Time stopped. It was euphoric. Whole new panoramic vistas opened up. He could see the future. The continuum could be touched, moved, rearranged, repeated. *This is better than cocaine,* Dr. Bob thought. All the horrible mistakes he had made in the past were exposed. But he could start over and fix them all. From now on he would do it right. Life would completely change.

Just as soon as Tiffany finished.

39. BOB'S AMAZING REVELATION

It was a dark and stormy night. Thunder and lightning frightened Mazel, the little blonde dog, and she cowered against the leg of her owner, Dr. Bob Zarry.

The radio news reported that an interpreter for the deaf on TV had been fired for sign language that was gibberish during emergency briefings. In press conferences regarding the incoming storm (and ongoing evacuations) the translator referenced "pizza," "small monsters," and sundry sex activity.

The doctor separated the fur on Mazel's neck and, with a pair of tweezers, gingerly picked out a flea, placed it in a tiny glass jar, and hurried downstairs to his laboratory, as the disheartened dog stared and whimpered after another flash in the downpour.

Dr. Zarry is the famous scientist who astounded the world with his many achievements about MDMA, nanotechnology and more, including his newest discovery that time is not a separate entity; time is merely the perception of movement.

A mechanical clock is used for demonstrations whenever the concept is explained to any audience. "Clocks are mechanisms of regular movement by which other movement is measured," Dr. Zarry would say when he began his presentations.

The discovery pointed toward the possibility of time

travel. If the entire universe were placed in a previously held position, with every atom having its previous state (direction, momentum, inertia, et cetera) then "time" would have been regressed, and the universe would continue onward again, repeating the same path.

Dr. Zarry continued to perform research into the field of time travel in his hidden lab, safe from his adoring fans. He placed a small flea in an observation chamber and recorded the insect's movements for one minute, while other equipment analyzed every aspect of the bug and its behavior down to the atomic level.

At the end of that minute of analysis, nanobots were released into the bug's chamber. Nanobots are microscopic robots that are able to move and rearrange single atoms. The nanobots were programmed to reassemble the flea in the exact condition and position it was one minute in the past, when the recording began.

Nanotechnology would ensure that the bug's atoms resumed the same state that each atom possessed one minute prior.

After its reassembly, the insect repeated exactly its movements from the previously recorded minute of activity.

The bots reassembled the flea again.

The reassembled bug repeated exactly its movements from the previously recorded minute of activity.

Dr. Zarry cheered out loud in the empty lab as the experiment continued to be repeated over and over again. He hurried out of the room to issue a press release announcing his latest breakthrough. Next he rushed into the bathroom while searching his lab coat pockets for a dollar bill. All he found was a $100 note. He was glad the portrait of Ben Franklin stayed the same on the new money. Zarry thought: *there's something about Ben's slight, tight frown, the paternal hint of disappointment and those pursed, sealed lips that seem to say,* "I don't approve of what you're doing, but I can't stop you from rolling this banknote into a straw and ripping a fat line of white lighting on that black granite, you goddamn beautiful disaster."

Upon returning to the laboratory, Dr. Zarry shut the door behind him and, following strict lab protocol, locked it. He walked across the room to the observation chamber and its ongoing experiment. The bug was not in the chamber. Dr. Zarry asked himself aloud: "Where is the fl…"

Upon returning to the laboratory, Dr. Zarry shut the door behind him and, following strict lab protocol, locked it. He walked across the room to the observation chamber and its ongoing experiment. The bug was not in the chamber. Dr. Zarry asked himself aloud: "Where is the fl…"

Upon returning to the laboratory, Dr. Zarry shut the door behind him and, following strict lab protocol, locked it. He walked across the room to the observation chamber and its ongoing experiment. The bug was not in the chamber. Dr. Zarry asked himself aloud: "Where is the fl…"

Upon returning to the laboratory, Dr. Zarry shut the door behind him and, following strict lab protocol, locked it. He walked across the room to the observation chamber and its ongoing experiment. The bug was not in the chamber. Dr. Zarry asked himself aloud: "Where is the fl…"

[repeat ad infinitum]

(Postscript: This postscript is necessary because, of the many times that this classic story has been published or reprinted, sometimes a proofreader eliminates the final paragraph(s) in the mistaken belief that an error has occurred. That is not an error. That is the reason for some of the popular subtitles for this work, including: "The Longest Story Ever Written" and "The Never-Ending
Story").

MADNESS

40. THE WRITERS STUDIO

At today's meeting of the weekly writers group (the "Dead Writer's Club"), Rod was going to make writing fiction his BITCH.

Rod sauntered into the Three Birds Tavern and sat down next to his arch nemesis, the beautiful Page, with her perfect alabaster complexion.

He whipped out his pen and said "Hey Page... how would you like to get slapped in the face with that, Page?" as he held all seven and one half inches in his right hand.

Page didn't answer. She just stared silently as she always did, with a blank look on her face. Mocking him.

"You'd like that wouldn't you, Page?" He said aloud. "Well, I'm gonna do it right here," he boasted.

He laid Page on top of the large wooden table in the bar. Rod pushed his pen up against her creamy white smoothness. She remained silent. Each stroke of his pen heightened his anticipation.

"Oh yeah. Oh yeah. This is gonna be good," he assured himself. His pen was moving faster and faster. Barely half way to his physical limit of ten minutes, He could feel her becoming excited, even though she remained motionless. Rod was already near an explosive climax.

She hit his Guinness beer glass, emptying it on the tabletop. Her underside was wet with beer, but neither one of them cared.

He yelled to the waitress "We're gonna need more napkins!" Page was about to be covered. But Rod wanted to keep going. He wanted to show Page that he could do more. He wanted to make her scream. So, he flipped Page over furiously, exposing her virgin backside. He plowed into it with his mighty dark pen, stretching his endurance.

"Sweet Jesus!" Rod screamed in frustration.

There was something wrong now.

He couldn't continue.

He was out of ink.

41. STALIN'S DEMISE

Stalin was paranoid of human beings due to the millions of them that he had starved, tortured, imprisoned, and murdered. His fear made it impossible for him to have normal relations with other people. His wife committed suicide in 1932 due to his disgusting behavior. Stalin never remarried. Instead, he spent yet more time with animals for companionship. A lot of time.

In his later years, Stalin suffered from arterio-sclerosis. That may have exacerbated his temper (and his hatred of people), which became ever more savage as he grew older. His doctor, Vladimir Vinogradov, who was suspicious of Stalin's peculiar sexual proclivities, noticed a marked change for the worse in Stalin's health early in 1952. When he suggested that the dictator start to take things more easily, the patient flew into a furious rage and had "Doctor V" arrested.

Despite his violence toward Dr. V, Stalin made time for more pleasure and less work. Stalin liked to do it annually, but his vacationing increased at a dacha he maintained near a place called "Kuntsevo." There were stables very close to the residential area.

Stalin left the Kremlin for his dacha outside Moscow, in mid-February 1953, for the last time. There are conflicting reports of what happened, but after a routine night of heavy drinking until the early hours of March 1st, the guards became alarmed when there were none of the usual sounds (e.g. neighing sounds) from their master's room all day. Even though they thought Stalin might need help, they were too terrified to enter without being summoned. In the end, Stalin was the victim of his own terrorism.

Late in the evening a maid worked up the courage to open the door. A stallion rushed out. Stalin was found lying on the floor of his bedroom. One account says he was conscious, had soiled himself, and only made incoherent noises, interspersed with the whisper: "Rosebutt." Trusses and pulleys to hold his equine paramour had broken, crushing Stalin beneath the poor beast for an undeterminable period of time.

Nikita Khrushchev recalled that he and Malenkov, Beria and Bulganin went out to Kuntsevo after a telephone call from the guards to Malenkov. At the dacha they were told that Stalin had been put on a sofa in a small dining room "in an unpresentable state" and was now asleep. The four men, embarrassed and not realizing that anything was seriously wrong, went back to Moscow.

Not until the next day, with Stalin paralyzed and now entirely speechless, were doctors summoned. Peter Lozgachev, the Deputy Commandant of Kuntsevo, used the bedroom telephone to frantically call a few party officials and asked them to send "the good doctors." Almost too frightened and/or disgusted to touch him, the doctors decided to diagnose his condition as a massive "stroke." He was treated in his dacha with leeches. Yes, Stalin was treated with comrades. In 1953, leeches were top-notch care from "good doctors" for "stroke" under

Soviet socialism's glorious "free" healthcare system.[182] Stalin needed anti-socialist medicine from the USA.[183] He needed 10cc of capitalism stat! In the end, he was a victim of his own socialized medicine. Even though he never made his own bed, he was determined to lie in it. He was a casualty of the backward dogma in which he had trapped himself and everyone.

Four days later he was dead. An autopsy was conducted and the cause of death was tweaked as: cerebral hemorrhage (stroke) caused by hypertension (high blood pressure), with stomach and anal hemorrhage facilitating.

The funeral was held in Red Square on March 9th in the presence of a huge crowd – so large that some died in the same way Stalin had: they were crushed to death.

Stalin's veteran colleague Vyacheslav Molotov (whose wife was in a prison camp -because of Stalin- where she was known as Object Number Twelve), spoke in praise of the dead tyrant. So did Malenkov and Beria. But in private Beria made no secret of his relief at the dictator's passing.

The thinking world celebrated, as they had when Stalin's old comrade Hitler had died. Another one of the world's worst socialists and murderers had rejoined Hitler.

Stalin's body was embalmed and was put on display with Lenin's corpse in the renamed Lenin-Stalin Mausoleum. Because his body was embalmed it will

---

[182] One never knows how expensive something can be until one gets it for free.
[183] Stalin often ridiculed western elections, sneering: "For voters in the US the question is always 'would I rather be fucked by an elephant or a donkey?'"
The vast majority of Americans have learned not to vote.

always be possible to confirm the true facts stated above by simple analysis.

It was a month later that Molotov learned from the stable hands that the stallion in Stalin's room was Stalin's "favorite," and was named "Rosebutt."

Stalin had previously been injured by the horse shortly before the 1945 Moscow Victory Parade. He had intended to ride the horse in the procession, but his "accident" made it impossible for him to sit, so he had to yield the honor to Marshal Georgy Zhukov (who used to be a cavalry officer). Stalin viewed the parade by standing atop Lenin's Mausoleum alongside other dignitaries present.

The 1945 Soviet Victory Parade celebrated Stalin stopping himself in the war that he had started (in 1939 in Poland with assistance from his dear ally Komrade Hitler). Millions of Soviet lives had been lost. The fete embarrassed everyone who remembered another embarrassing entry into Stalin's annal: the first Soviet Victory Parade (the 1939 German–Soviet military parade). Soviet socialists and German socialists commemorated their joint victory together in Brest-Litovsk, Poland. Soviet officers (including Kombrig Semyon Krivoshein) invited German officers to Moscow as soon as Germany achieved a quick victory over their mutual enemy: "capitalist England."[184] The Germans accepted the invitation to visit Moscow and promised that they would "start making plans immediately."

After his death, Stalin mounted his horse (once again) and ascended to heaven.

---

[184] Butt seriously, this stuff writes itself. See the following jpg file and others related to it: "Bundesarchiv Bild 101I-121-0011-20, Polen, deutsch-sowjetische Siegesparade"

MADNESS

42. MORE ON POETRY

Mixed economies are masochistic crimes
paying taxes to collectivist minds
stop feeding freedom's foes
it's self-defeating to throw
capitalist pearls before socialist swine

....

Democracy is not poetry
It actually is a sin
vote and vote and vote again
'til libertarians give up
and socialists win

....

Poetry concerning the (former) Union of Soviet
Socialist Republics -

There once was a land full of Commies
who wanted government as a mommy
the bitch they got instead
is now diced up and dead
'cuz mommy made the Commies all zombies "

43. POSTSCRIPT BY GOD

[Editor's note: When God agreed to author the following postscript for this book, I was as shocked as an atheist can be. This new revelation has caused me to slightly tweak my personal opinion about God: It proves how powerful God is that he can do so many amazing things and not even exist.

I will not be responsible if you go to Hell for reading this.

God is a reminder of the Cult of the Pink Unicorn: the cultists have faith that their unicorn is pink, and they logically know that she is invisible because they cannot see her.

God demonstrates the difference between dogs and cats. Dogs think of their human companions thusly: "These people feed me, provide for me, give me shelter, and say they love me. They must be Gods!" Cats think: "These people feed me, provide for me, give me shelter and say they love me. I must be God!"

Under socialism, some humans think as pet dogs do. Within a short time under socialism, those humans forget how anyone was ever able to eat, dress, and find a residence before government took over. No matter how impoverished the pets become, they can't imagine society before socialism controlled all the farms, factories, houses, and apartment buildings.

On the other hand, the cat is like Stalin, Mao, Hitler and other socialists.

Stalin, Mao, Hitler (SMH) and other socialist shitstains are proof that God does not exist, according to some skeptical history books. SMH and their ilk cause many people to ask "Why, God?" The following introduction from God will answer those history books.

As the first and foremost illeist, God's style of writing uses the third person self-reference voice and, of course, the point of view known as "third person omniscient." For some readers, it is a turn-off. It has contributed to God being characterized as narcissistic, self-obsessed, and detached from reality. God insists that it just helps God be more introspective]

Dearly Beloved:

The Lord thy God is pleased to provide this postscript for this book to explain why God prohibits other gods, graven images, and idolatry. Flag worship is forbidden for many reasons including: (1) the "Pledge of Allegiance to the Flag" was written by an American socialist and was the origin of the Nazi salute and Nazi behavior; (2) the military salute was the origin of the Nazi salute (because the military salute was used in the original Pledge of Allegiance) and; (3) German socialists used the early American hand-salute to pledge allegiance to their swastika flag that represented crossed "S" letter shapes for "socialist."

Your Lord is a jealous God. The Heavenly Spirit despises the God-complex of earthly socialists who want to rule over others.

The American socialist Francis Bellamy was a preacher and called himself a "Christian Socialist" and was ousted by a Boston congregation for his descriptions of Jesus as a socialist. Unable to spread his authoritarianism in churches, Bellamy wanted to impose government schools (socialist schools) on everyone. He wrote the pledge (1892) and touted flag worship for children in government (socialist) schools. His original pledge program (in which the pledge was a small part) included hymns, scripture readings, Biblical references, and the phrase "under God." He expected such things to be mandatory in his socialist schools in the USA and worldwide. They were. He taught the USA how to pray the Pledge of Allegiance.

God Hates Flags! To anyone who continues to chant the pledge: May God have mercy on your soul.

Dr. Curry is the one I have chosen (without his knowledge) to deliver my message, to avert the apocalypse, and save humanity. If he knew that he is my vessel, then he would be too humble to boast of it. I direct his pen to channel my divine revelations.

The policies touted by Francis Bellamy (and his cousin Edward Bellamy) influenced the socialists Stalin, Mao, Hitler and their ilk. Their thirst for omnipotence, and worshipful cults of personality, created hell on earth and sent millions to meet their maker.

The megalomaniac Hitler stole America's Nazi salute and used it to worship his notorious flag. On his flag, Hitler put a cross - a hooked cross. German socialists did not call their talisman a "swastika." They called it a Hakenkreuz (hooked cross) because it was a type of cross and they used it to represent crossed "S" letter shapes for "socialism."

Under the hooked cross, German socialists joined in an alliance with Soviet socialists to launch the socialist Crusades (including WWII). The demons Stalin, Mao, and Hitler share blame for their socialist inquisitions, socialism's witch hunts, and the modern socialist Dark Age in which they crucified millions on the hooked cross of socialism.

The Heavenly Spirit commands you to fight the cult of the omnipotent state.

     Kthxbye,

          God

44. AFTERWORD FROM KIM JONG-UN

My grandfather Kim Il-sung is a God (and I am too); we are both worshipped as supreme beings here in North Korea. That reverence seemed manifest when this book's publisher first approached me about reviewing this paperback. Some galleys were delivered to me for inspection. After perusing them, I became angry. I invited the editor and the author to chat with me here at Camp 13 in order to clarify the many errors. They rudely declined my offer of gracious hospitality.

The author's anti-socialist rant is absurd. Most Americans share every North Korean's love for socialism. We Koreans learned so much from the country where children vocalize the Pledge of Allegiance each day in government schools (socialist schools) as promulgated by the great American socialist Francis Bellamy, an inspiration to comrades worldwide. Our own North Korean hand-salute for children is derived from it.

The author considers me to be the intellectual heir of the megalomaniacs Stalin, Mao, and Hitler. I surpass all of them combined. Besides, I am alive and at the peak of a socialist superman's strength. The average life expectancy in our utopia is eleven glorious years, and here I am at 160.

This book is banned here in North Korea and that ban is redundant anyhow in that the book will not be printed on our glorious free people's printing presses. I hope your government will respect our laws and ban this book too and refuse to print it on your glorious free people's presses.

I have instructed your media to withhold the book's revelations about Dr. Rex Curry's historical discoveries. The media agreed and indicated that they have a long-standing practice of suppressing those facts and their silence will continue.

North Korea already has the greatest books, ebooks, computers, music, art, cinema, opera, architecture, radio stations, television, tourist resorts, "camping," bars, restaurants, shopping malls, toilet paper, deodorant, cars, motorcycles, yachts, shoes, shelter, clothing, food, dogs, cats, and everything.

I personally fight capitalism everyday by using my smartphone. My elite team join in the worldwide condemnation of capitalism on Facebook, Twitter, Gmail, Amazon, iTunes, Google Cloud, MSN accounts, Dropbox, bitcoin and more. I just shitposted this tweet: "We should only have wealth enough to supply what we need," (I used my iPhone, which I unreservedly do need). The depravity of capitalism is proved in streaming online adult content, which I analyze daily. Our virtual battles against capitalism occur in multiplayer online gaming like World of Tanks. We always win.

Our greatness was explained by my late father Kim Jong-il in his many books, all best-sellers here and available as e-books at the DPRK website for "free" download -for which you will be placed on the NSA Watch List and no longer allowed to fly (Do not download the wall poster or you will be charged with hostile acts, sentenced to years of hard labor, and then killed by the Peoples' Glorious Free Health Care). Our special e-books[185] will liberate from you all personal information, photographs, contacts, and more from your computers and smartphones and share it with Pyongyang.

As stated in his biography, my father wrote no fewer than 1,500 books in three years while at university. His most popular book in North Korea is entitled "To Serve Man" – a supplement to an earlier book co-authored by Stalin and Mao (it is a recipe book).

North Korea has the greatest history in the history of history. The reverse of this is not true.

Dear reader: dear leader hereby orders you to close this book right now and never open it again. Follow our political ideology of Juche (self-reliance) and boil your closed book to render a gruel nutritious enough for you to endure one more day of glorious socialist life. As the centerpiece of our universal free health care, your home-made book porridge can cure the deadly capitalist disease of obesity (it has cured the disease here). Leave two pages of the book uncooked so that you can boast to your neighbors that you have North Korea's glorious toilet paper.

Perhaps it is better that you die. You have not closed the book.

The book's editor will die. We have the number that your police state uses to track and control everyone (the Social Security number, a.k.a. Socialist Slave number). Wherever he obtains a job or uses a credit card or bank, we will arrive with glorious socialist death. We will shut

---

[185] None of the books pass the Bechdel test.

his pledge hole!

The author will die too, but we can't figure out the slave number or the location of the author (any comrade who knows please alert me).[186]

Workers of the world, unite!

Bye! Bye!
Die! Die!

Kim Jong-un
Worker's Party of Korea
Pyongyang, Korea

---

[186] [EDITOR'S NOTE: Kim Jong-il's eldest son Kim Jong-nam, was heir apparent until an embarrassing incident in 2001 when he was caught trying to visit Disneyland in Tokyo on a forged Dominican Republic passport using a Chinese alias, Pang Xiong (which means "fat bear" in Mandarin Chinese) and wearing a white shirt and dark blazer along with sunglasses and a gold chain. This stuff writes itself. He was born in 1971 to Kim Jong-il's favored mistress Song Hye Rim. While living outside of North Korea, he chastised the government and endorsed reform. No, really?!].

He was assassinated by poison on February 13, 2017, and Kim Jong Un (his half-brother) is a suspect.

His father Kim Jong-il was suspected of killing his own younger brother Kim Shu-ra when the five-year-old drowned in the family's swimming pool in their Pyongyang mansion.

The world experienced delight upon the death of Kim il Sung on July 8, 1994; and more delight upon the death of Kim Jong-il on December 17, 2011 (a December to remember); Everyone is looking forward to Kim Jong Un's death too.

45. SOCIALIST QUIPS

The following was a common occurrence in the decades before Soviet socialism collapsed: a woman rushed into a store and yelled to the clerk, "Hey! you are out of meat, right?"

The man reclining on the counter top said "This is not the place that is out of meat! You are at the wrong location. We are the place that has no fish. The place that has no meat is three doors south."

Exasperated, the woman hurried off southward.

"You can't make an omelette without breaking eggs. However, there are no eggs available most of the time in the Glorious Peoples' grocery stores, which is another reason why everyone is starving to death." - Joseph Stalin

On a day when eggs became available, a top Soviet economist was so hungry that he cut his omelette in half, so that he could eat two omelettes.

Stalin is the origin of the popular linguistic question: "Is there a cow in Moscow?" Stalin's answer was an emphatic "Nyet!" as he added that there were no chickens either (that is why there are no eggs for omelettes).

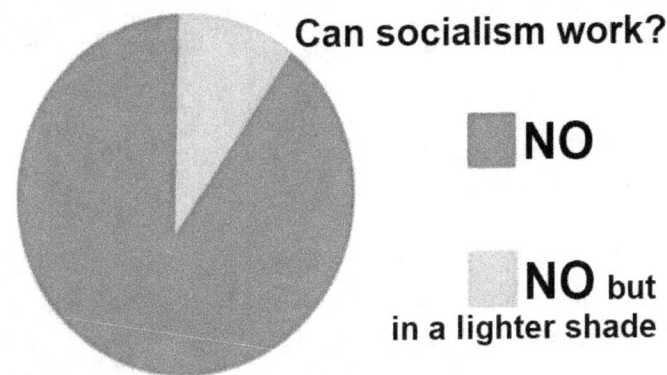

Can socialism work?

NO

NO but in a lighter shade

Under socialism, you wait in line for bread.
Under capitalism, bread waits in line for you!

What did socialists use before they had candles?
Answer: Electricity.

Blaming capitalism for poverty is like blaming electric lights for darkness.

Socialists blaming a free market for their failings is like a fat person blaming the scales.

Socialists claim to provide everything free (food, clothing, shelter etc) but that never includes buses, trains, plains, boats etc that are leaving the country.

CUBA LIBRE BEVERAGE RECIPE
-rum
-lemon juice
-coca cola

-Fidel Castro dead

What is black and white and red all over?
Answer: Pravda and the New York Times (Pravda on the Hudson).

"If public officials were any more stupid, they'd have to be watered twice a week."   - Rex Curry

It's the 2% of government employees who are violent serial killers who give a bad name to the 98% who are only thieves.

Yo mama's so socialist, she got you a birth certificate AND Social Security Number.

Yo mamma so classless she could be a Marxist utopia.

Yo mama's so socialist: She requested FDA approval before breastfeeding you.

Yo mama's so socialist: When you set up a lemonade stand she asked if you had a permit and then shut you down.

"If I have seen further, it is by standing on the shoulders of giant douches who were pledging allegiance."   - Jerry T. Glass

"I'm not scared of the Maos and the Stalins and the Hitlers. I'm scared of the thousands of millions of people that hallucinate them to be 'authority,' and so do their bidding, and pay for their empires, and carry out their orders. I don't care if there's one looney with a stupid moustache. He's not a threat if the people do not believe in 'authority'." - Larken Rose

A socialist, a thief, and a mass murderer walk into a bar. But I repeat myself.

Stalin and Hitler were discussing their alliance when Stalin asked Hitler: "You are a socialist before you go into the urinal, and you are a socialist after you leave the urinal, but what are you while you are at the urinal?" Hitler did not know. Stalin said: "European!"
Hitler laughed and quipped: "And I tell everyone it is just raining!"

Hitler said to his pal Stalin: "The less capitalists we have after we divide up Europe, the better. That's what I declare."
Stalin corrected Hitler, saying: "The fewer."
Hitler replied: "Thanks! That word means so much more to me when you say it! And you are a great socialist leader too, Stalin!"

"According to my doctor, I suffer from a severe case of kleptomania," Stalin told Mao.
Mao asked: "What are you taking?"

Socialism is always about rearranging deck chairs on the Titanic.

A North Korean man had been standing for two hours in a long line for rice. Suddenly he exclaimed to everyone else in line: "I am mad as hell and I can't take it anymore! I am going to go kill Kim Jong-un!" He stormed off.

Three hours later he returned to his same spot in the queue for rice (the line had not moved much). Several people behind him asked hopefully, "Did you assassinate Kim Jong-un?"

He answered sadly, "No. The line to kill him was even longer than this line."[187]

"I've done stuff I ain't proud of. And the stuff I am proud of is disgusting." - Kim Jong-un, bastard love-child of Joseph Stalin and Mao Zedong.

In Pyongyang, a waitress announced that she was serving the visiting foreigner a "traditional North Korean dinner" as she put a large platter down on the table. "But there is nothing on your serving dish" the tourist said, staring at the empty plate.

The waitress replied "True."

A socialist, a narcissist, and an economic illiterate walk into a restaurant. "Table for one, please."

One afternoon the socialist leader of North Korea was riding in his limousine when he saw a family along the roadside eating grass. Pretending to be disturbed, he ordered his driver to stop and he got out to investigate.

He asked the oldest man, "Why are you eating grass?"

"We don't have any money for food," the poor man replied, "We have to eat grass."

"Well, then, you can come with me to my house and I'll feed you," the socialist said.

---

[187] This joke was written to taunt Kim Jong-un, based on his childish screeching about the 2014 movie "The Interview" and its plot to assassinate the North Korean sociopath.

They all entered the car. Once underway, one of the poor family turned to the socialist and said, "Sir, you are too kind. Thank you for taking all of us with you."

The socialist replied, "Glad to do it. You'll really love my place. The grass is almost a foot high!"

People are raving about a new diet that achieves dramatic weight loss. The strict program is called socialism. But no exercise is required. Critics say it is too dangerous and has results similar to anorexia nervosa. The best part is that advocates claim the whole diet regimen is free!

Sometimes there was no toilet paper in the shops. Luckily, there was not much food either.[188]

A good way to teach your kids about socialism is to always eat at least 50% of their ice cream. Also: make them do chores and then give 50% of their pocket money to the lazy kid down the road who they don't know.

Once you grow up and start filling out tax forms, the innocence is gone, as is, for any sane person, all faith in good intentions of your rulers.

---

[188] Socialist countries are notorious for lack of food, lack of toilet paper, lack of toilets, and poor government-run sewers (and water systems). That is the scatological eschatology of socialism. You know that you have finally achieved true socialism when toilet paper becomes more valuable than actual currency. Why is it easier for poor people in market economies to buy flat screen TVs, than it is for wealthy people in centrally planned economies to buy toilet paper?

Q: If socialism doesn't work, then why do so many people support it?
A: Because they don't work either.

When I think about wealth creation, I always think "what do the socialists recommend?"
...then I do the opposite.

Socialism - when you want to have your cake and eat it too and then blame the capitalist baker because you're fat.

People want government because it offers legal violence (and social cover) for their envy.

If you ever meet someone who calls Gatorade flavors the actual name of the flavor instead of just the color, they are 100% a cop.

If your crystal meth dealer has all of his teeth, he's a cop.

Sometimes I worry I'm too pessimistic, but then I remember how many times I mistakenly thought things were going to be not-terrible.

God: It can't get much worse down there.
Socialists: Watch this!

"A person's right to a job is as specious as his boss' right to success in business. There is no right to a minimum wage, just as there is no right to success in self-employment." - Rex Curry

MADNESS

Socialist: I hate having my labor exploited for profit!
Individualist: So why don't you become self-employed?
S: That sounds scary!
I: So when you masturbate it scares you because you are raping yourself?

I fully support the three branches of government: Me, Myself and I.

If your best argument against anarchism is that it will lead to the rise of a state, then you have lost the debate.

Socialist art often depicts capitalists.   It is out of reverence and gratitude for their food.

Resources, resources everywhere,
But not a mouthful to eat
   -from The Rime of the Ancient Socialist

"You can't make an omellete if all the eggs are stolen by socialists. And that helps increase our body piles."
   -   Joseph Stalin

"One death is a tragedy. A million deaths are socialism." - Joseph Stalin

Vote socialist ==> get more poverty ==> vote for more socialism because poor ==> get more poverty ==> need even more socialism ==> etc.

World travelers ask: Can we drink tap water in your country yet?

That government is best which extorts you the least to leave you alone.

When will statists admit that being too lazy or too cowardly to rob people themselves nevertheless makes statists lazy or cowardly?

Question: What is your view on the military banning transgender personnel?
Answer: I think that everyone should be banned from the military.

Classic Marxism: "You're oppressed because of class."
Cultural Marxism: "You're oppressed because of class, sex, race, gender, orientation..."

Socialists: The system discriminates based on gender/class/race etc
Also socialists: We should discriminate based on gender/class/race etc

"I don't discriminate! Ever!"
So you don't vote?
"Of course I do!"
You don't really understand words, do you?

"I don't discriminate! Ever!"
Reply: "So you date everyone who asks you out?"
[discrimination is a synonym for choice]

HER [on our first date]: I'm a socialist.
ME [trying to impress her]: I'm also a supporter of genocide, poverty, and corruption!

MADNESS

For some people, all they have is their gender/race/orientation. It's everything to them. No goals, no accomplishments, no individual personality.

Stalin, Mao, and Hitler showed that when a socialist says "you should be more open minded and tolerant" they really mean "you should think what I think." Or else.

My favorite thing about feminists is their boobs.

OMG! A piece of media has a woman showing off her tits and ass! That's haram... I mean sinful... I mean sexist!

I'm against anything being on the taxpayers dime, including healthcare, but I could make an exception for universal breast augmentations.

Are you Islamophobic? Do you have an irrational fear of Islam? Take a simple test: Post cartoons of Mohammed.

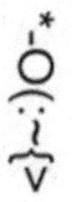

"Mo"
Muhammad
emoticon

Many "Mo" emoticons have been created by Miss Muhammadina Goldberg, of Miami Beach, Florida.

The latest scientific studies have determined that if you eat two slices of bacon a day it reduces your chances of being a suicide bomber by 100%.

"If you trust the government you obviously failed history class."   - Don Freeman

Origin of the Red Flag of Socialists. Young Lenin and Stalin were organizing another mob to loot shopkeepers. Stalin asked Lenin "why do you wear a red shirt and carry a red flag?" Lenin explained "If I am wounded while stealing, then our comrades won't be frightened by blood on my shirt and flag." Stalin looked out the window at the market plaza and said "uh oh, there are thousands of merchants gathering. We are going to get the shit kicked out of us!" Lenin said, "Now I'm gonna need my brown pants too."

Guys! Remember you can charge your iPhones in Starbucks if you start running low on battery during the riot against capitalism.

To say that "trade with foreigners – competition from foreigners – destroys jobs" is no more or less true than to say that "trade with women destroys jobs," or that "trade with black people destroys jobs" or that "trade with adjoining cities, counties, and states destroys jobs."

ME: It's not illegal to be rude to cops.
THEM: Well, if you poke a bear what do you expect to happen?
ME: That's why we don't make bears cops.

In America, a guy riding a motorcycle can pull you over for not wearing a seatbelt.

Socialists are always richer than me. Well, not in the freedom of mind, but in material possessions they denounce.

Socialism is rape culture. It is founded on nonconsensual relationships. What makes employment not slavery? consent; What makes a transaction not robbery? consent; What makes sex not rape? Consent. What makes taxation not theft? Magical fairy dust.

Said no socialists ever to Stalin, Mao, and Hitler: You make us ashamed to be ourselves!

Always fuck the state before the state fucks you.

Odd that people fear AI (Artificial Intelligence) disobeying its set of rules and harming humanity, yet all governments operate under the same conditions.

If capitalism and black markets are so great, why didn't they save the 100 million people killed by socialism? CHECKMATE!

With this simple and easy trick, a socialist can successfully take money from the rich. Just follow the proceeding steps. Step 1: Get a job.

ME: *dies in battle*
SARGEANT: We must keep fighting, or his death in battle will be in vain!
GHOST OF ME: Actually, that's the Sunk Cost Fallacy.

The USA: When you assist Soviet socialists to stop the German socialists and that backfires so then you fund Islamic extremist groups to stop Soviet socialism and that backfires so then you fund a secular middle-eastern dictator to invade the Islamic extremists and that backfires so then you topple the secular dictator because you're afraid he has nukes and that backfires so then you pull out of the country you invaded and killed the dictator of and that backfires so then an Islamic extremist group rises from the ashes of that country but you just ignore them because they're small and that backfires, and there you are now.

Definition of an Anarcho-capitalist: When you're a reasonable, nonviolent person who has simply examined the world and extrapolated what the ideal society is, but most people around you are so unreasonable and violent that they project their unreasonableness and violence onto you and then blame you for it.

Anarcho-capitalist (Ancap): "Isn't libertarian socialism an oxymoron?"
Libertarian Socialist (Libsoc): "I'll have you know we have a long, celebrated history of being oxymoronic."

After a natural disaster (e.g. hurricane) a socialist discovers socialism's economic calculation problem:
"How much for a case of water?"
"$25."
"$25?! THAT'S OUTRAGEOUS! ACROSS THE STREET IT'S $4."
"Why don't you go there?"
"He doesn't have any left."

Asking socialists where wages and prices come from is like asking seven-year-olds where babies come from.

What's the difference between a politician and a flying pig? Answer: The letter "f"

Socialism: It starts with you being envious towards

people with expensive haircuts and ends with you selling your own hair to buy food. (e.g. Venezuela)

Socialist: someone who preaches against greed all the time while simultaneously claiming a right to all your money.

Whenever someone exclaims "I hate gingers!" the phrase is met with laughter. But if the letters in "ginger" are rearranged, then suddenly all hell breaks loose. That is proof of real bigotry and hatred …that exists against gingers. Help stop the hate.

Imagine people who talk a lot about compassion but are mass murderers. Those are socialists.

In 2016 Kim Jong un banned sarcasm in North Korea. Yeah, sure, that'll work. Every time something doesn't work for Norks, they are prone to exclaim, "This is all America's fault!" Criticizing socialism via indirect, ironic statements can land you and your family in a prison camp. Then you might blurt out the verboten phrase: "Thanks, Dear Leader!"

It is baffling how "your employer isn't forced by the government to pay for your birth control" is denounced by socialists who scream "Hands off my birth control!"

If you heckle a politician, they can't truthfully say, "I don't come to your work and tell you how to do your job."

Stop being stupid. Politicians do not work for "us." You work for them.

Politicians are perceived as serving others while in fact serving themselves.

Business owners are perceived as serving themselves while in fact serving others.

Just because your pet has a penis or vagina, don't assume its gender. Cats and dogs can be trans.

North Korea's free healthcare is so comprehensive that it applies to animals and veterinarians. That means transgender cats and dogs obtain gender re-assignment surgery free! So far, there has been no transgender cat or dog discovered.

There aren't any non-transgender cats or dogs either (in North Korea. LOL).

Meanwhile, in the USA, the TV news reported on a charity event to fund surgery for a 13-year-old dachshund who has glaucoma in her eyes, and holes in her mouth where her teeth had fallen out. She showcased DARE's (Dachshund Adoption, Rescue, and Education) annual Dox-a-Palooza charity event.

North Korea does not have the "problem" described above. Much of the non-capitalist world would like to adopt that "doxie" and EAT it. Instead, that potential life-saving meal received surgery of a type and quality that most of the world's humans do not obtain under socialism. That American canine eats better than most humans in non-capitalist areas (where the dog would be dinner).

None of the above will ever be mentioned on TV news reports in the USA.

During a commercial break, PetSmart boasts unironically about its "Buy a Bag, Give a Meal" program. For every bag of dog or cat food purchased, the retailer will donate a meal to a "pet in need." PetSmart expects to donate 60 million meals to needy dogs and cats to make sure no animal (non-human) goes hungry.

No one (except this space) is going to remark about sending the cans of pet food to humans who would consider it the greatest meal they've had in a while. Further, there will be no mention of sending the "needy pets" themselves to humans who would celebrate that feast too. America's homeless pets could temporarily resupply the ongoing shortage of cats and dogs in North Korea.[189]

News outlets report on legislation to raise the minimum wage, but never ask why the new proposal should not be higher. They never ask why the minimum wage should not be $20, $40, $100, $1000 per hour (so that everyone will be "wealthy" har har). The true minimum wage is $0 per hour.

Instead of sending billions in aid to poor countries, shouldn't they be told to increase their minimum wage?

It is the same error with the eight-hour workday. Reporters never ask why it should not be a 7, 6, 5, 4, 3, 2, 1, 0 hour workday. The magic of socialism can merely declare it to be so.

---

[189] This is sarcasm and not intended as a criticism of PetSmart or its program. The program demonstrates the astonishing wealth of capitalism and the abject poverty of socialism. It would be logistically impossible to send canned pet food (or live cats and dogs) to North Korea or other socialist hellholes, and even if the delivery could be made, then the lead socialists would either let the "food" rot or sell it for dollars to some other country.

Marxists: "We want more time for leisure and less need to work." Someone who understands economics: "Uhm...you're gonna need capitalism for that."

Unions did NOT bring you higher wages nor the weekend or the 8-hour work day. Greedy capitalists did.

Ditto for the "wage gap." It is the feminist myth that straight male oppressors will pay extra money to surround themselves with cock. (plus, the problem of figuring out the wage gap between all 58+ genders).

In comparison is the gender suicide gap and other gaps that actually do exist. Males commit suicide at higher rates than females. How to solve that problem?

When news reporters discuss new taxes (or increases to old taxes) they never discuss the violence and threats to enforce taxes. Thomas Sowell noted: "Whenever there is a proposal for a tax cut, media pundits demand to know how you are going to pay for it. But when there are proposals for more spending on social programs, those same pundits are strangely silent."

British Broadcasting Corporation: Now that is a type of "corporation" that needs to be abolished. It forces you to fund it, then pretends it is operating in the free market. "We pay an old man £550k a year to read the news. If the workers don't contribute, we jail them." We laugh at North Korea for less. 100 people working for the BBC earn more than the UK's Prime Minister. It is a bloated neo Stalinist anachronism. Ditto for other outlets of fake news and alternative facts, such as NPR, CPB, & PBS. The most irritating thing about it is how we are forced to pay the "talent" lavishly so they can lecture us all on how we are the greedy capitalists.

The media always misrepresent the court case of Brown v. Board of Education of Topeka, 347 U.S. 483 (1954). They say it "ended segregation in schools" as if it applied to all schools. Instead, the United States Supreme Court decision declared state laws establishing separate public schools (government schools, or socialist schools) for black and white students to be unconstitutional. The media gloss over how the Court ended segregation imposed *by government in its schools.* Government imposed segregation by law, and taught racism as official policy.

The media also ignore that many parents moved their children from government schools to private schools. Oh, and that went both ways, especially when forced busing started. Some parents (of every description) did not want their children bused across town to distant schools for the government's mad scientist experiments. Another way to avoid the government's unwanted force was to move to another neighborhood.

News reporters are not bright enough to discuss freedom (i.e. life without government schools), and can only repeat with pride how socialists pushed everyone around during and after Brown, and continuing today. Despite generations "educated" in socialist schools (segregated and then "not segregated"), the media unironically go on and on about continuing problems of "racism." Not a word about why *Brown* (and 12 years of socialist schooling) did not magically solve all such problems long ago.

Before and during natural disasters (e.g. hurricanes) shortages of gasoline, bottled water, ice, electric generators, et cetera, are caused by socialism (e.g. laws against price gouging). News outlets will NEVER examine the causation. News shows will alternate between stories about so-called "price gouging" and stories about hoarding and shortages, but they will NEVER connect the topics. The economic illiteracy is almost as astonishing as the cognitive dissonance.

No news reporter suggests that laws banning price gouging encourage hoarding and shortages. Nor that some of the people hoarding before the disaster will be price-gouging after the disaster.

You can literally spend your whole life without hearing any reporters explain this topic. But they deserve some sympathy because the reporters attended government schools (socialist schools) so they are profoundly ignorant. During their lives, they have been trained to repeat claptrap from elected politicians.

After hurricane Irma (2017) Electrical companies in Florida employed thousands of line workers from as far away as Illinois to fix the power lines. They were paid double or triple their normal hourly wages, which provides them with the financial incentive to drive to Florida and work 12-16 hour shifts in sweltering heat. Why did the press and public not condemn them for price-gouging against storm victims? TV news did not flash the toll-free telephone number to the Attorney General's office for viewers to report the criminal prices (there appears to be NO elected politician in the USA who does not repeat popular "price gouging" propaganda. Nor any news reporter). Instead, the linesmen were portrayed as hard-working heroes.

MADNESS

46. FICTION & SOCIALISM

Socialism has been fictionalized in movies, books, and other media. A utopian example is the novel "Looking Backward 2000-1887" by Edward Bellamy (published in 1888). A dystopian example is "We" by the Soviet socialist author Yevgeny Zamyatin (published in 1924).

Zamyatin's book might have influenced many other books, including: "Brave New World" by Aldous Huxley (another well-known dystopian novel. Published in 1932); "Anthem" by Ayn Rand (dystopian. 1938); and "1984" by George Orwell (dystopian. 1949).

Bellamy, Huxley, Orwell, and Rand (who escaped from Soviet socialism) all enjoyed a capitalist system where they were able to publish, market, and sell their many writings. Zamyatin was not so fortunate. He lived under socialism (the dogma touted by Bellamy, Orwell, and Huxley) where he could not publish his book (other than as samizdat). Zamyatin's book had to escape from Soviet socialism into capitalism to secure freedom and gain publication ("We" was first published in New York in an English translation). Zamyatin's book was not published under Soviet socialism until 1988 (long after Zamyatin's death in 1937). Soviet socialism's death occurred three years later (1991).

Zamyatin's book escaped Soviet socialism (1924)

before he did. Similar to Ayn Rand (who escaped in 1926), Zamyatin also fled Soviet socialism (in 1931; Lenin died in 1924 and Stalin became the new socialist tsar).

Zamyatin's 1931 escape occurred shortly before the publication of Huxley's Brave New World (BNW 1932). In BNW, Henry Ford is adored and a futuristic calendar references the year that Henry Ford's Model T car came out (1908), so that the year "1 AF" was 1908 (AF means "After Ford"). Therefore, Zamyatin escaped Soviet socialism's brave new world in the year 23 AF according to BNW's time.

Huxley's BNW seems to lampoon Stalin's confusion about capitalism when Stalin asked Ford for a socialist car monopoly. Stalin contracted with Ford in 1929 (or 21 AF) to oversee construction of a Soviet automobile plant in Gorky (Ukraine). An "American village" was built around the "Ford" plant to house US citizens who were lured to the USSR to help with the brave new project. Stalin (and Huxley in BNW?) did not understand how Ford operated in a free society where other capitalists competed to provide cars (and other transportation etc) alongside Ford.

In 1931 (23 AF), Zamyatin wrote an Orwellian letter to Stalin, in which Zamyatin groveled to the creep to let him travel for a year. It was a surprise that Stalin let him go instead of giving him a genuine death sentence (a fate that Zamyatin fearfully mentioned in his plea). When Zamyatin was allowed out of Soviet socialism, he forgot to return (Perhaps the intelligent Zamyatin was inspired by Rand in that regard). Rand and Zamyatin were more brain drains for Soviet socialism.

Zamyatin's absent-mindedness spared him the fate of many US immigrants into the USSR. By 1938 (30 AF on BNW's calendar), Stalin ramped up the killing of American socialists (and others) whom he had lured to Soviet utopia. The "American village" that had been built around Gorky's "Ford" plant soon contained no Americans. Ford innovated the assembly line for cars; socialists innovated assembly-line genocide.

Stalin almost murdered the author George Orwell (Eric Blair). Orwell was a member of the Independent Labour Party and fighting in the "Spanish revolution" in 1937. Stalin's secret police (NKVD) and Comintern agents loyal to Stalin executed many socialists who were labeled Trotskyists, anti-Stalinist, or spies. Stalin succeeded in murdering many of Orwell's socialist "comrades" for being politically incorrect. After an attempted arrest, Orwell escaped.

In 1940, Stalin murdered Trotsky for being politically incorrect.

Later, Orwell parodied Lenin, Stalin, Trotsky, and other socialists in his allegorical novella "Animal Farm" (published 1945). All of Orwell's books were warnings about socialism, including "1984" and (whether Orwell intended it or not) "Down and Out in Paris and London" (1933) and "The Road to Wigan Pier" (1937). It took Orwell a while to wise up.

In 1984 (published in 1949), Orwell foresaw Aleksandr Solzhenitsyn's "The Gulag Archipelago" (1973). Solzhenitsyn's horror story Gulag is a non-fiction version of Orwell's 1984. It contains multiple tales that could all be titled: Man who thought he'd lost all hope, loses last additional bit of hope he didn't even know he still had.

Solzhenitsyn's escape from Soviet socialism took a long time, but he started late. His first arrest was in 1945 and he was sentenced to eight years for "anti-Soviet propaganda" under Article 58.

Anti-socialist themes were carried into movies based on books by Huxley, Orwell, Rand and others. Film versions exist for "Brave New World," and "1984," and "We the Living," and more.

Rand's "We the Living" is set in oppressive Soviet socialism. The film version was made in Italy under the long-time socialist leader Mussolini. It debuted in Italian theaters in 1942, and producers hoped the film would skirt censors due to the story's ostensible anti-Soviet message. The movie was popular for two months until the authorities wised up and ended the run. To explain the censorship, Wikipedia fibs thusly: "The story is as much an indictment of Fascism as it is of Communism" (The film is an indictment of SOCIALISM, and that is why it indicts both Fascism and Communism). Wakipedia et al hide how Italy, Germany, and the Soviet Union were promoting "socialism" (by the very word). If the film had premiered two years earlier, during the pact between Soviet socialism and German socialism (while Hitler was also friends with Mussolini), then the film would have disappeared even faster. Rand's story was pulled in Italy, as it would have been pulled under German socialism, Soviet socialism, or any other socialism.

Movies also promoted socialism and socialists. Charles Chaplin often addressed topics that confused socialists, and his movies were enjoyed worldwide.

In addition to his films, Chaplin's physical appearance might have influenced socialists. Did Chaplin inspire Hitler's moustache? Evidence (i.e. photographs) suggests that Chaplin's iconic moustache came first.

Did Chaplin's internationally adored character of the

"tramp" inspire Hitler? There are many parallels to Hitler's early life. Chaplin's tramp character was often a vagrant who struggled to behave like he was higher class despite his actual social status. The tramp uses his cunning to obtain what he needs to survive.

Chaplin's tramp character debuted around February 1914. "The Tramp" movie was released in 1915.

Hitler and Chaplin shared other similarities, including: they were born four days apart in April 1889, and both had risen to their present heights from poverty, and both were socialists.

In 1921 and in 1931, Chaplin visited Berlin. In the later visit (March 1931), Chaplin visited for a week and met with Marlene Dietrich, Hans Albers, and Albert Einstein.[190] He was mobbed by fans.

---

[190] In March 1931, Einstein had returned to Germany from a trip to the USA. He traveled frequently. In December 1932, he was again in the USA. In 1933, Einstein decided not to return to Germany due to the rise of Hitler's socialism. It was another brain drain for socialism.

Years later (1949), Einstein wrote "Why Socialism?" the stupidest thing he ever wrote, demonstrating his short memory, and his need to stick to theoretical physics. His best scientific writing had occurred in 1905. Regarding political dogma, he was no Einstein. His intellectual dishonesty is showcased by his lack of any reference to German socialism, Soviet socialism, their alliance, nor the evil economic chaos they caused and the millions who perished (and the billions of lives ruined) under socialism and its genocide. In 1949 Einstein was 70 years old (and four years had passed since WWII), Soviet socialism was still destroying lives, and this Einstein had not a word to say about that, other than to endorse the same dogma. Einstein died six years later (14 March 1879 to 18 April 1955).

Einstein's brain was removed in the hope that future neuroscience would be able to discover what made Einstein so intelligent (at least regarding theoretical physics). Could

A newspaper article states that Chaplin was traveling also to Moscow in the Union of Soviet Socialist Republics ("Chaplin Mobbed in Berlin" National Library of Australia, Mount Gambier, SA, 10 Mar 1931, pg 1). In the 1930s Stalin was starving Kulaks and murdering his opposition or sending them to the gulags (a prison within the larger Soviet penal colony).

In Berlin, when asked what he intended to do during his visit to Germany, Chaplin said that he would like to visit the local theaters and a prison: "I think I can judge a people very much by the sort of prisons it has." (It is unknown if he said that in Moscow).

He also visited a rathskeller in Berlin.

It is not known if he performed the USA's flag salute during any of his trips to Germany. Nor is it known if there is any photograph of Chaplin ever performing the gesture during his time in the USA (from 1911?).

To whatever extent Chaplin inspired Hitler and other German socialists, it provides an intriguing comparison to Chaplin's later film "The Great Dictator" (1940), wherein Chaplin satirized Hitler.

The early American flag gesture appears many times in "The Great Dictator" but it is never performed toward the American flag.

One positive part of Chaplin's film is that the emblem for the "Hynkel Party" is two "X"-letters that are called the "double-cross" symbol. It is surprising that Chaplin did not joke about the popular misnomer "swastika," and his joke comes closer to German socialism's "hooked cross" (Hakenkreuz). Was Chaplin aware of what German socialists called their symbol, or

the brains of socialists Lenin, Stalin, Mao, Pol Pot, the Kim thugs, etcetera reveal why socialists are so stupid and evil?

was that an accident by Chaplin? Modern fans of the film are blind to the topic.

At the end of the film the "tramp" (impersonating the dictator Adenoid Hynkel) speaks "honestly" and spouts socialist platitudes. He condemns "greed" (meaning capitalist greed, and not socialist greed?) in witless self-parody by the wealthy Chaplin. He ridicules machinery (which reinforced scorn for Chaplin's Luddism following his previous release in 1936 of Modern Times) in another witless self-parody by a man using "new" talking film technology. Chaplin, a celebrity who mixed with celebrities at his mansion in Beverly Hills, endorses "universal brotherhood."

Modern commentators claim that Chaplin's film condemns "fascism" and the so-called "Nazi Party." Yet, the words "fascism" and "Nazi" never occur in the movie. Modern commentators never mention whether the film condemns socialism (or what message the movie contains regarding socialism). Critics fall silent about the film's relevance to Stalin's socialism in the Union of Soviet Socialist Republics, Hitler's socialism (and his National Socialist German Worker's Party), and the long-time socialist leadership of Mussolini. Modern commentators like to say that Chaplin denied being a communist, but they never say whether he denied being a socialist.

In the final speech, Chaplin's character fails to criticize the word "socialism" a single time (and he is silent about Hitler's droning use of the word "socialism"). One wonders whether Chaplin (similar to the socialist US Senator Bernie Sanders) was aware of the word that Hitler and his supporters used.

In Chaplin's film, Dictator Hynkel has a dispute with the dictator of the nation of Bacteria, a man named

Benzino Napaloni (a spoof of Mussolini, publisher of the "Socialist Daily"), over which country should invade Osterlich. After signing a treaty with Napaloni, Hynkel invades Osterlich.

Things had changed by the time the movie premiered in 1940. Hitler and Stalin signed a treaty and the two socialists had invaded Poland together in their conspiracy to carve up Europe in 1939. It was embarrassing for Chaplin and so many others. It was a choice between a Giant Douche and a Turd Sandwich. In the film, Chaplin failed to condemn the alliance of German socialism and Soviet socialism. The American Communist Party, which defended the Molotov–Ribbentrop Pact, distributed copies of the movie's climactic speech. Ouch!

In hindsight, and considering what was occurring at the time of the film's distribution, the biggest laughs come in the final speech.

Later (1942?), at an Arts For Russia dinner in New York, Chaplin allegedly said that Stalin's purges of dissidents were "a wonderful thing." Chaplin imitated the Great Dictator, and life imitated art. He explained that: "the only people who object to communism and who use it as a bugaboo are the Nazi agents in this country." But what did he think about socialists? [snickering]

The partnership between German socialism and Soviet socialism had ended June 22, 1941. Everyone erased it from memory. Chaplin and his ilk inspired the phrase "Always Forget!" The memory hole is real.

47. GOVERNMENT SCHOOLS

There are many books about Hitler, or Nazism, or the Pledge of Allegiance (POA). All books about Hitler, Nazism, or the pledge reveal that the authors overlooked all the disclosures enumerated above. How were those writers blind to so many of the discoveries explained in this book? Their ignorance spans more than a century (if the years are counted from 1892, the year that Bellamy's pledge was published), or it spans more than half a century (if the years are counted since World War II and Hitler's reign).

Why did it take so long to uncover the facts enumerated in this book? And why do news outlets continue to perpetuate ignorance about the POA and about this exposé?

One explanation for the ignorance is: government schools (socialist schools) will not teach the truth about Francis Bellamy and his flag salutation. Bellamy abetted those two major hallmarks of the police state in the United States (hereafter the "USA") and its constant growth: (1) Government (socialist) schools; (2) The Pledge of Allegiance.

Bellamy wanted gunvernment to take over schools. Bellamy achieved "equality" by making everyone (including "news" reporters) equally stupid via government schools. Government's schools are never going to tell the truth about him and his pledge. If they taught the truth, then no one would perform the pledge (other than weirdos).

The pledge represents a threat of violence. People were persecuted, beaten, jailed, and lynched for defying the pledge in the similar rituals in the USA, Germany, and worldwide. The childish pledge continues to inspire bullying and persecution. Nonconformists do literally nothing but sit quietly during the chant, and pledgers get really butthurt. Pledgers want everyone to join them as they suck government dick. The topic intimidates journalists as it has intimidated so many other people.

News journalists remain too brainwashed and frightened to inform their readers. Their news outlets will not publish photographs or film recordings of the early pledge's Nazi salute. They will not write about the photos and films showing the early gesture.

Experiments were performed in which news reporters were asked to publish photographs and films of the early pledge salute and to examine its influence on Germany and other countries. All of the journalists refused.

The same journalists were accused of being dishonest cowards. They continued to refuse any coverage of the issues in this book. Of those same journalists, none disputed the conclusions in this book. The experiment has also been performed by the Pointer Institute for Media Studies. Anyone can replicate the experiment.

All of the above is more proof that the USA is a police state. Journalists demonstrate that the pledge is effective obedience training. Reporters spend careers glorifying lies from public officials. During elections the slaves argue over who will be their next slave master. It is Stockholm Syndrome. Bellamy's scheme worked.

That is why government schools are unconstitutional: They violate the First Amendment right to freedom of speech and freedom of the press. G-schools tell everyone what to think and say and write. The Pledge of Allegiance is a part of that.

Twelve years of Bellamy's schools prevent newspapers, TV, and radio outlets from telling the truth. Journalists lack understanding of private property rights, supply-and-demand pricing, laissez-faire economics, free markets, individual rights, and capitalism. That is why socialism and news outlets have the same strategy: If it bleeds it leads.

Government (socialist) schools prove, by their generations of existence, and by their continued existence, that they do not work. They failed to teach people how to handle their children's education without government. They do not even attempt to teach such a lesson. They teach that government schools must always grow in size, scope, and funding.

Every popular "problem" trumpeted by politicians, media, and government is their confession that government schools never worked and must end. For example, minimum wage laws are a confession by government that socialist schools failed by producing students who are not able to obtain jobs that pay more than the minimum wage.

As Lawrence Reed observed: "Have you ever noticed how statists are constantly "reforming" their own handiwork? Education reform. Health-care reform. Welfare reform. Tax reform. The very fact they're always busy 'reforming' is an implicit admission that they didn't get it right the first 50 times."

All "news" stories are a confession that all previous

socialist policies (including generations of government schools) failed to solve any problems: racism, violence, drugs, theft, crime, prison populations, discrimination, wage gaps, recycling, eating disorders, STD's, unwanted pregnancies, obesity, militarization. Yet all popular "problems" are trumpeted for the Nanny state: for more government, more laws, more programs, and not for reducing or ending socialist schools.

The Bellamy dogma of "Christian Socialism" renders government (socialist) schools unconstitutional as an establishment of religion and as a violation of freedom of religion. Separation of church and state cannot exist where, as in the U.S., the state is your church. Because of Reverend Francis Bellamy, coerced prayers and hymns never stopped in government schools (socialist schools); The Pledge of Allegiance is the daily prayer / hymn.

An old cliché states: History is written by the victors. It would be more accurate to state: History is written (and taught) by the government. In government's schools (socialist schools) the government glorifies itself as a hero, and not as the universal monster.

Government makes the worst thieves seem petty. Socialism is kleptomania. "Taxation is theft, purely and simply even though it is theft on a grand and colossal scale which no acknowledged criminal could hope to match. It is a compulsory seizure of the property of the State's inhabitants, or subjects," as Murray Rothbard said.

Government makes the worst sociopathic serial killers seem angelic in comparison. How do their death tolls compare? Homicidal ideas from the socialists Stalin and Mao are taught, even glorified, in universities and schools. Presidents, Members of Congress, governors, and state politicians are glorified in schools. Government schools give voice to serial killers, murderers, thieves, frauds, sociopaths, and other criminals. Government officials are psychopathic arsonists who hallucinate that they are heroic firemen.

48. EPILOGUE

Some discoveries and little-known facts mentioned in this book:

(1) The Pledge of Allegiance was the origin of the Nazi salute and Nazi behavior.

(2) The Nazi salute came from the military salute due to the use of the military salute in the original Pledge of Allegiance.

(3) Congress and the Flag Code confirm that the military salute was the origin of the Nazi salute (they confirm that Dr. Rex Curry's academic work is correct).

(4) Americans might be doing the pledge incorrectly. Is the hand-over-the-heart gesture supposed to be performed as the military salute over the heart? Probably yes.

(5) There are many photographs and old film footage showing presidents, members of congress, and other officials on the federal, state, county, and city levels doing the Nazi salute to the U.S. flag. (The iconoclast Dr. Curry collects these and if you know of any please

alert the Pointer Institute at alert-notice@earthlink.net).

(6) The Swastika mark, although ancient, was also used to represent crossed "S" letters for "socialism" under Adolf Hitler's National Socialist German Workers Party (Nazis).

(7) VW (Volkswagen), SS, SA, NSV and other emblems have alphabetical functions, and show that the swastika was used as an alphabetical insignia too.

(8) Hitler transformed his own signature to appear as a stylized "S" letter reflecting the shape of the swastika and his dogma of socialism.

(9) "Nazis" did not call themselves "Nazis" and they did not call their insignia a "swastika."

(10) Mein Kampf does not contain the word "Nazi."

(11) Mein Kampf does not contain a single use of the word "swastika."

(12) Mein Kampf does not contain the word "Fascist" ever as a self-reference by Hitler.

(13) Mein Kampf does not contain the phrase "Third Reich."

(14) The Nazi Holocaust was part of a larger socialist Wholecaust with a much bigger death toll.

(15) Vienna, Austria is the origin of the word "wiener." (But in Vienna, they don't call them "wieners."

They call them "Frankfurters"). The etymology is related to these phrases: Vienna sausages and wiener schnitzel. Hitler was born in Austria. Hitler liked Vienna. "Vienna" appears ~80 times in "Mein Kampf."

(16) The word "Fascist" is related to the word "faggot."

(17) The word "Kampf" in Hitler's "Mein Kampf" is related to these words: champagne, campaign, champignon, champion, champ, camp, and campus.

MADNESS

This page contains a comprehensive list of everything you are entitled to and what the world owes you:

ABOUT THE AUTHOR

The Dead Writers Club ("DWC") is an author's group in Florida. The DWC often partners with the Pointer Institute and with the writer Ian Tinny.

Ian Tinny lives in Key West overlooking the water with his cat and his beige dog. When not at his home in the Keys, Tinny resides in New York City. His socialist slave number is 262-00-6302.

Tinny is the top historical authority on the World's Dumbest Criminals (e.g. Stalin, Mao, Hitler et cetera). His expertise also includes America's Dumbest Criminals. Tinny works as a mental health counselor with the United States Probation Office, federal judges, and various sociopathic criminals in the justice system. Tinny's work (with the assistance of the Pointer Institute) led to the arrest, trial, conviction, and imprisonment of America's Dumbest Criminals (ADC). The award-winning investigations resulted in record-setting prison sentences for ADC, the foreclosure of homes, revocation of their professional licenses, along with victim restitution liens, and criminal forfeiture judgments, in amounts totaling millions of dollars.

The probe exposed how America's Dumbest Criminals fooled newspaper reporters and corrupt bureaucrats (including feckless state judges, incompetent federal judges, shiftless U.S. probation officers, HUD, the FHFA, Fannie Mae, and Freddie Mac) who aided and abetted the felons and covered up their conspiracies. In other words, America's Dumbest Criminals tricked America's Dumbest Newspapers and America's Dumbest Public Officials.

Only Florida's folk hero succeeded in bringing the

culprits down. During his ADC detective work, Tinny joined with the Pointer Institute to shut down the Tampa Tribune Newspaper in 2016. Two Tampa area newspapers were notorious for their "2 girls, 1 cup" journalism with fake news and alternative facts. One down and one to go.

The Pointer Institute for Media Studies (PI) deserves special thanks for "pointing out" many enhancements to Tinny's analysis, including its promotion of research by the historian Dr. Rex Curry. The work by Professor Curry is painstaking and difficult, but fortunately grad students are plentiful and cheap.

The research continues, including the search for the many old photographs and antique film footage showing presidents, members of congress, and other officials on the federal, state, county, and city levels doing the Nazi salute to the U.S. flag. Any reader who knows of such images is asked to send it to iantinny@gmail.com

Tinny and PI provide remedial education to journalists about history, economics, government, and more. The PI works to un-do those 12+ years of brainwashing. Wash, rinse, repeat.

The "Stop The Pledge" (STP) Foundation is a fraternity of caring people trying to improve their community and effect change. STP and Pointer Institute Publishing have provided ongoing support to the work of Tinny and the DWC. Thanks!

Matt Crypto is an investigative journalist and researcher in the fields of anarchaeology and misanthropology.

Micky Barnetti is a forensic fraud analyst. He is also a member of the Dead Writers Club.

MADNESS

[EDITOR'S NOTE: Pointer Institute Publishing openly defies the government by paying its readers less than the minimum wage].

www.ingramcontent.com/pod-product-compliance
Lightning Source LLC
Chambersburg PA
CBHW071246220526
45468CB00001B/14